Little, Brown Series
in Clinical Pediatrics

Nutrition and Feeding
of Infants and Toddlers

Nutrition and Feeding of Infants and Toddlers

Edited by

Rosanne B. Howard, M.P.H., R.D.
Director of Nutrition Training, Developmental
Evaluation Clinic, The Children's Hospital,
Boston, Massachusetts

Harland S. Winter, M.D.
Assistant Professor of Medicine, Harvard
Medical School; Assistant in Gastroenterology,
The Children's Hospital; Assistant in Pediatrics,
Massachusetts General Hospital,
Boston, Massachusetts

Foreword by
Harry Shwachman, M.D.
Professor of Pediatrics Emeritus, Harvard
Medical School; Senior Associate in Medicine,
Senior Associate in Cystic Fibrosis,
and Chief Clinical Nutrition Division
Emeritus, The Children's Hospital,
Boston, Massachusetts

Little, Brown and Company
Boston/Toronto

Contents

Foreword

Many nutritional practices have developed since I arrived as a house officer at The Children's Hospital in 1937. At that time, Dr. Harold Stuart was preparing growth charts of weight and height percentiles based on a local pediatric population. These charts, which became an essential component of every child's medical record, made us consider the infant's growth and nutritional status. Today, these charts have been standardized and are based on a larger heterogeneous pediatric population. They remain the first step in the nutritional assessment of infants and children.

Another advance in hospital-based nutrition was the disappearance of the formula room on the infants' ward. The preparation of standardized, sterilized infant formulas was more easily and less expensively done by commercial companies that specialize in nutritional products. They produced formulas not only for the normal neonate but also for the child with special needs. Soy-based formulas became readily available for infants with cow's milk protein intolerance; medium chain triglyceride (MCT) was added for children with fat malabsorption; and of special importance to me, formulas became available with MCT, glucose, and hydrolyzed protein for infants with cystic fibrosis.

We have come a long way in discovering the significance of nutrition in infant development and the use of nutrition in the treatment of disease but not so far in making nutrition an integral part of child care. The theory of nutrition is often left unapplied. This is what makes *Nutrition and Feeding of Infants and Toddlers* unique—it is applied nutrition. This book emphasizes the practical but also presents the scientific basis for nutritional therapy, information that can be used by the primary health provider.

Within these pages nutrition is integrated with the practical aspects of feeding as well as with child development. Several chapters devoted to the infant feeding experience discuss developmental feeding milestones and feeding issues. Also, special attention is given to nutritional risk—nutrition for children with renal disease, congenital heart disease, cystic fibrosis, infectious diarrhea, liver disease, prematurity, and other medical conditions that place the child in nutritional jeopardy. The special problems of children with oral-facial anomalies and neurological handicaps are also included in conjunction with a discussion of feeding equipment, specialized feeding techniques, and positioning. It is evident that the authors of these chapters are nutrition practitioners and have practical experience with the types of feeding problems faced in a pediatric practice.

Nutrition and Feeding of Infants and Toddlers combines the theory and practice of nutrition. It is edited by a pediatric gastroenterologist and a nutritionist, a registered dietitian who is experienced in translating nutrition into child feeding advice for parents. Together they make the practice of nutrition easier for the busy practitioner.

Harry Shwachman

Preface

In the nineteenth century, industrialization and the introduction of safe cow's milk ushered in the era of big business in infant feeding. The safety and convenience of formula won over mothers and physicians alike, who had little scientific data on the merits of breast-feeding with which to answer the proponents of the formula and baby food industry. In addition, the need for women to work outside the home, as well as the American emphasis on speed and efficiency, hastened the trend in bottle-feeding. While infants were switched from the breast to the bottle, baby foods were introduced earlier. Prior to the 1930s solid foods were seldom offered before one year of age, yet in the past fifty years, more than 400 different varieties of infant foods have been produced for consumption.

Today, the widespread use of infant formula and the early introduction of solid food are in the process of critical review. Also under scrutiny is the American diet: a diet low in fiber and laden with fat, salt, and sugar; a diet promulgated by the mass media. Families must now sort through the advertisements that urge them to buy candylike cereals or salt- and sugar-filled snack foods as they make their food selections from the ten thousand or so items on their supermarket shelves. Their decisions are further modulated by the demands imposed by day-care centers, work schedules, changing family roles, and single-parent homes. It is in this complex environment that decisions are made about infant feeding. These decisions, which may ultimately affect health and longevity, are unfortunately often made with little guidance from health professionals.

In the pages that follow, we present information on the techniques of infant feeding along with the behavioral implications and nutritional requirements. Our intention is to communicate an approach that not only combines the science of nutrition with the art of infant feeding, but also considers what is fed as well as how the infant is fed.

R.B.H.
H.S.W.

Acknowledgments

We wish to thank

Our associates who shared their time and valuable opinions: Stuart Berman, M.D., F. Sessions Cole, M.D., William J. Eichelberger, R.Ph., Susan Laramee, M.S., R.D., Allen C. Crocker, M.D., Frederick Mandell, M.D., Margarite J. Queneau, M.S., R.D., Dorothy M. MacDonald, and especially Frances J. Rohr, M.S., R.D.

Our colleagues who provided technical skills: Robert A. Weinstein, Mary Boston, and Shirley Lerner.

Our friends and family for their encouragement and love: Beatrice M. Howard, the John E. Howard family, Leo and Kay McLaughlin, Natasha L. Vogdes, Madeline and Milton Winter, Elsie Brizzi, William Price, and especially Susan Weinstein Winter.

Contributing Authors

Marvin E. Ament, M.D.
Professor of Pediatrics, University of California, Los Angeles; Chief, Division of Pediatric Gastroenterology and Chief, Nutritional Support Services, UCLA Center for Health Sciences, Los Angeles, California

Jeffrey A. Biller, M.D.
Instructor, Tufts University School of Medicine; Assistant Pediatrician, New England Medical Center, Boston, Massachusetts

William G. Bithoney, M.D.
Instructor in Pediatrics, Harvard Medical School; Medical Director, Comprehensive Child Health Program, The Children's Hospital, Boston, Massachusetts

T. Berry Brazelton, M.D.
Associate Professor of Pediatrics, Harvard Medical School; Chief, Child Development Unit, The Children's Hospital, Boston, Massachusetts

Thomas E. Cone, Jr., M.D.
Clinical Professor of Pediatrics Emeritus, Harvard Medical School; Senior Associate in Clinical Genetics and Medicine, The Children's Hospital, Boston, Massachusetts

William H. Dietz, Jr., M.D. Ph.D.
Assistant Professor of Pediatrics, Tufts University School of Medicine; Director of Clinical Nutrition, New England Medical Center, Boston, Massachusetts

Robert L. Gatson, M.D.
Assistant Professor of Pediatrics, Loyola University Stritch School of Medicine, Maywood, Illinois

Rosanne B. Howard, M.P.H., R.D.
Director of Nutrition Training, Developmental Evaluation Clinic, The Children's Hospital, Boston, Massachusetts

Julie R. Ingelfinger, M.D.
Assistant Professor of Pediatrics, Harvard Medical School; Director, Hypertension Clinic, The Children's Hospital, Boston, Massachusetts

Judith A. Lothian, M.A., R.N.
Nursing Consultant, Division of Nursing, New York University, New York, New York

Dorothy M. MacDonald, B.S., R.N.
Head Nurse, Surgical Outpatient Department and Nursing Coordinator, Maxillofacial Program, The Children's Hospital, Boston, Massachusetts

Janis Maksimak, M.D.
Private Practice, Williamsport Pediatric Associates, Williamsport, Pennsylvania; Formerly Senior Fellow in Ambulatory Pediatrics, Harvard Medical School and The Children's Hospital, Boston, Massachusetts

Martin Maksimak, M.D.
Pediatric Gastroenterologist; Geisinger Medical Center, Danville, Pennsylvania; Formerly Fellow in Pediatric Gastroenterology, Harvard Medical School and The Children's Hospital, Boston, Massachusetts

Celeste Martin Marx, Pharm.D.
Assistant Professor of Clinical Pharmacy, Massachusetts College of Pharmacy and Allied Health Sciences; Clinical Pharmacist for Obstetrics, Gynecology and Neonatology, Brigham and Women's Hospital, Boston, Massachusetts

Thalia Metalides, M.S., R.D.
Pediatric Nutrition Consultant, Boston, Massachusetts

David H. Perlmutter, M.D.
Instructor in Pediatrics, Harvard Medical School; Assistant in Gastroenterology, The Children's Hospital, Boston, Massachusetts

Patricia M. Queen, M.M.Sc., R.D.
Assistant Director, Clinical Nutrition, The Children's Hospital, Boston, Massachusetts

Frances J. Rohr, M.S., R.D.
Nutritionist, Developmental Evaluation Clinic, The Children's Hospital, Boston, Massachusetts

Harry Shwachman, M.D.
Professor of Pediatrics Emeritus, Harvard Medical School; Senior Associate in Medicine, Senior Associate in Cystic Fibrosis, and Chief, Clinical Nutrition Division Emeritus, The Children's Hospital, Boston, Massachusetts

Harland S. Winter, M.D.
Assistant Professor of Pediatrics, Harvard Medical School; Assistant in Gastroenterology, The Children's Hospital; Assistant in Pediatrics, Massachusetts General Hospital, Boston, Massachusetts

Nutrition and Feeding
of Infants and Toddlers

1. Infant Feeding:
A Historical Perspective

Thomas E. Cone, Jr.

Appreciation of the practice of infant feeding requires a view, even if fleeting, of the historical background of this subject.
Grover E. Powers (1935) [41]

Prior to a century and a half ago, the successful practice of infant feeding consisted almost entirely of the use of human milk, either from the mother or from a wet nurse. Animal milks, broths, pap, honey, and wine were the main food substances used in hand feeding; these rarely led to the development of a healthy child if they were the exclusive sources of nourishment, unless some human milk also was fed to the infant. For example, in London in the early part of the nineteenth century, less than one in eight infants who were not breast-fed survived their first year [16].

The most complete account of infant feeding and hygiene from antiquity is that of the Greek Soranus of Ephesus who studied medicine in Alexandria and practiced in Rome between A.D. 110 to 130. In his discourse on diseases of children, which formed part of his treatise *On Diseases of Woman*, he wrote [13]:

After the infant has been swaddled . . . it should rest and receive no food at least for the first two days, for the child is apt to be in continual motion during all this time and its body is still amply provided with nourishment derived from the mother, which it first must have time to digest before it is ready for new food. The case is altered should it develop premature appetite . . . For this purpose, slightly boiled honey is much more to be recommended . . . During the first twenty days the mother's milk is, as a rule, unfit for consumption by the child, being thick, cheesy and difficult to digest, a wet nurse is preferable.

Soranus, like his predecessors, thought that as long as the infant was breast-fed, all diseases that required internal treatment were to be treated by remedies, dietetic or otherwise, given to the nursing mother or wet nurse. He wrote [48]: "In general so long as the infant is fed on breast milk we prescribe a regimen to the nurse appropriate to the disease of the infant."

The fact that Soranus did not mention artificial foods as either a supplement to human milk or as a substitute for human milk does not necessarily suggest that artificial foods were unknown to the ancient Greeks or Romans. In fact, the existence of many infant feeding devices in terra-cotta, clay, and even glass from as early as the second or third centuries A.D., some almost identical in size and shape with modern versions, is evidence that artificial foods were used. The use

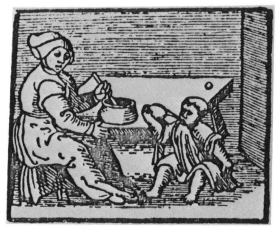

Figure 1-1. Woodcut illustration in the Regiment der Gesundheit *(1549) for a poem by Heinrich von Louffenburg. (Courtesy of the Wellcome Institute for the History of Medicine, London.)*

of such vessels was not confined to the ancient world as is shown by a thirteenth-century illuminated manuscript with an illustration of a woman feeding an infant in her arms by means of a horn and as described by a poem written by Heinrich von Louffenburg in 1429 about the care of the body that was reprinted in the 1549 edition of the *Regiment der Gesundheit für die Jungen Kinder* [38]. This edition contains a woodcut illustration of a child feeding from a bottle similar in shape to that of some of the Roman clay vessels (Fig. 1-1).

INFANT FEEDING IN EUROPE (1487–1800)

Renaissance literature before the fifteenth century contains nothing concerning the feeding of infants. The fifteenth-century books *The Book of Nurture, The Babees Book,* and *The Book of Curtasye* that describe the most intimate particulars of adult life during this period do not even mention infant feeding [48]. It was not until late in the fifteenth century that anything about the feeding of infants was written in medical treatises. The first treatise concerning infant feeding was published in 1472 by Paolo Bagellardo and was entitled *Libellus Egritudinibus Infantium* [16]. Begellardo wrote that a wet nurse is to be procured for the feeding of the newborn infant, but "if the infant is a child of the poorer class let it be fed on its mother's milk" [48].

The earliest English book that mentioned infant feeding appeared in 1545, when Thomas Phaire [35] published his *Boke of Chyldren.* He described a method of testing breast milk, which was first described by Soranus, by observing the behavior of a drop of milk placed on a fingernail. Interestingly enough, Phaire described this method 1500 years later in almost the exact words of Soranus [48].

That mylke is goode that is whyte and sweete; and when you droppe it on your nayle and do move your finger, neyther fletheth abrod at every stiring nor will hange faste upon your naile, when ye turne it downeward, but that whyche is betwene bothe is beste.

Even as late as 1910, more than 1800 years after Soranus, Henry E. Koplik, in his *Diseases of Infancy and Childhood,* wrote [26]: "The milk should with gentle pressure flow freely from the ducts. A drop is caught on the nail of the thumb. This time-honored test will bring out the color of the milk, whether too watery, yellow or white to the experienced eye."

Artificial feeding as a substitute for the breast was not even suggested until the eighteenth century [50]. The social and economic records of the common people provide an understanding of the feeding habits of the time.

The only sources of information available to us about infant feeding prior to the eighteenth century are collections of family letters. Unfortunately, children were mentioned only on a broad level in these letters and fine details such as their feeding habits were rarely discussed. Beyond exacting implicit obedience, parents appeared to have shown little interest in the ordinary incidents of their children's daily lives [16].

One can assume that the ways in which infants were reared changed little, if at all, during the three or four centuries before the reign of Elizabeth I. Each generation accepted the tradition handed down by the one preceding it [12]. Breast-feeding was practically the only means of nourishing an infant. Feeding bottles had not been invented yet and artificial foods were limited to bread and pap (usually bread soaked in milk). Cow's milk rarely was mentioned as a substitute for breast milk during the seventeenth and early part of the eighteenth centuries [7, 8].

During the sixteenth century, many odd beliefs centered around the wet nurse. Phaire, like his contemporaries, believed that various characteristics—both good and bad—could be transmitted through the breast milk. For example, an ill-tempered woman could transmit vice in her milk; a treacherous mind and temper might be transmitted through the milk of a redheaded woman.

In conjunction with wet nurses were baby farmers, who flourished chiefly during the reign of Elizabeth I. Mothers unwilling to nurse their own children (and there seem to have been many of them) would send them to nurses in the country known as baby farmers. For generations, these notorious baby farmers plied their trade. The parish records of England show that many infant deaths due to improper feeding were reported by them [36].

On the dangers of artificial feeding Phaire (1545) wrote [35]: "I intend to write somewhat of ye nourse and of ye milke with ye qualities and

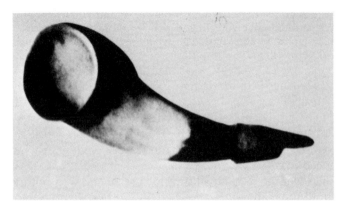

Figure 1-2. A sixteenth-century cow's horn used as an infant-feeding device.

complexions of the same. Phavorinus [an early Roman writer] affirmeth that if the lambes be nourished with the milk of goates, they shall have course woole lyke the heare of goates; and if kiddes in lyke manner sucke upon shepe, the heare of them shall be soft lyke wolle." No doubt the "goate and shepe story" frightened many. If a lamb grew a beard from suckling a goat, what would befall a child if fed on cow's milk? This, we may be sure, was duly debated, and the claims of cow's milk were not even considered. Another objection to the use of cow's milk was due to the frightful sanitary conditions existing in the large cities. Fortunately, artificial feeding, which would have greatly increased the wastage of infants, was not practiced.

Simon de Vallambert, the author of the first pediatric work written in France (1565), claimed that one of the best foods to add to the infant's diet after the age of three months (or even earlier) was cow's milk. He advised the addition of cow's milk or goat's milk (the latter he thought more suitable) with semolina, flour, or crumbled white bread in it, sometimes even adding an egg yolk. He gave one of the first descriptions of a baby-feeding apparatus in sixteenth-century texts: "a horn with an opening at both ends, one end being made into the shape of a teat, through which the infant sucks the pap just as it sucks breast milk by the nipple" [48] (Fig. 1-2).

Omnibonus Ferrarius, a sixteenth-century Italian physician, also discussed infant feeding in his widely read *De arte medica infantium* (1577) [48].

We must now speak of feeding from the beginning of teething up to the age of two years or as long as the nurse feeds the infant; for some follow the view of Galen and nurse up to the third year after birth, some, according to the advice of Avicenna, for two years, and some for twenty months, but before the complete eruption of all the teeth it is unfitting to take the infant from the breast milk, for he should be able not only to bite up solid food but also to chew it carefully . . . When the child is seven months old and the first central and lateral incisors have appeared and are fully cut, then it is good for the infant to accustom himself to more solid food but without giving up the milk. And first chewed bread is to be put into the baby's mouth, and later vegetables previously cooked, and chewed by the nurse and then meat and the like.

Early in the eighteenth century a number of changes were becoming apparent concerning infant feeding. If the mother could be supplanted by a wet nurse, perhaps the wet nurse also could be supplanted. Why not employ some food other than human milk? In the middle of the eighteenth century, it was finally considered safe to feed the infant water-pap as soon as the first tooth had appeared. The use of cow's milk, however, generally was still not acceptable. The breast was not withdrawn completely until the child was two years old, and for the first time in recorded history, mixed feeding was employed. Because of the success of water-pap made from bread and baked flour, other foods were developed and used. Weak broth was given with the first tooth; with the second tooth, the minced wing of a chicken was fed. For the first time, sugar was added and given with bread boiled in water [48].

Michael Underwood, the most advanced writer on diseases of children in the eighteenth century, considered cow's milk the most proper food to use when breast milk was unavailable and was baffled by the weird mixtures that were fed to infants in the past. He wrote [49]:

It was indeed been a wonder to me how the custom of stuffing newborn babies with the such like could become so universal, or the idea first enter the mind of a parent that such heavy food could be fit for babies' nourishment at the age of six or seven months. This food may be justly considered a poison, which, if not puked up, or very soon voided by stool, may occasion sickness, gripes (inward fits), and all the train of bowel complaints, which may terminate in Worms, Convulsions, Rickets, Scrofula, Slow Fevers, Purging and a fatal Marasmus.

Underwood recognized the importance of choosing a milk with a composition as close as possible to mother's milk. In the fourth edition of his treatise (1799), he included two comparative analyses of the milk of women, cows, goats, asses, sheep, and mares. Underwood believed that cow's milk was best suited for the healthy infant, but for the very young or for those with diarrhea, the milk of an ass was recommended because it had fewer curds than other milks. He also suggested adding barley water as a diluent to cow's milk. (This was the beginning of milk dilution.) Some years later, other diluents were mentioned in writings; the preferred one was a small quantity of light jelly made from hartshorn shavings and boiled in water to the con-

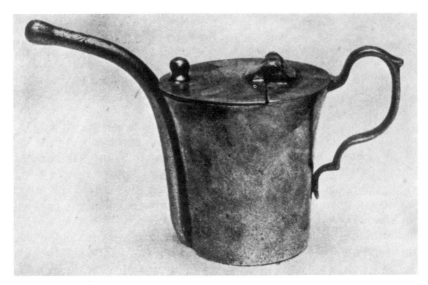

Figure 1-3. Bubby-pot baby-feeder described by Hugh Smith in 1777. (Courtesy of the Wellcome Institute for the History of Medicine, London.)

sistency of cold veal broth. A little Lisbon sugar or loaf sugar was then added.

Underwood was also the first person to mention the importance of cleansing the milk receptacle. He suggested the "new" pot invented by Dr. Hugh Smith [46] (Fig. 1-3) and recommended that it be cleansed carefully and scalded at least once a day, and the spout thoroughly rinsed, "lest any sour curds should stick about it."

As the nineteenth century began, mixed feeding was in general use. A variety of concoctions was recommended for breast-fed infants just a few weeks old. Water-pap still figured prominently, while oatmeal, rice, or barley boiled in cow's milk was given at the end of the first month. Herb tea and beer soup were also advised by Churchill [6].

One of the major reasons for the difficulties encountered in artificial feeding was the lack of suitable feeding utensils. A suitable vessel was needed from which a child could take its food by the natural act of sucking. Naturally, a cow's horn was suggested. This was followed by the baby-feeder first described by Filippo Baldini in 1784. The neck of the baby-feeder terminated in an expansion devised to admit a sponge, which projected like a nipple (Fig. 1-4).

INFANT FEEDING IN COLONIAL AMERICA

The mortality that usually accompanied the artificial feeding of infants in seventeenth- and eighteenth-century England made breast-feeding

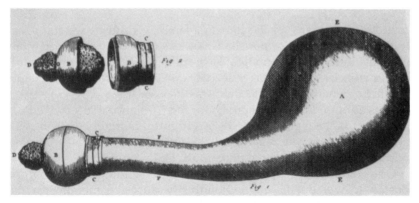

Figure 1-4. Baby-feeder with sponge for sucking described by Filippo Baldini in 1784. (From Still, G. F. The History of Paediatrics. *London: Oxford University Press, 1931.)*

essential to the survival of the race, yet the technique of such an important custom seldom was mentioned by the early American colonists. There is ample evidence that nearly all infants were breast-fed, but little was written about breast-feeding in either printed or manuscript material. According to Demos [10], the most knowledgeable historian of the period, there are occasional incidental references to breast-feeding in the records of Plymouth Colony. For example, Lidia Standish, testifying in a fornication trial, spoke of herself as "a mother of many children my selfe and have nursed many" [8].

The study of birth intervals at Plymouth Colony presents some indirect evidence that breast-feeding commonly was used. In the average family, children were spaced roughly two years apart (or a bit longer near the end of the wife's child-bearing years). This pattern is consistent with the practice of breast-feeding a child for about one year because lactation normally presents a biological impediment to pregnancy. Demos claims [10]: "The exceptions can nearly always be explained in the same terms. When one finds an interval of only twelve or fifteen months between two particular deliveries, one also finds that the older child died at or soon after birth." Hence there would be no period of breast feeding to speak of, and hence nothing to delay the start of another pregnancy.

WET-NURSING

Although wet-nursing was a well-accepted seventeenth-century custom in Europe, it is difficult to find definitive evidence of its widespread use in seventeenth-century America. By the eighteenth century, however, there were many references in colonial newspapers, according to Guerra [20], to the availability of wet nurses.

Despite its faults, wet-nursing was thought to be far superior to "dry-nursing" or artificial feeding. In court cases in America involving foundlings, orphans, or illegitimate infants, wet nurses were supplied to the county, town, or parish. This was sound policy because infant mortality in the Paris Foundling Hospital in the late eighteenth century where artificial feeding was practiced was 85 percent of 32,000 infants; in Dublin, where artificial feeding was also practiced, only 45 in 10,000 infants admitted to the hospital between 1775 and 1796 survived—in other words, 99.6 percent died. This frightful mortality explains why artificial feeding was regarded with suspicion and why it was not popular during the eighteenth century [48].

One common practice was the custom of sending infants born in Boston to wet nurses in the country because it generally was acknowledged that infants thrived better in country air. The farming out of babies to be nursed, as noted previously, had become a well-established custom in seventeenth-century England; as Caulfield wrote [5]: "This practice received some scientific support in the eighteenth century when Jonas Hanway [21], after comparing the infant survival rate of London parishes with that of country parishes, attributed 'the differences to the salubriousness of country air'." In the United States, Benjamin Rush [5] had found that moving infants with cholera infantum to the country was the best of all treatments. "Bad air" became the accepted explanation for the spread of diseases from person to person.

In view of the paucity of original American instructions for feeding infants "by hand," it may be assumed that most mothers used feeding techniques described by English folk customs or in popular English medical books such as those by Nicholas Culpeper and William Cadogan [12]. These English authors, notably Cadogan [4], had an ingrained prejudice against boiled cow's milk and strongly advocated feeding nothing but breast milk until the child was 3 to 6 months old. After that age, but only when absolutely necessary, one could feed "thin light toasted bread and water boiled almost dry and then mixed with fresh milk, not boiled" [4].

INFANT FEEDING IN THE NINETEENTH CENTURY

A sad fact of nineteenth-century pediatrics was that the first years of a child's life were by far the most treacherous. Most deaths were attributed to improper bottle feeding. How to overcome this formidable cause of infant mortality became the primary mission of pediatricians for the six decades between 1870 and 1930. It was not until the very end of the nineteenth century that changes were made in the empiricism and dogmatism that had dominated infant feeding techniques for almost the entire century.

Many nineteenth-century reports indicated that among infants who were not breast-fed, as many as 80 to 90 percent died. In the New York Infant Asylum, where bottle-feeding was practiced in 1886, the deaths kept pace with the admissions; in the New York Foundling Asylum, bottle-fed infants were kept by themselves in a room known as the ward of the dying babies [33]. In the foundling home located on Randall's Island in New York City, only one bottle-fed infant admitted to the hospital over a period of a year and a half reached the age of one year [47].

Throughout almost the entire nineteenth century, pessimistic opinions about the fate of bottle-fed infants prevailed. Near the end of the century, Job Lewis Smith, one of the founders of pediatrics in America, wrote [47]:

In the large cities, if I may judge from our New York experience, this mode of alimentation (artificial feeding), for young infants should always be discouraged. It generally ends in death, preceded by evidences of faulty nutrition. A considerable proportion of those nourished in this manner thrive during the cool months, but on the approach of the warm season they are the first to be affected with diarrhoea (the so-called summer complaint) . . . In my opinion, based on a pretty extended observation, more than half of the New York spoon-fed infants, who entered the summer months, die before the return of cool weather, unless saved by removal to the country.

Before bottle-feeding could be considered on a rational basis, it was necessary to determine the precise composition of human and cow's milk. Simon [45] was the first to perform accurate milk analyses and his studies may be considered the first real landmarks in the science of infant metabolism as a basis for rational infant nutrition. His studies, published in 1838, passed unnoticed for about 30 years.

Simon scientifically analyzed and compared the constituents of human and cow's milk. His results showed that the casein in cow's milk amounted to 7.2 percent and in human milk to 3.4 percent. He found that cow's milk contained 2.8 percent sugar and human milk 4.82 percent. It is obvious that his figures for protein were too high, and for sugar, too low. One reason for this error was that he included all protein, including lacto-albumin, under the term casein. He did not miss the point, however, that cow's milk contains more casein than human milk. These chemical studies, as well as others, supported the concept that various constituents of cow's milk were harmful to infants. These studies also provided incentive to try to replicate human milk. Such attempts were exemplified with the production of numerous milk mixtures, now obsolete, and in the various cream and top-milk mixtures.

Biedert [3] is usually considered the originator of the scientific study of artificial infant feeding. He published one of the first scientific treatises on infant nutrition in 1869 and in 1878 he described "fat diarrhea." In his treatise he included his observations that the protein content of cow's milk was approximately twice as high as that of human milk.

Biedert also studied the effect of acid on the consistency of the curd and suggested that casein curds were responsible for digestive difficulties. He maintained that the casein of cow's milk was less digestible than that of human milk; he thus suggested that instead of cow's milk, a series of graduated mixtures of cow's milk, water, and milk sugar should be used. Biedert's milk formula mixture was the parent of Rotch's concept of percentage feeding [40].

THOMAS MORGAN ROTCH AND THE
PERCENTAGE METHOD OF INFANT FEEDING

Rotch's percentage feeding (also called the laboratory or American method) was based, as was Biedert's mixture, on the idea that the protein of cow's milk is the food element that is difficult to digest and, on the other hand, that the fat and sugar of cow's milk are comparatively harmless and easy to digest [40].

The fact that all infants cannot be fed on the same mixture of cow's milk, water, and sugar was the pivotal point of Rotch's method. Taking into consideration the composition of human milk, each infant must be considered separately while designing a formula, which within certain limits, would be most suitable to the infant's needs. It further assumed that in feeding an infant the important thing in modifying the food was to offer the infant an exact percentage of protein, carbohydrate, and fat. Rotch contended that what is good for or adapted to one infant may not be suitable for another. In his own words: "What is one infant's food may be another's poison" [39].

Rotch [40] taught that not only the proteins, but the fats and sugars of cow's milk as well, may be the cause of disturbance in an infant's digestion. He was unquestionably the father and greatest proponent of the method of infant feeding commonly used in this country from 1890 until 1915—the *percentage method*. This method was further elaborated upon by Holt and Koplik [7]. All three of these pediatricians taught that the basic factor underlying the modification of milk was that cow's milk contains more casein than human milk. Thus, cow's milk must be diluted to lower the percentage of casein. Unfortunately, reducing the percentage of casein also reduces the amount of sugar and fat to a level below that found in breast milk. Consequently, besides the water or cereal diluent added to reduce the casein level, cream and sugar were added.

Rotch [40] had pointed out that percentage feeding is a method of calculation rather than a method of feeding; he often wrote that "no one can satisfactorily prescribe food for an infant who does not have knowledge of the composition of that food." From the analyses available at the time, Rotch assumed that the average composition of human milk was about 4 percent fat, 7 percent sugar, 1.5 percent protein, and 0.2 percent ash.

Rotch wanted to provide a way to ensure that the composition of food was equal to the digestive capacity of the individual infant. Rotch saw more clearly than had Biedert that tolerance of cow's milk varied enormously according to age. He grew to believe that minute variations in the composition of food, perhaps as little as 0.1 percent variation in a single food element, could make the difference between its being digested or not. The percentage system of feeding insisted upon the very careful gradation of the size and composition of the feedings from week to week, with the result that milk was prescribed with the same accuracy and precision as dangerous drugs.

A well-managed milk laboratory was needed in order to determine accurately the composition of formulas as demanded by the percentage method. Such a laboratory became the cornerstone of Rotch's method [40]. He pointed out that "the actual modification (of milk) in many instances could not but be improperly done by mothers and nurses and what was needed in milk modification was a perfection of technique. This perfection could only be done in a special milk laboratory." Rotch further commented that "just as the pharmaceutical laboratories represented perfection of technique, so should there be milk laboratories where perfection of technique could be carried out in dealing with foodstuffs, and so only could the real value of these foodstuffs be determined."

Although most of Rotch's contemporaries agreed that the positive results produced by percentage feeding were better than anything that had been accomplished previously concerning infant feeding, one wonders how much of the success was due to Rotch's requirement for a very pure quality of milk and how much of the success was due to the percentage system itself.

Rotch's method had been adopted almost universally by American pediatricians by the end of the 1890s, although it found little favor abroad, being considered too complicated and artificial. By the end of the first decade of the twentieth century, the popularity of percentage feeding was waning, largely because of mounting criticism by American authorities [8]. Furthermore, as the twentieth century began, the far more scientific calorimetric method of infant feeding, as developed by Rubner and Huebner, had made its appearance [41].

Koplik [26], although an early advocate of the percentage method, gradually came to view this method as overly refined and essentially artificial, not taking into consideration the normal variations in human milk. He satirically commented on "the idea of trying to benefit a sick infant by offering him a food that is fundamentally unsuitable, yet figured out to amazing nicety" [26].

By 1915 many pediatricians had begun to discard the whole rigamarole of top milk and percentages. They began to return to simpler methods that had proved themselves at least as successful, but were abandoned because they did not achieve the impossible, namely to make cow's milk an equal substitute for human milk [8].

Today, the minutiae of percentage feeding seem amusing; nevertheless, the focus on the composition of milk and the teachings of Rotch and his colleagues unquestionably advanced our knowledge in the area of infant nutrition.

CALORIMETRIC METHOD OF INFANT FEEDING

Rubner and Heubner's [41] classic monograph on metabolism and average daily caloric needs of normal and atrophic infants appeared in 1898. These studies provided the information needed in order to feed infants according to their caloric requirements. These studies also were the starting point of all modern studies concerning infant metabolism.

Isaac A. Abt described these investigations [7]:

Thus it was possible for the first time to estimate the complete metabolism and energy quotient in infants in various conditions; it was also determined that only a small amount of protein was required for infant nutrition. The activity of the alimentary canal in infants suffering from digestive disturbances, the utilization of the food consumed and the variation of water elimination in rest or activity of the infant were investigated, and the carbohydrate metabolism and other problems were also studied. These observations conducted over a period of time (with Rubner's help) led Heubner to a new conception of energy quotients. He learned that the food requirements of infants of various ages could be calculated which proved to be of practical and fundamental value in infant feeding.

SANITARY MILK SUPPLY

Despite the important contributions by Rotch and others concerning the practice of infant feeding, no contribution was more valuable than the campaign for a sanitary milk supply. As early as 1830 Robert Hartley [22] began a drive to improve the purity of the milk supply. A pure milk campaign started soon thereafter as a by-product of the temperance movement. Although Gail Borden started the first sanitary inspection of milk in 1857, it was not until late in the nineteenth century that the campaign culminated in success. Linnaeus E. LaFétra described New York City's milk supply of 1882 as follows [27]:

More than half of the milk used in the city came from cows fed on distillers' mash. At Ninth Avenue and 18th Street, adjoining a distillery, were sheds containing 2,000 cows. The stables were rented at five dollars per cow and mash supplied at nine cents a barrel. City tramps were the milkers, being paid for their labor by night shelter in the stables. The cows were diseased and the milk filthy.

Even in the early twentieth century, "dirty" milk usually was found in all large American cities. Abt [1] vividly described the odorous tin cans in which it was sold, "with flies festooning the open containers and customers carrying the milk home in open pitchers or pails in the hottest months." Then once it had been taken home, Abt [1] wrote, "the milk container was set out in a hot room on a table because there were no ice boxes."

It was not unusual for a city administration to sell its garbage to a farmer who promptly fed it to his cows. Distilleries also kept cows and fed them distillery wastes producing what was called "swill milk." This particular liquid, from which babies purportedly felt the effects of the alcohol, caused a scandal in New York in 1870; it was revealed that some of the cows, cooped up for years in filthy stables, were so enfeebled from tuberculosis that they had to be raised on cranes in order to be milked [2].

PROPRIETARY (ARTIFICIAL) INFANT FOODS

The studies of the chemist Justus von Liebig, a pupil of François Magendie, on the chemistry of food had a great influence on the feeding of artificial foods to children. Not only did Liebig devise and market a patented infant's food, but he also developed a biochemical classification of organic foodstuffs and the processes of nutrition. The beginning of the proprietary food industry might be dated 1867 when Liebig marketed his "perfect" infant food [7].

LIEBIG'S MIXTURE

The formula Liebig devised was a mixture of wheat flour, cow's milk, and malt flour, cooked with a little bicarbonate of potash that was added to reduce the acidity of wheat and malt flour. Liebig's mixture was the first to take into account the infant's supposed physiological needs (caloric feeding was developed about 30 years later). Two years after Liebig introduced his infant mixture, it was widely advertised in America as "the most perfect substitute for *mother's milk*" [7].

Liebig's mixture was the first of an almost endless variety of infant foods that appeared during the last quarter of the nineteenth century. Often, totally unwarranted claims were made for these foods. They consisted either of dried milk or a cereal alone or in combination with dried milk, with or without the addition of a malt preparation of some kind. Many of the infant foods contained nothing but a dry, carefully prepared cereal.

The proprietary foods sold in the United States could be divided roughly into three groups. The first group contained dried cow's milk in combination with some cereal and sugar. Nestlé's Food, which contained much unchanged starch, and Horlich's Malted Milk, in which the starch was largely converted into soluble carbohydrates, such as maltose and dextrin, were examples of the first group. These foods were intended to be the sole foodstuffs in the infant's diet and were severely criticized by leading pediatricians. The second group contained some form of malted carbohydrate in which the starch was completely changed to dextrin and maltose. The most widely used food in this group was Mellin's Food, which was a desiccated malt extract. The third group of infant foods were those composed of a pure cereal to be used with fresh cow's milk. Eskay's Food, Imperial Granum, and Robinson's Patent Barley were the best known brand names [7]. Great harm resulted from the use of these foods because they were often used as the infant's only form of food. Because most of them contained little more than concentrated carbohydrate, they usually produced disastrous results such as persistent diarrhea, anemia, and failure to thrive.

During the nineteenth century, infants customarily received nothing but milk until about the age of 10 months. Holt's feeding regimen [23] during the first year was similar to those published by his contemporaries.

1. Nothing but milk until the infant was 8 or 9 months old.
2. Beginning at 10 months, beef juice starting with one tablespoon and increasing to 4 to 6 tablespoonsful daily by 12 months of age.
3. Also at 10 months of age, gruel made from the grains of oats, wheat, or barley, or from farina or arrowroot; 1 to 3 tablespoons may be added to each feeding.

Infants were not given solid animal food substances until they were nearly one-year-old through the late 1920s. Even before 1839 when Sylvester Graham [19] and his followers advocated vegetarianism, there was widespread fear of giving too much animal food to children. Dewees [11] had written, "Children should never make animal substances a principal part of their food, until the age of puberty."

As the nineteenth century ended, many foods continued to be interdicted for children under the age of 4 years such as bacon, liver, tomatoes, beets, and bananas, as well as all canned, dried, and preserved fruits [7]. Jacobi [25] advised: "Before children are 2 years of age no vegetables in any quantity should be given to them. Small quantities may be given later on; they will be acceptable and readily digested."

Rotch [39] was as emphatic as Jacobi about the age at which to offer solid foods to a child. He permitted baked potato at 17 months or later and vegetables at 30 months (easily digested ones only such as squash, young peas, and young beans). Rotch, as well as Holt and Jacobi, did not recommend fresh fruits in the child's diet until the third year of life, probably because of the fear that fruits and vegetables might be responsible for "the summer diarrheas."

INFANT FEEDING IN TWENTIETH CENTURY AMERICA

During the early 1900s American pediatricians were confronted with several widely conflicting hypotheses about the causes of nutritional disturbances from infant feeding. Biedert [3] claimed that the difficulty of digesting casein was a prominent cause of infantile digestive disorders; Finkelstein [14] opposed Biedert's theory that casein was harmful; Czerny [9] claimed that fats were injurious to the digestive tract; and, as mentioned before, Rotch believed that protein was the cause of disturbance in infant digestion. Finkelstein and Meyer [14] advanced the theory of an alimentary fever caused by sugar or salt; this led Finkelstein to develop his protein milk, *Eiweissmilch*. He showed that proteins per se were not necessarily harmful. However, his theory of salt-and-sugar fevers was opposed so strongly that he ultimately abandoned his dogmatic position concerning the supposed pyrogenic action of carbohydrates. He finally accepted Czerny's view that fats are more harmful than casein in a bowel previously irritated by sugar fermentation.

By 1917 the concept of caloric feeding had become universal in America; however, there was an occasional dissenter. For example, Morse [34] in 1935 wrote: "To me it [caloric feeding] still seems as irrational as it ever did to base any scheme or system of infant feeding solely on the caloric needs of babies or on the caloric values of food." Holt and Howland in 1917 described the caloric needs of infants as follows [24]:

From numerous observations the nutritive needs of an infant of average size and weight in health have been shown to be 100 or 110 calories per kilo (daily) (45 to 48 per pound) of body weight for the early months of the first year; gradually diminishing to 70 to 80 per kilo (30 to 35 per pound) (daily) by the end of the year.

These caloric intakes of 1917 are only slightly less than those given by the Food and Nutrition Board of the National Academy of Science—National Research Council in 1980 (see Appendix 1).

INFANT FORMULAS

Soybean Formula

John Ruhräh [42] published the first paper on the soybean in infant feeding in 1909; his was a pioneer contribution of considerable historical interest. He devised several preparations, including soybean milk, which he suggested might be used "as a substitute for milk in diarrhea, in intestinal and stomach disorders, and in diabetes mellitus" [42]. He also said that he "had hoped to be able to make a more complete clinical report . . . but . . . my first crop was eaten by rats, my second moulded in the pods owing to some unusually damp weather, and insects ate about two-thirds of my last crop" [43].

Two years later, in 1911, he published a second paper on the use of the soybean in cases of summer diarrhea and in cases in which milk disagrees with the infant [43].

By the late 1920s Lewis Webb Hill and his colleague, H.C. Stuart, were recommending the use of soybean milk in cases of infantile eczema [7]. However, it was not until the 1950s that formulas with protein derived from soy flour were widely utilized in the United States as milk substitutes. Although these formulas were more satisfactory than most other milk substitutes available at the time, parents often complained that soy formulas caused loose, malodorous stools and excoriation of the diaper area. By the mid 1960s formulas with protein from water-soluble soy isolates had become so popular that they had almost replaced soy-flour formulas.

Evaporated Milk

The idea of commercially preserving milk by evaporating most of the water and preserving it with sugar (condensed milk) dates back to 1853 when Gail Borden was granted patents in the United States and England for his vacuum-evaporation method, the principles of which still apply in modern methods of condensing milk [7].

The process of preserving unsweetened condensed milk, now known as evaporated milk was introduced by Myenberg in 1883, who sterilized the evaporated products by using steam under pressure; this method is still used today. Heating produces certain alterations in the chemical and physical properties of milk. The casein undergoes alteration and the curd is much finer than in raw, pasteurized, or quickly boiled milk. However, this milk was not really considered acceptable for feeding infants until 1927 when Marriott [28], in particular, first recommended the use of unsweetened evaporated milk instead of ordinary cow's milk in the preparation of his lactic acid milk formulas. Marriott [28] pointed out that evaporated milk was already sterilized and heated sufficiently to ensure the formation of very fine curds when lactic acid was added. Evaporated milk had a lower buffer value than ordinary cow's milk because of the conversion of part of the calcium and phosphate into a form of insoluable calcium phosphate. Also, the fat in evaporated milk was homogenized. In addition, evaporated milk was inexpensive and easily obtained [29].

Marriott [28] recommended a formula of equal parts of evaporated milk and an acid-sugar mixture (corn syrup, 90 ml; lactic acid, U.S.P. 5 ml; water to 250 ml) for all healthy infants during their first 6 to 8 months. The amount of corn syrup was decreased after cereal was given to the infant (in 1927, this was usually not until the infant reached the age of 9 months).

Marriott and Schoenthal [31] found that evaporated milk (without the addition of lactic acid), when fed to 752 young, healthy infants, resulted in an average weight gain exactly equal to that of babies fed exclusively on breast milk or on formulas prepared from bottled, pasteurized milk.

During the 1930s and 1940s, evaporated milk became the most widely accepted and versatile milk used in infant formulas [30]. By 1960 it was estimated that 80 percent of bottle-fed infants in the United States were fed either on evaporated milk or on some kind of prepared milk marketed in evaporated form. The former prejudices of "canned" milk had been overcome [37].

Single-Formula Mixtures (Humanized Milks)

Partly as an outgrowth of the complexity of the percentage feeding method, the search for a single formula food, or humanized milk, has always seemed alluring.

At the meeting of the American Pediatric Society in 1915, Henry J. Gerstenberger and colleagues [17] were the first to describe an artificial milk or food that was "in all possible respects similar to human milk." Gerstenberger imitated the fat of human milk by using a combination of various homogenized animal and vegetable fats. This mixture contained roughly 4.6 percent fat, 6.5 percent sugar, and 0.9 percent protein. Four years later Gerstenberger and Ruh [18] reported the use of this food in about 300 cases and gave it the name Synthetic Milk Adapted, or SMA. This descendent of illustrious ancestry long maintained the lead in the years devoted to the goal of producing a one-formula milk with which normal babies could be fed successfully (see Chap. 5).

SOLID FOODS

During the first quarter of the twentieth century, infants usually were not offered solid foods until they were about 1 year old. But by 1925 McLean and Fales wrote [32]:

There is still much controversy regarding the age at which a varied dietary should be commenced. Many pediatrists (pediatricians) still believe it inadvisable to introduce significant amounts of solids into the diet of the infant of less than 1 year of age. Many others are convinced that better results are obtained by giving part of the food requirements of infants of 6 months of age in solid form.

By the mid-1930s Brennemann [7] suggested that 6 months was the proper age at which to introduce solid foods and in 1953 Sacket [44] claimed that he offered infants "solid foods on the second day of life on a 6-hour schedule" and that they were well tolerated. There is no actual proof that there is any nutritional or psychological benefit in introducing solid foods so early in the infant's life. On the other hand, proof of harm caused by the early introduction of solid food is lacking.

One development that made the feeding of vegetables and fruits easier for mothers was the beginning of the canned baby food industry in the late 1920s. This industry played a role in the promotion of earlier solid feeding.

The age at which solid foods should be introduced into the infant's dietary regimen continues to be a subject of controversy (although far less passionate now) in the pediatric community. The general tendency had been to introduce solids at an increasingly early age. Intense peer pressure on the mother for early introduction of solid foods also has had a great influence.

A major objection to the early feeding of solids is that the practice may encourage overfeeding, which may lead to infantile obesity. Because an adequate intake of all essential nutrients can be provided without solid foods, there seems to be no advantage in introducing solid foods during the first three or four months of life.

CONCLUSION

Until almost this century, the successful practice of infant feeding consisted almost entirely in the use of human milk from the mother or from a wet nurse. Hand or artificial feeding consisted largely of animal milk, pap, panada, and broths, and rarely led to the development of a healthy child if they were the only sources of nutriment.

By the 1870s accurate analyses of both human and cow's milk led to the development of scientific infant feeding. American contributions in this area were of extraordinary significance. The fight for clean, wholesome milk, combined with the biochemical and clinical studies of milk by investigators such as Jacobi, Rotch, Holt, and Koplik during the early 1900s, finally made it feasible for bottle-fed infants to be reared in good health.

During the twentieth century infant feeding has become so simple and safe that we are likely to forget the long and dangerous road that had led to this accomplishment. We have now emerged from a chaos of complexity to a chaos of simplicity. A review of even the highlights of the history of infant feeding in America will remind us of our enormous debt to those who preceded us. But consideration of the incidence of childhood obesity, iron deficiency anemia, and dental caries reminds us of the work in infant nutrition that still needs to be done.

For a number of years it appeared that infant feeding practices were influenced more by the marketing techniques of the infant formula and baby food companies than by the scientific community. Breastfeeding was discouraged and baby foods were introduced at very early ages. Recently these practices have come under critical review (see Chap. 5). Trends are changing in infant feeding as a more holistic approach is developed. This approach is discussed in the pages that follow.

REFERENCES

1. Abt, I. A. *Baby Doctor.* New York: McGraw-Hill, 1944.
2. Bettman, O. L. *The Good Old Days—They Were Terrible!* New York: Random House, 1974.
3. Biedert, P. *Untersuchungen ueber die Chemischen Unterschiede der Menschen— und kuhmilch* (dissertation). Giessen: W. Keller, 1869.
4. Cadogen, W. *An Essay upon Nursing and the Management of Children from their Birth to Three Years of Age.* London: J. Roberts, 1748.
5. Caulfield, E. Infant feeding in colonial America. *J. Pediatr.* 41:673, 1952.
6. Churchill, F. *On the Diseases of Infants and Children.* Philadelphia: Lea & Blanchard, 1850.
7. Cone, T. E., Jr. *200 Years of Feeding Infants in America.* Columbus, Ohio: Ross Laboratories, 1976.
8. Cone, T. E., Jr. *History of American Pediatrics.* Boston: Little, Brown, 1979.
9. Czerny, A., and Kleinschmidt, H. Ueber eine Buttermehlnahrung für schwache Säuglinge. *Jahrb. Kinderheilkd.* 87:1, 1918.
10. Demos, J. *A Little Commonwealth.* London: Oxford University Press, 1970.
11. Dewees, W. P. *Treatise on the Physical and Medical Treatment of Children.* Philadelphia: Blanchard & Lea, 1853.
12. Drummond, J. C., and Wilbraham, A. *The Englishman's Food: A History of Five Centuries of English Diet.* London: Jonathan Cape, 1939.
13. Duncum, B. M. Some notes on the history of lactation. *Br. Med. Bull.* 5:253, 1947–1948.
14. Finkelstein, H., and Meyer, L. F. Ueber "Eiweissmilch": Ein Beitrag zum Problem der künstlichen Ernährung. *Jahrb. Kinderheilkd.* 71:525, 1910.
15. Fomon, S. J. What are infants fed in the United States? *Pediatrics* 56:350, 1975.
16. Forsyth, D. The history of infant feeding from Elizabethan times. *Proc. R. Soc. Med.* 4 (part 1):110, 1910–1911.
17. Gerstenberger, H. J., et al. Studies in the adaptation of an artificial food to human milk. *Am. J. Dis. Child.* 10:249, 1915.
18. Gerstenberger, H. J., and Ruh, H. O. Studies in the adaptation of an artificial food to human milk. II: A report of three years' clinical experience with the feeding of S.M.A. (synthetic milk adapted). *Am. J. Dis. Child.* 17:1, 1919.
19. Graham, S. *Lecture on the Science of Human Life.* Boston: Marsh, Capen, Lyon & Webb, 1839.
20. Guerra, F. *American Medical Bibliography, 1639–1783.* New York: Lathrop C. Harper, 1960.
21. Hanway, J. *An Earnest Appeal for Mercy to the Children of the Poor.* London: T. Cadell, 1766.
22. Hartley, R. *An Historical, Scientific and Practical Essay on Milk.* New York: Leavitt, 1842.
23. Holt, L. E. *The Care and Feeding of Children* (2nd ed.). New York: Appleton, 1899.
24. Holt, L. E., and Howland, J. *Diseases of Infancy and Childhood* (7th ed.). New York: Appleton, 1917.
25. Jacobi, A. *Infant Diet.* New York: Putnam, 1885.
26. Koplik, H. E. *Diseases of Infancy and Childhood.* Philadelphia: Lea & Febiger, 1902.

27. LaFétra, L. E. The development of pediatrics in New York City. *Arch. Pediatr.* 49:36, 1932.
28. Marriott, W. McK. Preparation of lactic acid milk mixtures for infant feeding. *J.A.M.A.* 89:862, 1927.
29. Marriott, W. McK., and Davidson, L. T. Acidified whole milk as a routine infant food. *J.A.M.A.* 81:2007, 1923.
30. Marriott, W. McK., and Jeans, P. C. *Infant Nutrition* (3rd ed.). St. Louis: Mosby, 1941.
31. Marriott, W. McK., and Schoenthal, L. An experimental study of the use of unsweetened evaporated milk for the preparation of infant feeding formulas. *Arch. Pediatr.* 46:135, 1929.
32. McLean, S., and Fales, H. L. *Scientific Nutrition in Infancy and Early Childhood.* Philadelphia: Lea & Febiger, 1925.
33. McNutt, S. A. The Babies' Hospital—a summer's work. *Med. Rec.* (N.Y.). 35:234, 1889.
34. Morse, J. L. Recollections and reflections of forty-five years of artificial feeding. *J. Pediatr.* 7:303, 1935.
35. Phaire, T. *The Boke of Chyldren.* Edinburgh: E. & S. Livingstone, 1957.
36. Pinchbeck, I., and Hewitt, M. *Children in English Society,* Vol. 1. London: Routledge & Kegan Paul, 1969.
37. Powers, G. Infant feeding: Historical background and modern practice. *J.A.M.A.* 105:753, 1935.
38. Poynter, F. N. L. The story of artificial infant-feeding. *Br. Med. Bull.* 5:254, 1947–1948.
39. Rotch, T. M. Infant Feeding—Weaning. In J. M. Keating (Ed.), *Cyclopaedia of the Diseases of Children, Medical and Surgical,* Vol. 1. Philadelphia: Lippincott, 1889.
40. Rotch, T. M. An historical sketch of the development of percentage feeding. *N. Y. Med. J.* 85:532, 1907.
41. Rubner, M., and Heubner, O. Die Natürlich Ernährung eines Säuglings. *Z. Biol.* 36:1, 1898.
42. Ruhräh, J. The soy bean in infant feeding. *Arch. Pediatr.* 26:496, 1909.
43. Ruhräh, J. Further observations on the soy bean. *Trans. Am. Pediatr. Soc.* 23:386, 1911.
44. Sackett, W. W., Jr. Results of 3 years experience with a new concept of baby feeding. *South. Med. J.* 46:358, 1953.
45. Simon, J. F. *Mother's Milk and Its Chemical and Physical Properties* (Latin dissertation), Berlin, 1838.
46. Smith, H. *Letters to Married Women on Nursing and the Management of Children* (6th ed.). London: C. and G. Kearsley, 1792.
47. Smith, J. L. *A Treatise on the Diseases of Infancy and Childhood* (2nd ed.). Philadelphia: Henry C. Lea, 1872.
48. Still, G. F. *The History of Paediatrics.* London: Oxford University Press, 1931. P. 30.
49. Underwood, M. *A Treatise of the Diseases of Children.* London: J. Matthews, 1784.
50. Wickes, I. A. A history of infant feeding. *Arch. Dis. Child.* 28:232, 1953.

2. The Infant Feeding Experience

Rosanne B. Howard

Trends in infant feeding have changed from the breast to the bottle and back again to the breast, but the interpersonal aspects of feeding have remained constant. From birth, feeding is intermingled with emotions.

The infant makes the biological need for food known through crying and motor restlessness. The response of the maternal figure to these needs satisfies the infant's hunger and provides the first interpersonal experiences. While the infant is cradled and suckles, biological as well as emotional needs are met. The infant simultaneously experiences the pleasure of satiety with solace, warmth, comfort, and communication. As feelings of intimacy are transmitted, food and the process of eating become associated with security. Gradually, the biological need for food becomes entwined with emotions.

Thus, nourishment initiates a process that has a profound effect on development and extends well beyond infancy. This chapter explores not only the feeding skills and behavior of developing infants, but also the effects that feeding has on the developing infant.

INFANT DEVELOPMENT AND FEEDING

Over the years, a large body of research has been devoted to human development. Many alternate ways of studying development have evolved in which feeding plays varying roles. Each theory contributes toward the understanding, prediction, or guidance of behavior. Depending on the theoretical perspective, feeding can play a role in personality development, cognition, perception, and interpersonal relations. People tend to follow a particular theory because it blends with their own philosophy of life or helps them understand their past experiences. Health professionals offer many different philosophies concerning feeding. As a result, there is a range of answers to questions on weaning, feeding, and other problems, depending on whether the advice comes from one who advocates a psychodynamic, behavioral, organic-maturation, or other viewpoint.

During the late nineteenth century, the psychodynamic view of human development emerged. Sigmund Freud theorized that as infants mature their instinctual sexual energy (libido) is invested sequentially in biologically predetermined areas of the body. In each stage, one body organ predominates the mode of the infant's interactions; first, the mouth; second, the anus; and finally, the genital organs. In the first year, the infant is said to be orally dominated. All feelings including pleasure, hostility, and aggression are expressed with the

mouth. Freudians consider either excessive or inadequate oral gratification as instrumental in the development of an oral personality that
is characterized by passivity, dependence, eating problems, and
speech disorders [17]. According to their viewpoint, the early experiences of the child form the roots of the adult personality. Therefore,
an infant's oral experiences are considered to be the foundation of
personality development.

In the mid-1900s Freud's psychodynamic view was translated by
Erik Erikson into a more relevant format to meet the needs of the
American culture of the time. While drawing heavily from Freud, he
stressed the need for social integration. He looked for components
that fostered growth, whereas Freud looked from the origin of pathology. Erikson divided the life span from birth to senescence into
eight stages, each with a developmental crisis. Partial resolution of
each crisis is essential before the next stage may be entered. Between
birth and 12 to 18 months, the establishment of trust is the crisis. The
infant prepares for the next developmental level, autonomy, by ov-
ercoming a sense of mistrust. Because infants' initial contact with their
environment is with their mouths, they learn trust from feeding and
from oral exploration of their surroundings [14]. Infants develop trust
after their cries of hunger have been consistently met and satisfied
by their caregivers. Interestingly, some ancient tribes were rumored
to withhold food from their infants so that they would develop a sense
of mistrust and become aggressive warriors. In our own culture, it is
interesting to speculate on the effects on infants who are denied the
opportunity to learn trust through feeding, because they are fed by
gastrostomy or hyperalimentation for long periods, or because of
neurological impairments that impede sucking. These children are at
risk for developing a sense of mistrust concerning feeding because of
their undeveloped feeding skills (which may cause them to gag and
choke). This is often complicated further during hospitalization by
multiple caregivers with different feeding techniques. Whether this
ultimately influences personality development is open to question;
however, food resistance and negativism often outlast the phases of
organic insult [25].

In opposition to the global and intangible theories presented by the
psychodynamic school are the theories of the behaviorists. The stim-
ulus-response theory was postulated on the assumption that all physical and mental acts can be reduced to physical phenomena and can
therefore be observed and measured. The basic premise is that all
behavior is learned. Therefore, behaviorists consider the relationship
between feeding and development to be a learning experience and
also consider food as a positive reinforcer [4]. Thus, as the infant re-
lieves hunger pain and gains pleasure, behavior is learned. This behavior is repeated in future states of heightened drive and transferred

from one learning situation to another. If food is withheld and/or the feeder is distant, the infant is conditioned negatively by the feeding experience. This negative response may become generalized and produce distress in the infant and conflict with the mother figure. Because behaviorists consider feeding to be a learned behavior, food habits can be formed or changed simply by changing the reinforcement. For example, to promote good eating habits, a behaviorist would praise a child for eating vegetables and ignore the child when the food is spit out. Unfortunately, the opposite approach is usually taken at family mealtime. Parents often fail to recognize the inconsistencies of their mealtime expectations. Children often receive attention (or reinforcement) for spilling or playing with food and do not receive much attention for good mealtime behavior. This is a point to explore with a family whose child has feeding problems.

To those with an organic-maturation point of view, child development is autogenic. The mastery of skills is seen as self-generative toward higher levels of achievement. In Jean Piaget's theory of cognitive development, the individual's basic goal is to learn to master the environment (both external and internal). The pleasure of mastery spurs curiosity, problem solving, imitation, practice, and play activities. There are four developmental periods, each of which is characterized by specific interaction patterns with the environment. Feeding is the focus during the first, or sensorimotor period. From birth to age 2, development proceeds from the reflexive activities of the neonate to sensorimotor activities for problem solving. Children's intellectual experiences consist of observing and adaptively manipulating themselves and their environments [20]. Feeding provides the earliest sensorimotor experience (the suckling infant is held, tastes, smells, and feels milk). The infant gradually becomes able to organize this information, mentally coordinate the several related components of the feeding experience, and repeat the behavior. The result of this learning is an organized series of movements that the infant repeats in order to reinstate the feeding event. Thus, according to the organic-maturation view, as their body systems mature, infants learn a series of increasingly complex skills and have the opportunity to practice them.

Following the organic-maturation perspective, Arnold Gesell made very detailed, longitudinal observations of infant and child development [18]. He proposed the theory that maturation of the neuromuscular system allows for progressive organization of behaviors. From this research, a set of norms was developed to indicate when motor, adaptive, language, and personal-social behavior patterns typically appear in children from birth to the age of 16. With respect to feeding, characteristic patterns develop following physiological and neurological maturation. The infant progresses from a totally de-

pendent eater to an independent eater with the sequential development of head, trunk, gross, and fine motor control. Gesell regarded
feeding behavior as a major key to understanding infant personality.
He felt that the fields of clinical pediatrics and infant psychiatry should
take into account the personality symptoms displayed in appetites,
activity rhythms, physiological fluctuations, food preferences, food
resistances, and the methods by which a child learns self-feeding.
According to Gesell's theory, an inquiry into the usual food intake
and feeding atmosphere can give insight into a child's behavior. For
example, a 2-year-old child who is drinking only from the bottle (refusing the cup) may be having separation problems.

In this brief overview of some human development theories, it can
be seen that feeding plays an important role that, when questioned
theoretically, remains elusive. The association between a good early
feeding relationship and healthy adaptation has been observed from
differing research points such as attachments [7], mothering patterns
[9], and styles of interpersonal relationships [24]. Undoubtedly, the
pleasurable interaction of giving and taking provides the child with
a secure base from which to explore the world. Whether breast- or
bottle-feeding provides a more gratifying experience continues to be
an unanswered question.

FEEDING GRATIFICATION: BREAST- AND BOTTLE-FEEDING

The achievement of a gratifying experience involves a successful interaction between the caregiver and the infant, synchronized with the
infant's ability to suckle, swallow, and coordinate breathing. The significance of the differences in gratification offered in breast- versus
bottle-feeding are difficult to measure (Fig. 2-1). This does not imply
that infants or their mothers have the same experiences breast-feeding
as they do bottle-feeding. The experiences differ in regard to a number
of psychosocial and psychophysical variables. The differences become
more manifest when unrestricted breast-feeding (as practiced in
preindustrial countries) is compared to bottle-feeding.

Recent work in Africa with the Kun San, a hunter-gatherer group
in the Kalahari Desert, gives an interesting insight into the effects of
unrestricted breast-feeding [28]. Infants are breast-fed for an average
of three years. Small portions of the premasticated adult diet are introduced at the age of 1 month. As teeth appear, soft adult foods are
premasticated, and then coarser foods are provided; however, considerable breast milk consumption continues through the first year.
The infant nurses for 30 seconds to 5 minutes, with an average time

*Figure 2-1. A, B, and C. When there is a high degree of feeding synchrony, the
subsequent attachment of infant and caregiver is strong whether breast- or bottle-
fed.*

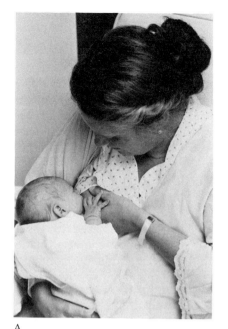

A

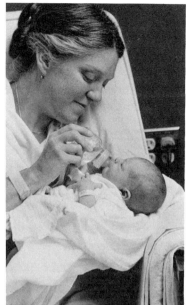

B

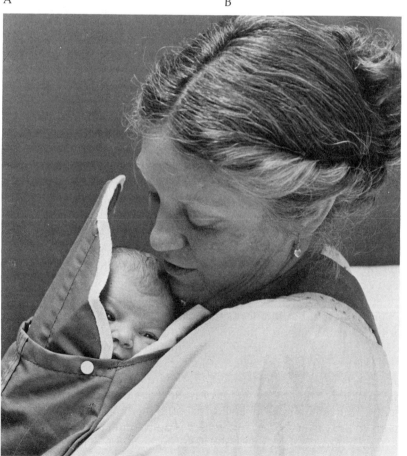

C

of 1 minute every 10 to 20 minutes of the waking hours. The infant sleeps with the mother and presumably can nurse throughout the night. Births are spaced 3 to 4 years apart. Apparently, maternal gonadal function is suppressed by the suckling pattern. Thus, breast feeding every 15 to 20 minutes appears to provide some hormonal protection against conception.

The feeding practices of the Kun San demonstrate patterns of infant care that have existed in the human species for more than one million years. In contemporary industrialized societies, unrestricted nursing and continuous physical interaction have been replaced by token breast-feeding or bottle-feeding with more limited contact. Infants spend less time in social contact with the feeder and lie horizontal for many hours of the day. Although generations have survived these practices, their evolutionary impact on development and mother–child interactions remains unknown [29].

The difference between token or "episodic" breast-feeding and unrestricted breast-feeding begins with the initial feeding experience. Token breast-feeding is characterized by severe limitations of sucking with rules regarding the number of feedings, duration, and the amount of mother–infant contact. Because of the limited contact, mothers initially may experience milk engorgement and pain. Infants who cannot grasp the nipple due to the engorgement may become frustrated. Alternatively, unrestricted breast-feeding stimulates the flow of milk and prevents engorgement. With bottle-feeding, there is usually no difficulty establishing milk flow. However, bottle-feeding does not usually allow the infant as much control, self-regulation, and synchronized interaction as breast feeding [1, 32]. The data of Crow and associates suggest that breast-feeding allows the infant to have more control during the feeding, whereas the mother has more control in bottle-feeding [12].

Many physiological changes occur in the mother who is breast-feeding, including rise in mammary skin temperature, rhythmical uterine contractions, and nipple stimulation (see Chap. 5). It also has been observed that women practicing unrestricted breast-feeding are not subject to the mood cycles connected with ovulation [32].

Similarities and differences exist between breast- and bottle-feeding for the infant. Breast-fed infants feed longer and spend a greater proportion of time with the nipple in their mouths [6]. With bottle-feeding, a rubber nipple delivers milk without much effort on the part of the infant, whereas with breast-feeding, the infant must put more effort into sucking. The assuagement of hunger is immediate with breast-feeding but sometimes delayed in bottle-feeding because the milk needs to be warmed first. The mouth-nipple contact of breast-feeding ensures a proximal mother-child feeding position, whereas there is more variation in positioning with bottle-feeding. An en face position (eye to eye and face to face) can promote proximity in bottle-feeding and increase the opportunity for social interaction and a rhythmical flow between the infant and feeder.

The mechanism of oral gratification related to sucking motions differs with breast- and bottle-feeding. With breast-feeding, infants suck with a compression action of lips, gums, and cheek muscles. The infant's tongue is thrust first forward and then backward as the nipple and areola are pulled back into the posterior oral cavity. With bottle-feeding, the rubber nipple requires a tugging response, flanging the lips into a large "O" and relaxing the cheek muscles [32]. The tongue, which moves forward to control the flow of milk into the esophagus, may at times be impeded by the rubber nipple.

The significance of the differences in suckling technique on behavior in later years is unclear. Caldwell's review concluded that feeding method per se has not been demonstrated to have reliable and consistent effects on behavioral development, although such effects have not been ruled out [11]. Most studies that attempted to determine the impact of breast- versus bottle-feeding were done on populations in which only token or short-term breast-feeding was present or in which the type of breast-feeding was unknown. Also, because of attitudinal and personality factors, no groups of breast- and bottle-fed infants are likely to be equal; psychological comparison may show differences due to uncontrolled covariables rather than to a cause-effect relationship determined by the method of feeding [32].

FEEDING AND ATTACHMENT

By feeding, infants develop attachments to parents that are fostered by the infant's instinctual survival responses of clinging, sucking, following, crying, and smiling [7]. During feeding, tactile stimulation that enhances the infant's ability to relate is promoted [23]. The process of attachment, like feeding, is a reciprocal balance of giving and taking between the caregiver and the infant. Reciprocity between the feeder and the infant is described as having a rhythmical quality; an ebb and flow. Brody reported that an infant's satisfactory weight gain is positively correlated with a mother who is sensitive, consistent, attentive, and able to accommodate to the needs of her infant [9]. Brazelton found that the mother's ability to be sensitive to her infant's capacity for attention as well as to the infant's need to withdraw from her after a period of attention is the most important factor in maintaining the rhythm. A mother's behavior during feeding was found to be an indicator of her overall behavior toward her infant [8].

Observation of the infant's temperamental pattern and the caregiver's response during feedings provides insight into the attachment

Table 2-1. Assessment of Feeding Synchrony

Assessment Area	Questions Asked
Timing of feedings	Does mother or infant determine feeding time?
Amount of food	Does mother or infant determine the amount of food and the end of feeding?
Rate of feedings	Who sets the pace of feedings?
Determination of food preference	Is there tact in handling the infant's food preference?

Data from Ainsworth, M. D. S., and Bell, S. M. Some Contemporary Patterns of Mother-Infant Interaction in the Feeding Situation. In L. Ambrose (Ed.), *Stimulation in Early Infancy*. New York: Academic Press, 1969. Pp. 133–170, and Ainsworth, M. D. S., et al. Individual Differences in Strange Situation Behavior of One-Year-Olds. In H. R. Schaffer (Ed.), *The Origins of Human Social Relations*. New York: Academic Press, 1971. Pp. 17–52.

process during the infant's first three months. When there is a high degree of feeding synchrony between the mother and child, subsequent attachment is strong [2, 3].

Synchrony can be assessed by observing the timing of feedings, the amount of food fed, the pace of feedings, and whether or not consideration is given to the infant's food preferences. During feedings, infants' social communication is composed of cries, whimpers, and open eyes (Table 2-1).

Observations of infant feeding indicate that it occurs in five distinct steps [33].

1. *Prefeeding behavior.* The level of arousal shown before feeding that indicates hunger.
2. *Approach behavior.* The predominant physical mode or reaching out to food or showing readiness to eat.
3. *Attachment behavior.* Activities occurring between the time the nipple touches the mouth and the time the infant is successful in nursing from it.
4. *Consummatory behavior.* Sucking and swallowing.
5. *Satiety behavior.* The infant's acts that indicate that the infant has finished.

Within the consummatory phase of eating, newborn infants have a natural, regular, rhythmic sucking pattern consisting of bursts of sucking followed by a pause of 4 seconds [27]. The length of bursts appears to be related to the milk flow, whereas the pauses are related to the mother-child interactions. Stimulation of the infant (e.g., jiggling the bottle) during the pauses reduces the likelihood of the infant's immediate return to a burst pattern of sucking; however, stopping the stimulation somewhat increases the speed of the infant's return to sucking. The mother's stimulating actions do not succeed in getting the infant to take more. In fact, Crow and coworkers found that the greater the mother's response, the less milk the infant consumed [12] (see Chap. 3). As mutual awareness of synchrony develops over the first few weeks of life, mothers are reported to change the way they stimulate their infants during the pause phase of sucking [27]. They stimulate the infants briefly and then wait for the infants to respond instead of stimulating until the infant begins to suck again.

The ability of the mother and infant to achieve feeding synchrony influences intake. The data of Pollitt and Wirtz suggest that intake during feeding depends in part on the behavioral synchronization of both the mother and infant. If the mother and infant repeatedly display behaviors that interfere with satisfactory feeding, they may imperil the growth of the infant. Also, data on infant communication shows that infants are active participants, not just passive recipients, making a significant contribution to the determination of the total volume of intake [36]. When infants are malnourished, they are less active and responsive; they elicit less response or stimulation from their mothers. This affects the infants' behavior and learning abilities [34] and ultimately affects the process of attachment. Other conditions that interfere with feeding synchrony potentially can jeopardize the attachment process. For example, the stress of prolonged hyperbilirubinemia and the use of phototherapy can result in a loss of control over normal sleeping and waking rhythms. Infants afflicted with this condition can offer misleading feeding cues and sleep through feedings. Infants with respiratory distress who stop eating due to their inability to coordinate breathing and feeding also give misleading cues to their caretakers and make synchrony difficult to achieve. Thus, in the feeding dyad, the condition of the infant, as well as the emotions of the feeder, contributes to the successful achievement of synchrony.

For some time, the effects of the emotional state of the feeder on infant feeding behavior has been recognized. Escalona studied the effect of emotional strain on the behavior of fifty babies ranging from 10 days to 24 months old [15]. The infants were in a nursery in a women's reformatory. Feeding difficulties and reduced intake were greater on parole days and holidays when the moods of mothers and attendants were more labile, although the routine was the same. During the 20 months of study, the prevailing emotional atmosphere became a sensitive indicator of the eating behavior of the infants. When formula was offered by a substitute caregiver, intake improved considerably. Thus, the feeding problems seemed to be associated with maternal behavior.

A lack of synchrony between the feeder and the infant causes confusion in the infant's conceptual awareness. For example, an infant who appears hungry irregularly can be overfed or underfed depending on the feeder's interpretation. The feeder may attempt to placate the infant with more milk or withhold milk while trying to place the infant on a schedule. Thus, infants come to rely on cues emanating from the feeder to know when and how much to eat, and they lose their own sense of control. The ability to control is considered to be an important ingredient of cognitive development; without it, there are regulation problems. Infants become unable to recognize hunger or satiety or differentiate the need for food from other sensations (i.e., thirst). The inability to recognize hunger and other body sensations, along with a lack of sense of individual control, are traits often found in individuals with obesity or anorexia nervosa. According to Bruch, the early histories of these individuals often fail to give evidence of gross neglect, but do indicate inappropriate responses, whereby mothers superimposed their interpretations of the needs of the infants rather than interpreting the cues offered by the infants [10].

When there is a lack of feeding synchrony and lack of attachment, feeding problems are common. Infants with growth failure due to sensory deprivation tend to be fussy eaters; however, sometimes they have insatiable appetites and are willing to eat anything. They often spit, vomit, or turn away from their feeder. They may fall asleep during feedings and have foul-smelling stools or abdominal distention [13]. In Pollitt's study, families of failure-to-thrive infants reported significantly lower caloric intakes and more feeding problems with their infants than families of thriving infants. Smaller, less regular meals and poorer responses to food were observed [35] (see Chap. 9). Also, Gunther found profound anxiety and depression in mothers who experience difficulty in feeding their babies with subsequent disturbance of the mother-child relationship [21].

The infant who requires long-term hospitalization and is fed by gastrostomy or life support line (i.e., tracheoesophageal fistula) often is missing a gratifying feeding experience and the opportunity to develop close attachments. Practitioners must be alert to possible sensorimotor deprivation in these high-risk infants and should enlist mothers and primary care nurses to provide the appropriate oral, motor, and environmental stimulation. Infants should be held (condition allowing) as frequently as a breast-feeding infant. Prior to food introduction, oral stimulation with pacifiers dipped in formula to accustom the infant to taste and play that encourages hand-to-mouth activity should be encouraged. Because parents are constrained in feeding, other avenues of parenting must be found. Parents of children with feeding problems need ongoing professional support and help in dissociating feeding failure from their overall parenting ability.

For the infant, the task in infant feeding is to produce clear feeding cues and respond appropriately to the feeder. The parents' tasks are to respond to the infant's cues, alleviate distress, and provide growth-fostering situations [5]. Growth-fostering situations include social, emotional, and cognitive activities. They depend on the parents' available energy as well as their knowledge and skill. Parents must be aware of the child's level of development and adjust their behavior accordingly in order to play affectionately and engage in social amenities associated with feeding while reinforcing desirable behaviors. They must feed their infants according to cues emanating from the infants and adapt food and utensils to their infant's developing feeding skills.

INFANT FEEDING SKILLS

The natural course of learning to eat progresses from breast- or bottle-feeding to assisted spoon-feeding in combination with finger-feeding, and then to the independent use of utensils. These eating skills develop simultaneously with the development of head, trunk, gross, and fine motor control.

During the first 3 to 4 months, the normal infant participates in feeding with cries of hunger and oral reflexive responses. The reflexes of rooting, sucking, swallowing, and biting are the basic movement patterns of infant feeding.

Two responses incorporate the rooting reflex and may be elicited from the touch stimulus: the side-to-side turning reflex and the directed head-turning response [26]. The infant's head initially will turn toward the stimulus and then toward the other side. For a few seconds, head turning from side to side occurs in arcs of decreasing size, and then the fulcrum of turning is gradually oriented toward the stimulus so that the infant's lips make a brushing contact with it. The directed head-turning response is a single, well-directed, purposeful looking movement of the head that results in the infant's mouth being brought into contact with the nipple. The side-to-side response predominates for the first 2 to 3 weeks and wanes as the directed head-turning response becomes easier to elicit.

The rooting reflex occurs when tactile stimulation is given at the upper lip, lower lip, or the corners of the mouth. This response begins to disappear sometime around the age of 3 months. The rooting reflex is stronger before a feeding, and when the child is in the position associated with feeding. With breast-feeding, the rooting may persist for a longer period of time than with bottle-feeding.

The early infantile way of sucking is called suckling and is observed during the first 5 to 6 months; it involves a definite extension-retraction movement of the tongue. Milk is obtained by a rhythmical licking action of the tongue on the nipple combined with the opening and closing of the jaw [30]. Suckling includes both a lip reflex and the actual sucking reflex. The lip phenomenon is composed of involuntary movements of the lips towards a stroking stimulus placed on or about the mouth and their subsequent closure and pouting. Sucking may or may not follow. As soon as the mouth gets close enough to the stimulus, the tongue retracts and the lips are closed. Usually, swallowing follows and the infant makes sucking movements. Between 6 to 12 weeks of age, infants learn to breathe easily through their mouths and their swallowing pattern changes [26]. The tongue ceases to come forward as the mouth opens, and there is a more definite jaw movement. In a small percentage of infants, tongue protrusion persists beyond this age.

Initially, the suck and swallow reflexes work in a chain reaction. The infant can initiate a swallow only after the suckling reflex has occurred. Presumably, suckling throws saliva back into the reflexogenic zone and triggers the swallowing reflex. An upward movement of the hyoid bone indicates swallowing.

A true suckling pattern gradually is achieved, usually by the age of 6 to 8 months [30]. The tongue action of the true suckling pattern consists of raising and lowering the body of the tongue. There is less jaw movement than in the previous suckling patterns. Also, a greater amount of tongue tip elevation is found with a firmer approximation of the lips. The liquid is pulled into the mouth due to the negative pressure created by the combined closure of the lips and the lowering of the tongue.

The bite reflex is a rhythmical bite and release pattern of jaw openings and closings that occurs because of stimulation to the gums. The infant bites vertically until the stimulus is released. The bite reflex continues primarily as a reflexive behavior until 3 to 5 months of age. It is replaced by a more volitional bite that becomes a munching or early chewing pattern somewhere between the age of 6 to 9 months [30].

Usually, the gag reflex is present from birth to adulthood. It occurs with a stimulus to the posterior tongue or soft palate that causes constriction of the posterior oral musculature in order to bring the stimulating substance forward. Stimulation of the posterior half of the tongue or the pharyngeal area causes gagging. This protective response allows the return of food from the back of the mouth to the front. It consists of lowering the jaw forward and also downward movements of the tongue. Gagging elicited by the stimulation of the lips or front of the tongue is abnormal. Frequent gagging in a child may be caused by hypersensitivity of the gag or by swallowing difficulties or may be voluntarily induced by some to gain attention. As chewing begins, the gag reflex becomes weaker [31].

For feeding to be successful, all the reflexes must be integrated and merge imperceptibly with one another. Also, they must be coordinated with other activities of the infant. Of particular importance is the co-ordination of sucking and swallowing with respiration. The coordi-nation of sucking and breathing at 60 to 100 times per minute with swallowing occurring every 2 to 3 sucks places demands on the infant [22]. Swallowing is best performed at the end of inspiration or ex-piration and does not interrupt respiration for any more than 0.2 or 0.3 second. Breathing always takes precedence over feeding. (The in-fant experiencing breathing difficulties will stop feeding. In some in-fants, this marks the beginning of feeding refusals [25]) (see Chap. 11).

Successful feeding also requires that infants adapt their behavior and reflexes to their environment. For example, infants must adapt to either the breast or bottle with different movements of the mouth. Failure to adapt or disturbances in feeding behavior are symptoms found in infants who may later evince mental retardation or cerebral palsy [26]. The observation of spontaneous behavior provides more information than the examination of the individual feeding reflexes. Observations of feeding behavior can give information about the child's level of motor, linguistic, adaptive, and social maturation (see Chap. 11). However, the examination of individual feeding reflexes

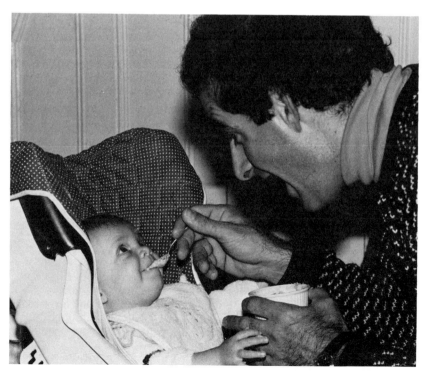

Figure 2-2. Infant's first foods are introduced (4 to 6 months).

gives relatively little information about the state of maturation of the infant's nervous system because feeding reflexes can be demonstrated in even the smallest of fetuses. (Lip reflexes are present in fetuses as early as age 9½ weeks and swallowing reflexes as early as 12½ weeks) [16]. Also, the ease with which feeding reflexes can be elicited varies even among healthy infants.

As the reflexive behavior of infants becomes voluntary, they learn to chew and swallow (rather than suck and swallow food) and to drink from a cup (Fig. 2-2). They also acquire all the manipulative skills that are necessary for independent feeding. Table 2-2 summarizes this transition.

Table 2-2. Development of Feeding Skills

Age	Oral and Neuromuscular Development	Feeding Behavior
Birth	Rooting reflex (retention = 3–5 months)	Stimulation to oral area (corners of mouth, upper and lower lip) causes lips, tongue, and finally the head to turn toward stimulus
	Suckle-swallow (retention = 5–6 months) interferes with taking solid food	A stimulus introduced into the mouth elicits vigorous sucking followed by a swallow if liquid is present
	Bite reflex (retention = 6–9 months)	Stimulation to gums elicits a rhythmical bite and release pattern
	Gag reflex (retention into adulthood)	Stimulation to the posterior tongue or soft palate causes constriction of the posterior oral musculature to bring stimulating substance forward
6–10 weeks		Recognizes feeding position and begins sucking and mouthing when placed in position
6–12 weeks	Infants learn to breathe through mouths	Swallowing pattern changes and tongue ceases to come forward. As the mouth opens, there is a more definite jaw movement, a sign of beginning readiness for solid food

Table 2-2. Development of Feeding Skills (*Continued*)

Age	Oral and Neuromuscular Development	Feeding Behavior
3–6 months		Drooling starts in normal infants at 3 months and disappears before 12 months; it increases with teething
	Beginning coordination between eyes and body movements	Explores world with eyes, fingers, hands, and mouth
4 months	Brings hand to mouth. Reaches for objects but overshoots	Finger sucking
5 months	Voluntary grasp	Palmar grasp
6–8 months	Sucking pattern	A true sucking pattern with less jaw movement
	Lateral jaw movements	Enables munching or early chewing. Can approximate lips to cup and cup-drinking begins. However, liquid dribbles from corners because tongue is projected before swallowing
6 months	Sits erect with support. Eyes and hands working together	Feeds self teething biscuit. Bangs cup and throws feeding utensils
	Reaches for and grasps object on sight	Reaches for food and feeding utensils
7–8 months	Sits alone without support	Freer to reach and grasp. Grasp has increasing finger-thumb opposition
9–12 months		Holds onto bottle and finger feeds
12 months		Uses cup independently with two hands. Beginning of independence with spoon. However, the spoon is grasped with the hand in pronation. Chews well (but not yet mature chew pattern)

Data from Gesell, A., and Ilg, F. *Feeding Behavior of Infants*. Philadelphia: J. B. Lippincott, 1937.

FEEDING BEHAVIOR: A DEVELOPMENTAL PERSPECTIVE

Within the first few weeks of life, the primary caregiver is able to interpret the infant's signals for feeding versus holding or the infant's need for non-nutritive sucking. (Non-nutritive sucking appears to help infants to quiet themselves. It seems to help contain them as much as holding does.) A reciprocity develops as feeding patterns become established. Between 8 to 12 weeks of age, infants regard their mother's faces for prolonged periods during feedings [19]. By 3 months of age, a social repertoire (looks at face at 4 weeks old, smiles at 8 weeks old, coos at 12 weeks old) has been added to feeding times [19]. Lip smacking noises join the growing mealtime resonance by age 22 weeks [19]. During this period, there is a major shift in the infant's organizational state with longer nighttime sleep patterns and more predictable alert states. Crying periods diminish, and feeding schedules become more regular. Infants express their needs with more differentiated cues that facilitate reciprocal exchange with their caregivers.

Between age 4 and 9 months, infants develop new feeding skills (see Table 2-2) and a broader awareness of the environment changes the way the infant approaches feeding. The first signs of autonomy develop almost simultaneously with the acquisition of the reaching skill (reaches for an object on sight and grasps it at 24 weeks old). Extraneous stimuli (e.g., noise) now capture the infant's attention and can interfere with feeding. This change can be puzzling to parents, who may interpret this behavior as disinterest in feedings or even in them, while in fact, infants are becoming more interested in the world apart from their parents. (Sometimes, parents experience a sense of loss because most parents find the dependence of the infant gratifying.) It is at this time that more active participation of the child in the feeding should begin even though the child will continue to vacillate between autonomy and dependence. Finger foods promote involvement as children learn to sit alone, develop eye-hand coordination, and hold their own bottles (see Chap. 5). Food and utensils become interesting objects. Smearing, poking, or spitting out food, and banging or throwing utensils represent exploration, not necessarily rejection. The developing sense of spatial awareness, permanency of objects, and casual connections creates in infants a sense of awareness of the utility of feeding utensils apart from play.

Between age 10 and 12 months, infants become even more vocal in their continuing bid for autonomy. Different kinds of vocalizations now accompany mealtimes. During feedings, infants will demand a play object (at age 40 weeks), throw bottles to the floor (at 44 weeks), and even hand the bottle to the feeder (at 48 weeks) [19]. Although infants are able to drink from a cup (4 to 5 swallows or more at age 40 weeks), they will continue to spill from the corners of their mouths while drinking liquids [19]. Although they will raise cups to their lips with assistance, they will tilt the cup instead of tilting their heads. Given free rein, they will throw the cup instead of putting it down. A grasp with a well-defined thumb opposition (at age 44 weeks) further refines finger-feeding and paves the way for spoon-feeding [19]. Some infants will allow parents to fill the spoon but insist on bringing it to their own mouths. With favorite foods, lip-smacking sounds can be heard. Although infants are chewing well by the age of 44 weeks [19], a good rotary chewing does not develop until 18 to 36 months. (As a result, undigested food is often found in the stool of normal infants at this age.)

With more independence through cruising (at age 48 weeks) and walking with support (at 52 weeks), as well as more proficiency with the spoon (52 to 64 weeks) [19], food idiosyncrasies begin to appear and infants' jabbering expresses their needs. Infants often refuse to be fed anything and may be unwilling to try new foods. Some are willing to eat only three or four foods and one or two meals per day. This behavior becomes more pronounced in the first half of their second year (see Chap. 6). This food negativism represents infants' differentiation of themselves from their environment and a true passage to feeding autonomy.

CONCLUSION

For most infants, being loved and fed comes to be associated as the repetitive cycle of emotional and nutritional gratification becomes integrated with the mother figure. During infants' first few months of life, the focus of activity is on their mouths. The overriding principle of care is total gratification of need. The mouth is a channel of feeling and taste that infants use to explore their environments.

All infants have unique feeding experiences due in part to the interpersonal interactions they are exposed to during feeding. Their genetic backgrounds influence their ability to feed and taste food and also make their feeding experiences unique.

Calm and comfortable feeding management forms a sense of security in the developing infant. Whether the infant is breast- or bottle-fed, the reciprocity of the adult-infant relationship should be the overriding feeding principle.

REFERENCES
1. Ainsworth, M. D. S. *Infancy in Uganda*. Baltimore: Johns Hopkins Press, 1963.
2. Ainsworth, M. D. S., and Bell, S. M. Some Contemporary Patterns of Mother-Infant Interaction in the Feeding Situation. In L. Ambrose (Ed.), *Stimulation in Early Infancy*. New York: Academic Press, 1969. Pp. 133–170.
3. Ainsworth, M. D. S., et al. Individual Differences in Strange Situation Behavior of One-Year-Olds. In H. R. Schaffer (Ed.), *The Origins of Human Social Relations*. New York: Academic Press, 1971. Pp. 17–52.

4. Bandura, A. *Principles of Behavior Modification.* New York: Holt, Rinehart and Winston, 1969.
5. Barnard, K. E. A perspective on where we are in early intervention programs. Adapted from a keynote address at a conference, "The Nursing Role in Early Intervention Programs for Developing Disabled Children," sponsored by the University of Utah College of Nursing, Division of Continuing Education, and Utah State Division of Health, Denver, Colorado, Feb. 1976.
6. Bernal, J., and Richards, M. P. M. The effects of bottle and breast feeding on infant development. *J. Psychosom. Res.* 14:247, 1970.
7. Bowlby, J. *Attachment and Loss.* Vol. 1. New York: Basic Books, Inc., Harper Colophon Books, 1969.
8. Brazelton, T. B., et al. The Origins of Reciprocity. In M. Lewis and L. Rosenbaum (Eds.), *The Effects of the Infant on its Caregiver.* New York: Ivan Wille and Sons, 1974.
9. Brody, S. Patterns of Mothering. *Maternal Influences During Feeding.* New York: International Universities Press, 1956.
10. Bruch, H. *Eating Disorders: Obesity, Anorexia Nervosa and the Person Within.* New York: Basic Books, Inc., 1978.
11. Caldwell, B. M. The Effects of Infant Care. In M. L. Hoffman and L. W. Hoffman (Eds.), *Review of Child Development Research,* Vol. 1. New York: Russell Sage Foundation, 1964. Pp. 9–89.
12. Crow, R. A., et al. Maternal behavior during breast and bottle feeding. *J. Behav. Med.* 3:259, 1980.
13. English, P. Failure to thrive without organic reasons. *Pediatr. Ann.* 7:774, 1978.
14. Erikson, E. *Childhood and Society* (2nd ed.) New York: W. W. Norton, 1963.
15. Escalona, S. K. Feeding disturbances in very young children. *Am. J. Orthopsychiatry* 15:76, 1945.
16. Fitzgerald, J. E., and Windle, W. F. Some observations on early human fetal movements. *J. Comp. Neurol.* 76:159, 1942.
17. Freud, S. *Three Essays on the Theory of Sexuality.* New York: Avon, 1962.
18. Gardner, H. *Developmental Psychology: An introduction.* Boston: Little, Brown, 1978.
19. Gesell, A., and Ilg, F. *Feeding Behavior of Infants.* Philadelphia: J. B. Lippincott, 1937.
20. Ginsberg, H., and Opper, S. *Piaget's Theory of Intellectual Development.* Englewood Cliffs, N.J.: Prentice-Hall, 1969.
21. Gunther, M. Instinct and the nursing couple. *Lancet* 268:575, 1955.
22. Halverson, H. M. Mechanism of early feeding. *J. Genet. Psychol.* 64:185, 1944.
23. Harlow, H. F., and Zimmerman, R. R. Affectional responses in the infant monkey: Orphaned monkeys develop a strong and persistent attachment to inanimate surrogate mothers. *Science* 130:421, 1959.
24. Heinstein, M. I. Behavior correlates of breast-bottle regimens under various parent-infant relationships. *Monogr. Soc. Res. Child Dev.* 344:919, 1963.
25. Howard, R. Feeding intervention for the tube-fed infant with food aversion. Unpublished manuscript, 1984.
26. Ingram, T. T. S. Clinical significance of the infantile feeding reflexes. *Dev. Med. Child Neurol.* 4:159, 1962.
27. Kaye, K. Towards the Origin of Dialogue. In H. R. Schaffer (Ed.), *Studies in Mother-Infant Interaction.* New York: Academic Press, 1977.

28. Konner, M., and Worthman, C. Nursing frequency, gonadal function, and birth spacing among the Kung hunter-gatherers. *Science* 185:932, 1974.
29. Lozoff, B., et al. The mother-newborn relationship: Limits of adaptability. *J. Pediatr.* 91:1, 1977.
30. Morris, S. E. A glossary of terms describing the feeding process. Workshop, Boston, Massachusetts, May, 1978.
31. Mueller, H. Facilitating Feeding and Prespeech. In P. Pearson and C. Williams (Eds.), *Physical Therapy in the Developmental Disabilities*. Springfield, Ill.: Charles C. Thomas, 1972. Pp. 286–288.
32. Newton, N. Psychologic differences between breast and bottle feeding. *Am. J. Clin. Nutr.* 25:993, 1971.
33. O'Grady, R. Feeding behavior in infants. *Am. J. Nurs.* 71:736, 1971.
34. Pollitt, E. Behavior of infants in causation of nutritional marasmus. *Am. J. Clin. Nutr.* 26:264, 1973.
35. Pollitt, E. Failure to thrive: Socioeconomic, dietary intake, and mother-child interaction data. *Fed. Proc.* 34:1593, 1975.
36. Pollitt, E., and Wirtz, S. Mother-infant feeding interaction and weight gain in the first month of life. *J. Am. Diet. Assoc.* 78:596, 1981.

3. Developmental Feeding Issues

T. Berry Brazelton, Robert L. Gatson, and Rosanne B. Howard

AN OVERVIEW OF FEEDING ISSUES DURING THE FIRST THREE YEARS

For most parents, feeding a child is equated to loving that child. So deep-seated is the feeling of responsibility for nurturing that parents consider any deviation from an optimal intake on the part of their child a reflection of their incompetence as parents. Some feel that their job is to get food into their baby, no matter what happens afterward. Dogged with the feeling that "my child never eats enough," parents may overlook the child's actual nutritional requirements. If this underlying feeling of responsibility is accepted as normal, professionals interested in helping parents avoid feeding problems will better understand the inevitable resistance as they try to divert parental anxiety from the issue of feeding. Anxiety about feeding cannot be diverted, but it can be accepted by parents who understand the reasons for the tension. Then and only then can they be led to an understanding of the forces in the child that are interfering with their own goals as parents who want to "feed the child."

Just as feeding is a critical area of concern for parents, issues of autonomy and of establishing one's own controls in feeding are critical for children in their own development. Unless children can establish feelings of mastery in feeding, the chances are great that feeding will not be a rewarding experience, but rather one of anxiety and conflict.

As babies or small children achieve each new step in development, their recognition of having completed a desired step leads to a vital sense of competence. Figure 3-1 schematizes the forces that interact during child development. As the central nervous system matures, it forces children to abandon any homeostatic state they might have achieved and to take more ambitious steps toward maturity. Two sources of reward fuel this rather demanding process: external reinforcements from the environment are carefully balanced by the need for the internal feedback of self-achievement. Recognition of self-achievement is critical so that children can experience feelings of self-competence. External reinforcement for accomplishment from parents and others heightens their pleasure in achievement. It is essential that a child experience the feeling of "I've done it myself!"

It is during this period of maturation, coincident with the burgeoning attachment of parents to the child, that parents must rec-

This chapter was written while R.L.G. was partially funded by the Robert Wood Johnson Foundation, Carnegie Corporation, the Saul C. and Amy S. Cohen Foundation, and the National Institute of Mental Health.

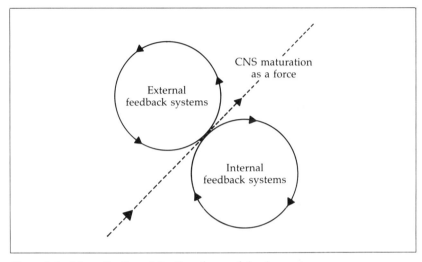

Figure 3-1. Schematization of the three forces of development.

ognize the child's need for detachment, or autonomy. This becomes the most difficult conflict in parenting. To achieve a balance between dependence and independence in the area of feeding is probably one of the hardest tasks parents will face. Parents must be helped to sort out their own needs for nurturing and hovering from those of the child who is hurtling toward independence in this important area. Professionals interested in preventing feeding difficulties must help parents accept their child's need for independence, despite the parents' longing for dependence. These issues may be painful for both the parents and the child to accept. The professional must be patient and understanding, as well as supportive in order to prevent the besieged parent from having a continuous confrontation with the child. Parents must be made to understand that the inevitable overfeeding struggle is an issue of autonomy rather than one of raw resistance on the part of the child.

FEEDING ISSUES IN THE FIRST YEAR

The decision to breast- or bottle-feed becomes the first feeding issue for new mothers. Most young women have a deep-seated bias for one mode or the other, based on past experiences in their lives (usually the way they were nurtured by their own mothers). Women who have seen their own mothers breast-feed a younger sibling are more likely to be successful at breast-feeding their own infants. Unfortunately, the trend for smaller families decreases the likelihood of this type of observation. However, the increasing bias in young parents toward the breast as a safer, more appropriate way of feeding is adding societal pressure to try to breast-feed. If breast-feeding is rewarding for the mother, she can create a pleasurable, rewarding atmosphere around feeding that will ultimately be rewarding for the baby as well. An intimate reciprocity of feelings, as well as of cognitive and affective cues, will certainly enhance the pleasure derived from this experience.

Kaye and Brazelton [5] studied the burst-pause sucking pattern into which small infants lapse after they are initially satiated. After a few minutes of intense sucking, a small baby is likely to start a burst of sucks that alternate with short pauses. This burst-pause pattern is a normal one for both nutritional and non-nutritional sucking. When a mother or a nurse feeds a baby, she will react by jiggling the bottle or the baby at the breast, speaking, touching, or looking down at the child during approximately 50 percent of the pauses. If an observer asks the adult who is feeding why she responds by stimulating the baby during the pauses, she will say, "I want him to keep going. I want him to get his food. If I let him stop he won't eat properly." We measured the length of pauses when the adult responded with a stimulus and compared those against the length of the pauses when the baby was not stimulated. The baby responded by prolonging the pause when she did react and shortening the pause when she did not. In other words, the baby's agenda seemed to be that of eliciting social interaction as well as food during feeding. We thought that this burst-pause pattern represented an ethological adaptation to elicit social stimuli and to hold the mother's attention at the time of the feeding. If a mother is breast-feeding, she is more likely to be acutely in tune with her baby's pauses than if she is bottle-feeding. However, if she does not find breast-feeding rewarding, her unconscious biases and resistance may transmit to the baby and result in an unhappy feeding situation. Hence, no mother should be pressed to breast-feed against her wishes.

We do not feel that a professional should put pressure on a mother who is deeply ambivalent about her ability or desire to breast-feed. This ambivalence often reflects unfortunate experiences in her past or a deep-seated fear of the inability to nurture her baby successfully. It would be more in the baby's best interest to support the mother fully in whatever decision she makes. As professionals we should provide a mother with the knowledge we have about the relative merits of each type of feeding and help her to understand her feelings in this area, which could interfere with successful feeding regardless of the technique chosen (see Chap. 5).

Frequent feeding is too often used as a way of trying to quiet a fussy or unhappy baby, especially in the first weeks or months after birth while parents are learning about the baby's cycles of consciousness, sleep, and fussy states. All new parents feel that a quiet baby is a happy baby, and that crying is a plea for help. Parents believe that if they do the right thing, the crying will stop. If fussing or crying continues, it must be a reflection of their inadequacy as parents. In fact, the desperation that parents experience when faced with an inconsolable infant may drive them to behave frantically and thus actually increase the baby's crying. Unfortunately, the most common reaction of the parents during these periods is to feed the child, hoping that sucking will quiet the child. This temporary solution may lead to overfeeding and may cause additional intestinal discomfort. Feeding can overstimulate an already exhausted infant, and parents should understand that sometimes an infant simply needs to fuss. After experiencing this with a first child, parents rarely try to use feeding as a cure-all with second or third children. This vicious cycle of fussing at the end of an active day, which many of us see as a discharge phenomenon, can be the etiological basis for so-called colic in the first 3 months. Parents should be warned not to overreact, since 80 percent of babies experiencing fussy periods do not have true colic.

Just as some parents overreact to an infant's needs, some ignore the infant's need for other sources of stimulation. By 6 weeks of age, a baby may need to have visual, auditory, or kinesthetic stimulation from an environment that persists in feeding him at every waking period. Parents who are primarily concerned with feeding their infant may be exposing the infant to an understimulating environment. By the same token, a baby may fail to thrive if exposed to an overloading or overstimulating environment. Even in what appears to be a nurturing environment, an insensitive parent may be reacting in ways that are inappropriate for the child. During feeding, many infants regurgitate or spit; if weight gain is inadequate, parents should look closely to see if they are responding appropriately to their child's eating difficulties (see Chap. 11). The baby often is hypersensitive to environmental stimuli and his or her hyperactive intestinal tract may be a reflection of a misfit with the environment. The gastrointestinal tract is a real mirror of psychological well-being or disturbance in the small infant.

Autonomy Issues

Babies learn about their world at feeding times. Absorbing and utilizing social information during feeding times is just as critical to their well-being as the food is and provides a way for them to learn about themselves. Children learn early that they can manipulate their environment. By refusing food, they can create concern about themselves. By crying, they can call their parents to feed them. By age 5 months, infants learn that they can manipulate the feeding by refusing to eat and by paying attention to the events surrounding them. Mothers are confused and upset by these interrupted feedings. If the child is being breast-fed, the mother may feel her milk is inadequate. If bottle-fed, she may feel the baby's refusal is a sign of teething, illness, or negativism.

Parents must realize that there are developmental reasons for interrupted feedings and for their child's half-hearted interest in being fed. The baby's sudden surge in awareness of environmental stimuli increases his or her sensitivity to sights and sound. The infant may pay more attention to the surrounding stimuli than to satisfy hunger. At such times, a parent can be advised to feed the child in a quiet, darkened room. Of course, this may not be feasible except in the early morning or late at night if there are other children or people around. Parents should be assured that two good feedings are probably enough to maintain the baby's caloric needs and will stimulate a mother's milk production successfully, even if the other daytime feedings are short and interrupted. Hence, this period of autonomy can be survived without causing conflicts in the area of feeding.

The next developmental stage, in which fine motor skills develop, brings with it new feeding methods and problems. At 8 months, coincident with the advent of the pincer grasp, infants are ready for feeding soft bits of food to themselves. If this new stage of development is not recognized by the caregiver, infants will begin to grab for the spoon or may refuse to be fed. Gently at first, they will act distracted or mildly negative during feedings. If parents ignore these pleas for autonomous participation in feeding, infants will begin to adamantly resist feedings. Mothers will report that their 9- or 10-month-old infants are likely to shake their heads at feeding times, already resisting being fed. A feeding problem can develop if mothers are not aware of the child's interest in self-feeding. A child wants to be allowed to hold onto and brandish a spoon or a piece of food at feeding times. A child's excitement about the new acquisition of the use of fingers in self-feeding is so great that it will surmount the need for food. Parents should be urged to offer soft finger bits of food to their 8-month-old so the baby can try out the newfound accomplishment (see Chap. 5). By one year, children now being introduced to solid foods are sure to be resistant to feedings in which they are not allowed to be an active participant. Parents who have allowed self-feeding at 8 or 9 months will have already overcome the problems of resistance to being fed. Mothers need this kind of explanation in order to be alert to the autonomy issue in their 8- or 9-month-old babies.

At the age of 1 year, coincident with the independence of walking and of making decisions for themselves, toddlers are likely to become extremely negative about being fed. If they have been given the chance to self-feed, they will be less resistant to being fed. If not, they are likely to begin to develop a feeding problem. As their resistance to being fed increases, parents' anxiety will mount. The two resistant forces could ultimately lead to a real crisis concerning feeding.

Parents often worry that if a child is self-feeding, he or she may not be receiving an adequate intake. They must be reassured that a reduced intake will tide the toddler through this negative period (see Chap. 6). Parents should be told that this period of negativism about feeding is part of a necessary and expectable stage of development, and that a child's need to self-feed is more important than the amount of food consumed.

FEEDING PROBLEMS

Feeding problems are usually based on a struggle between the parent and child. Respecting the child's need for autonomy in feeding can prevent many major crises. parents need to be prepared and to be given an explanation of feeding development as well as guidelines for a reasonable amount of food in a form easy to self-feed during the toddler years (see Chap. 6). Problems are more likely to develop when feeding is thwarted by illness, when the child has congenital anomalies that interfere with feeding, or when normal feeding has been delayed by prematurity. Parents are bound to become more anxious because of these problems and may not allow the normal progression of feeding skills.

Because of their anxiety and overprotectiveness, parents can interrupt the progression from the breast or bottle to the cup and from strained foods to table foods. The developmental feeding readiness of sick or impaired children can be overlooked if the child offers misleading cues in the feeding area or if parental concern about the illness takes precedence. Parents of sick children inadvertently overprotect or push them beyond their limits. Parents need help interpreting the effects of illness on their children's feeding behavior. In many instances, dietary restrictions cause additional stress in an environment already emotionally charged by illness or handicap. If parents equate the giving of food with the giving of love, their parenting ability may be threatened if they are not able to give food freely (see Table 6-3).

Illness and Feeding Behavior

All types of illness affect behavior, whether acute, chronic, major, or minor. Parents may become worried and feel guilty if their children are frightened. They may behave insensitively at such times and push a child to be "grown up" at the very time that the child needs to be treated as an infant. They push too hard—not because they don't care, but because they care too much and are frightened. The feeding area often becomes a battleground at such times.

Chronic illness can drain children and their families. Parents and children cope with disease as they try to live "normal" lives in environments filled with loss, grief, and stress. The children must confront the stresses of disease or of surgery while facing the normal challenges of maturation. Children's fears may be exposed during mealtime. They may regress back to the bottle or insist on being fed. In addition, parents and children must cope with the restrictions placed on diets, modes of feeding (e.g., hyperalimentation, gastrostomy), and impaired activity. Although each condition may impose specific limitations on feeding, some management issues are universal.

Striving for independence creates an added stress for ill children. For example, the negative 2-year-old usually wants everybody else's food, wants to self-feed, and does not want to be different. When diets or alternative feeding methods (e.g., gastrostomy) are imposed, crisis may arise. Parents worried about their child's poor growth and refusal of food may begin food battles. However, if they view the toddler's developing feeding autonomy as a major opportunity to promote the child's self-development and competence, they can avoid such a situation. They can allow the child to make food choices (e.g., milk or juice), allow the child to engage in self-feeding, or allow flexibility in meal schedules. Parents need anticipatory guidance. They must be helped to understand the normalcy of toddler negativism, independence, and autonomy and realize that these are not necessarily disease-related so that they will be able to plan strategies and relieve mealtime pressure.

When a different mode of feeding is required (e.g., gastrostomy, hyperalimentation) the developmental progression of feeding can be thwarted. For example, infants on long-term gastrostomy feedings may be reluctant to resume oral feedings. However, oral stimulation provided during the course of illness may make resumption of feeding more likely. Thus, giving infants a pacifier during gastrostomy feedings or hyperalimentation allows more active participation and will help promote autonomous feeding in the future (Fig. 3-2). Other avenues of sensorimotor stimulation also should be encouraged in these children to avoid deprivation states. As children return to normal feeding, feeding expectations should approximate their developmental ability (see Table 2-2).

With repeated hospitalization, feedings usually become difficult. Children must fit into regimented feeding schedules. Medical examinations or tests often interrupt mealtimes. Also, medications can alter appetite and taste. Finicky appetites or anorexia related to illness, as well as nausea and vomiting, will certainly interfere with feeding patterns. Because nutritional status is important for recovery, every effort should be made to maximize food intake. During hospitalization, parents need to communicate to the staff about their child's food preferences. They need to value and foster the child's independence during feeding. At discharge, they must learn to guide rather than to push food and to understand the possibility of regression in feeding behavior.

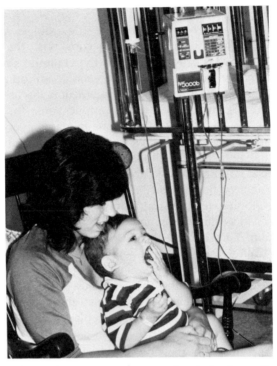

Figure 3-2. Child with pacifier being held by mother during hyperalimentation.

When evaluating chronically ill children for feeding problems, the improvement of nutritional status should be the primary consideration. Next, developmental level of feeding (e.g., finger-feeding) and the degree of feeding regression should be considered, as well as the child's idiosyncrasies. Anorexia-associated conditions must also be noted. Once all of these factors have been considered, a feeding plan can be developed to fit the child's level of psychological and motor function. Periodically, as the illness recedes and feeding behavior changes, the feeding plan must be updated. During rehabilitation, there may be testing behavior. The already weaned child may regress to a bottle. The child who has already accepted table foods may want only baby foods. If parents accept this behavior, children will gradually return to normalcy as they recover from the stress of hospitalization. In an accepting environment, feeding problems need not occur [3].

Acute illness imposes a different stress on usually healthy children and their families. Although acute illness can be time limited, it can have lasting effects, especially when superimposed on chronic illness. Children and their families must deal with the impact of sudden hospitalization, loss of health, and even the threat of death. Segal and Gagnon demonstrated that when parents thought their child might die, disturbed psychosocial behavior developed in the child [6]. Children unprepared for hospitalization are reported to go through predictable stages of grieving characterized by depression, helplessness, hopelessness, and turning inward. Bowlby [2] describes three stages of hospitalization in small children. The initial stage is that of *protest*, in which the child is likely to fight all attempts to be nurtured. The second stage is that of *despair*, in which the child begins to give up on the battle for autonomy and self-assertion. Without intervention, regression to an earlier stage of development is likely to occur. But there is still energy for recovery and reconstitution if the child's depression is respected and efforts are made to nurture the child in ways other than feeding, as well as in the feeding area. The child must be given an opportunity for play and mastery, which can be greatly enhanced by a single caregiver who can play a pivotal role. The third stage is of *turning inward* in every modality. In the affective mode, the child is likely to become severely withdrawn, negative, and unreachable. Cognitive processes are likely to level off, stop, or even regress. Motor development, which usually parallels cognitive development, may also cease or regress. Even autonomic and psychosocial processes such as those involved in feeding regress in efficiency. The child is likely to refuse adequate calories, and even if they are forced by gastrostomy or nasogastric tube, the child's growth may plateau. A severe form of failure to thrive can ensue, and psychosocial recovery becomes less likely.

During hospitalization, children sometimes find that food is their only vestige of control and use it to manipulate anxious parents and staff. Caretakers who force food reinforce children's regressive and negative behaviors and guarantee the perpetuation of feeding problems long after the illness has been resolved. Because illness and hospitalization can alter feeding behavior, those children whose earliest feeding experiences were difficult are at particular risk for problems later. All those concerned need to understand that finicky appetites and sometimes impossible food demands are part of the condition. Anxieties about food intake need to be minimized. The feeding environment needs to be normalized as soon as possible and children need to be given some control.

When an acute illness (e.g., gastroenteritis) is treated at home, there is a temporary interruption in mealtimes. Sick children who are irritable and lethargic can panic parents by refusing food. Parents need to understand the nature of the illness and its effects on appetite. They need to realize that poor food intake over the course of the illness will not do harm. Small and frequent amounts of clear fluids with salt or sugar to ease nausea should be a priority. When the child refuses liquids, gelatin and Popsicles can be used in the place of fluids. During this period of finicky appetite, parents must not fall into the trap of giving their children junk foods "just to get something into them." Also, they must not use food to bribe their children to take their medicine. This communicates to children that food can be used to bargain with and can pave the way for difficult feeding behavior after the illness.

Feeding Behavior in Premature and Small-for-Gestational-Age Children

The premature infant often has an initial feeding experience quite different from the full-term infant. When introduced to oral feeding, uncoordinated suck-swallowing movements and possible difficulties in coordinating breathing with feeding make feeding difficult and unpleasant for infants and parents alike. Instead of being held in warmth and comfort and gently suckled, these infants are placed in incubators (Isolettes) and possibly gavage-fed or maintained on hyperalimentation. They are denied the normal feeding experiences in which attachment is fostered (see Chap. 2). Caretakers should be encouraged to hold and interact with these infants as frequently as they would with infants on normal feeding schedules. These infants should be given pacifiers during such sessions. They should be stroked or sung to with an awareness of the level of stimuli that is appropriate for the premature infant. A low threshold for stimulation usually accompanies prematurity. Thus, it is easy to overload these infants and cause them to withdraw from communication.

In order to promote growth, small, frequent, energy-dense feedings are usually required and place extra demands on infants and parents. Much of the focus of parent-child interaction is on consumption. Poor intake and growth can escalate parental concern. Also, some infants offer misleading feeding cues, often complicated by disturbed wake-sleep cycles. Frequent behavioral and developmental assessment of these infants help anticipate their needs and determine appropriate support.

By the time some of these premature infants are ready to have their gastrostomies or hyperalimentation lines discontinued, their feeding skills may be developmentally delayed. They will need to go through a gradual feeding progression from one stage to another (e.g., strained food to table food); however, the time between stages depends on their developmental abilities rather than their age (see Chap. 2). Some infants prefer to go right to the cup because of earlier difficulties they might have had in coordinating their respiration with bottle-feeding. To them, bottle-feeding may mean choking or gasping for air. Other infants, if developmentally able, prefer to self-feed because they often have been threatened by lack of control, having had so many lines and tubes thrust upon them. Any effort to make feeding experiences more positive in the sensory and affective areas will enhance intake.

The small size of premature infants and small-for-gestational-age (SGA) infants leaves indelible imprints on parents concerning treatment. Parents often continue to see their infants as fragile and weak. Developmental delays in these children also reinforce these feelings. Unfortunately, parents sometimes view feeding as the area in which they can help these children make up for their delays. Parents must understand their children's growth patterns and constitutional limitations (see Chap. 7). They must realize that SGA infants appear to have real differences in their ability to assimilate all cues and stimuli from the environment. These children show differences in reactions to nurturance and to information from the environment. They score low on examiner scores of attractiveness, need for stimulation, interactive processes, and motor processes [1]. Parents describe them as difficult to live with, easily overstimulated, continuously on the go, unpredictable in their sleep and eating patterns, and generally highly reactive. This hyperactivity and unpredictability can cause disruption at mealtimes. When these behaviors and their growth patterns are understood as part of their condition, parents will feel more relaxed. Food should be offered in quiet, nonstimulating environments (i.e., without television, radios, telephones). Expectations for food intake should be made appropriate for the child's *size*, not the child's age.

In addition to differences in size and temperament, Fitzhardinge found that SGA children had increased problems in school (e.g., failing, needing special education) even though their I.Q. scores were normal [4]. Also, these childen had EEG abnormalities and speech defects (immaturity of reception and expression). These subtle learning disabilities may alter feeding. For example, such a child may have some difficulties learning to self-feed or understanding feeding commands. This is accentuated when household mealtimes are busy and when parents have difficulty maintaining the consistent approach necessary for the child with learning difficulties.

WEANING

Although premature infants and children with chronic illnesses are at special risk for feeding problems, all children present with transitory feeding problems during the weaning period. By definition, weaning means to accustom a child to the loss of mother's milk. Because feeding by either breast or bottle is an interactive process, both parents and children are in transition during the weaning period.

Weaning is a critical point in child development. It is during this time that the infant moves to a different developmental level. The infant becomes more independent as he or she learns new motor skills and masters many new tasks in a short period of time. For example, the toddler faces new demands as he or she learns to walk, talk, eat more adult-type foods, and meet new social requirements. The child is placed under a good deal of stress if forced to separate from the primary caretaker at this time.

Parents have their own set of problems and expectations to confront during the weaning process. Breast-feeding mothers may feel particularly sad about weaning, especially when it is initiated by the infant. Mothers may feel rejected and no longer of use to the infant. It is important to help mothers view weaning as a developmental process.

Weaning is an interactive process between mother and child. The breast and bottle serve other functions besides providing nutrition. It is important to understand these other functions when weaning begins. The bottle may have been used to quiet and to soothe the child as well as a means for inducing sleep, separate functions from nutrition but equally important. The mother must use her resources to introduce other ways to accomplish tasks previously accomplished with the bottle. For example, children who are cranky and tired may need help in quieting themselves. If the bottle had been used for this purpose prior to weaning, it may mean that mothers will have to take the time and energy to provide a quiet environment, a toy, or themselves rather than the bottle in order to soothe their children.

The exact timing of weaning varies according to local custom and individual preferences. The influence of cultural weaning practices cannot be overlooked (see Table 5-14). Some infants wean themselves early (see Chap. 5). Certain breast-feeding groups promote breast-feeding for long periods. This may cause dental caries (see Fig. 6-2) and prolonged mother-child interdependence. Sometimes children offer clear cues for weaning only to be ignored by mothers because of their own unfulfilled needs. The mother should be encouraged to express her ideas, desires, and needs concerning weaning in an open-ended, nonjudgmental atmosphere in order to help her begin the separation process.

Weaning begins with the introduction of food (at 4 to 6 months of age) and cup (infants can approximate their lips to the rim of a cup at 5 months). Sometimes infants refuse to drink their formula from a cup and insist on their bottles. This can delay the weaning process because parents may feel they must give a bottle to ensure formula intake. This is especially true for infants on special formulas (e.g., some infants with phenylketonuria [PKU] refuse to drink their special formula Lofenalac from a cup because of the odor of the formula, which is not as evident with a capped bottle). Although some children refuse the cup, they eventually will accept it when thirsty. Unfortunately, disturbed children may deny their thirst and refuse the cup completely. Thus, the child's psychosocial development and feeding behavior, not age, must be considered carefully when making weaning suggestions.

Weaning may be delayed due to illness or developmental delays. As the condition resolves or as the child progresses, weaning should be encouraged and will serve to foster development and growth. Weaning is a process that should take place over a prolonged period, not overnight. It should be regarded as a large developmental step for both infants and parents.

CONCLUSION

The years 1 to 3 are a time of first discovery, then of learning about self-mastery, independence, and, finally, separation from the mother. As the infant establishes "self," there is the ambivalence of separation. Infants are caught between wanting to continue their dependence and wanting to begin the process of separation. In the feeding area, children experience loss of the breast and bottle but replace this loss with the achievement of feeding themselves. While parents take pleasure in their children's newfound autonomy, they may experience a feeling of loss of control, due not only to the loss of their infants' dependence, but also to the kind of tortured exploration and refusals that accompany their children's newly found independence. These first years are a period of change, and feeding is often one of the major areas of conflict.

All parents have the feeling that getting food into a child is their job. If they are good parents, the children will eat well; if their children do not eat well, they regard themselves as failures. Unfortunately, parents derive a sense of accomplishment from their children's clean plates, and with this, they measure their children's developmental advances. Children perceive their parents' concern and respond accordingly, often choosing to manipulate their parents' wishes. Feeding is the first area where control is an issue, and for this reason, feeding plays a major role in child development.

Feeding is a time for learning new skills. It is a time for social interaction, for mastery, and for separation. Problems that arise around feeding affect growth and development. Certain children, because of prematurity, congenital anomalies, environmental deprivation (see Chap. 9), or illness, are at risk for feeding problems. Chronic and acute illnesses affect feeding behavior. Alterations in feeding behavior may occur at any phase of the illness and may even outlast the organic phase. When feeding behavior changes, all environmental factors must be explored (see Chap. 11). The task is to normalize feeding behavior. This takes time and support.

Providing parents with anticipatory guidance decreases the likelihood of chronic feeding problems associated with illness and prematurity. As quickly as possible, children should be nourished in the normal way and encouraged to resume feeding skills appropriate to their developmental level. An overprotective or developmentally inappropriate approach to feeding the ill, premature, or at-risk child fosters dependence and perpetuates the image of a sick child. This image makes normal growth and development difficult and turns feeding into a continuing problem.

REFERENCES

1. Als, H., et al. The behavior of the full-term but underweight newborn infant. *Dev. Med. Child. Neurol.* 18:590, 1976.
2. Bowlby, J. Grief and mourning in infancy and early childhood. *Psychoanal. Study Child* 15:9, 1960.
3. Brazelton, T. B. *Infants and Mother; Toddler and Parents.* New York: A Delta Special, Delacorte Press/Seymore Lawrence, 1972.
4. Fitzhardinge, P., and Stevens, E. The small-for-date infant II. Neurological and intellectual sequelae. *Pediatrics* 40(1):50, 1972.
5. Kaye, K., and Brazelton, T. B. Etiological Significance of Burst Pause Patterns in Infants. Presented at Society of Research in Child Development, Minneapolis, Minn., April, 1971.
6. Segal, J., and Gagnon, P. Effects of parents' and pediatricians' worry concerning severe gastroenteritis in early childhood and later disturbances in child's behavior. *J. Pediatr.* 87(5):869, 1975.

4. Development of the Gastrointestinal Tract

Harland S. Winter

The newborn infant thrives because of complex physiological mechanisms of ingesting and digesting nutrients. The maturation of the infant's gastrointestinal tract begins in utero when the yolk sac can be distinctly identified from the gut. Understanding the development of this system provides insight into appropriate patterns of feeding [19].

The purpose of this chapter is to define the role of the various organs in digestion and then to explain the functional intrauterine and extrauterine development of the gastrointestinal tract. This background is fundamental in understanding the rationale behind feeding the premature and the full-term infant. Although much physiological information and many important advances have been provided by animal experiments, the following discussion, with few noted exceptions, will be limited to that which is known about the human fetus and infant.

PHYSIOLOGY OF DIGESTION

Most of this book deals with the types of foods that should be given to the infant in the first three years of life. The common sense that tells us to avoid offering pepperoni pizza to neonates is supported by physiological constraints on absorption. Before discussing the development of mature gastrointestinal function, one must appreciate the organization of digestion and the role that each digestive organ plays.

Nutrients are masticated by teeth, if present, and shaped by the tongue and mouth into a consistency that can be swallowed. Digestion of starch and fat begins in the mouth with the secretion of amylase by the salivary glands and of lingual lipase by Ebner's glands at the base of the tongue. This specialized lipase is bile salt, independent and active at the acid pH of the stomach [13]. The base of the tongue, acting as a piston, pushes the bolus of food into the oropharynx, where the peristaltic activity of the esophagus propels it distally. The sole functions of the esophagus are to transport food to the stomach and, once there, to prevent its regurgitation. The lower esophageal sphincter, which is tonically contracted, relaxes when the cricopharyngeal muscle contracts. It remains open until the peristaltic wave passes and then contracts with a force greater than the resting pressure. Controversy exists regarding what the function of the normal lower esophageal sphincter is in a neonate. The frequency with which healthy neonates regurgitate suggests that the gastroesophageal junction is not competent in infancy. This may be related not only to an inadequate intrinsic pressure in the sphincter, but also to the decreased mechanical advantage afforded by the acuteness of the angle between the stomach and the esophagus (the angle of His). These two factors are responsible for preventing reflux. As the infant grows, the stomach changes shape and the angle of His becomes more acute. This allows for more of a mechanical advantage so that when the stomach becomes distended after a meal, there is a valvelike mechanism to prevent gastroesophageal reflux. This lack of anatomical advantage in the neonate may explain why the lower esophageal sphincter pressure needs to be so high and subsequently declines with growth.

Once in the stomach, food is mixed with hydrochloric acid, intrinsic factor, pepsinogen, mucus, fluid, and electrolytes. No absorption occurs, but small boluses of the particulate suspension are squirted through the pylorus into the duodenum. Pancreatic enzymes, bicarbonate, bile salts, lecithin, and cholesterol are added, and absorption begins. Throughout the duodenum, jejunum, and ileum, complex carbohydrates, fats, and proteins are broken down to monosaccharides, fatty acids, and amino acids, respectively, and absorption takes place. Some nutrients, such as vitamin B_{12}, are absorbed at specific receptor sites, mainly located in the ileum, whereas others, such as lactose, are absorbed throughout the small intestine wherever lactase is located on the brush border of the enterocyte. Bile salts, which have been secreted into the duodenum from the liver and gallbladder, are reabsorbed in the terminal ileum and recycled by the liver for further use.

In humans, the colon does not play a major role in the absorption of nutrients. Some carbohydrates can be converted into volatile fatty acids and absorbed, but the main function of the colon is to reabsorb water and electrolytes. Thus, the colon is not essential for digestion.

The orderly process by which the intricate digestive system matures will be presented by focusing first on the intrauterine development and finally on the extrauterine development of a gastrointestinal system capable of supporting the growth of a child.

INTRAUTERINE DEVELOPMENT

Interest in the development of the human infant dates to the early writings of Aristotle and Hippocrates, who thought that some of the physiological functions of the newborn were present in utero. Investigators in the eighteenth and nineteenth centuries hypothesized the existence of a continuum of function between the fetus and the newborn by showing that some of the physiological functions of infants were present in the fetus [9]. We now understand that the anatomical differentiation of the gastrointestinal tract results from a number of twists, bends, and rotations that occur throughout gestation. The foregut and hindgut become distinctly separate from the yolk sac at about 3½ weeks of gestation. Most anatomical structures are in place by the second trimester. During the last trimester, the gastrointestinal tract increases in mass and matures physiologically [10] by mechanisms that are poorly understood [8].

Odontogenesis, the development of the teeth, begins in utero at 6 weeks. Two weeks later, tooth buds for all 20 primary teeth are present. By 40 weeks of gestation, the tooth buds of the permanent first molars are present and calcification of the primary teeth is in progress. Nutritional sufficiency, especially of vitamins and minerals, plays an important role in the intrauterine development of teeth. The crystal and matrix of the tooth contain both calcium and phosphorus, whose absorption is regulated in part by vitamin D. Should the fetus have an inadequate supply of calcium during tooth development, enamel hypoplasia and irregular dentin formation will result. Because dentin will accrue calcium preferentially over bone, signs of vitamin D deficiency will be noted in alveolar and long bones first. Vitamin C, vitamin A, and protein also play a major role in the development of enamel and dentin, and deficiencies may lead to abnormal development of teeth. Because the fetus is very efficient in acquiring the necessary minerals and nutrients, these deficiencies, even when present in the mother, may not be evident in the newborn.

The esophagus is a simple tube that connects the oropharynx to the stomach. It is differentiated from the stomach during the fourth week of gestation. At 7 weeks, longitudinal channels develop and form a lumen. The ganglion cells are differentiated by 13 weeks and the esophagus is thought to be capable of peristaltic activity at this time. Swallowing is present as early as 16 weeks in utero [1, 21]. Polyhydramnios (increased amniotic fluid volume) is found frequently in infants in whom swallowing has been impaired in utero. This is most commonly a sign of anencephaly, esophageal atresia, or upper gastrointestinal atresias. The role of swallowing for the regulation of amniotic fluid volume is not clear, and the reason for normal volumes in some children with obstruction remains obscure. Amniotic fluid volumes range from 2 to 46 ml at 10 weeks of gestation to 500 to 1,100 ml at term [2]. It is estimated that the term fetus swallows approximately 450 ml of amniotic fluid per day [21]. The nutritive value of the amniotic fluid and its effect upon the development of the gastrointestinal tract is unclear. Much work has been done to define the glucose, protein, and lipid content of amniotic fluid, but the nutritional contribution of these components is undefined. Various gastrointestinal enzymes and hormones also have been identified, but their role in digestion is similarly obscure. Delayed development of the intestinal tract has been noted in children who have atresias in utero and in whom the bowel has not been exposed to amniotic fluid. This has been attributed to lack of function in utero, but the role of trophic factors in the amniotic fluid remains to be more clearly defined.

In addition to transporting amniotic fluid from the mouth to the stomach, the esophagus contains a specialized high-pressure zone at its distal end whose eventual role is to prevent aspiration or regurgitation of gastric contents. Although a high-pressure zone is present in the term fetus, little is known regarding the in utero development of lower esophageal sphincter function. Nevertheless, even premature infants have a distal high-pressure zone, which relaxes with deglutition. The fetus is capable of swallowing in utero, but the function of the lower esophageal sphincter in this activity is unclear. Because peristalsis in the body of the esophagus of the premature infant is disordered, with simultaneous contractions and biphasic wave forms, one assumes that similar motility patterns are occurring in utero [12, 16]. Waves appear to travel along the esophagus and continue through the stomach, implying that, initially, the esophagus and the stomach function as a unit as far as motility is concerned.

By 4 weeks of gestation, the stomach begins to differentiate in the foregut. Beginning in the neck, it descends into its final position by 7 weeks and begins to assume the characteristic shape. The ventral surface grows more slowly than the dorsal surface, which elongates to become the greater curvature. At 6 weeks, rotation occurs and the lesser curve becomes positioned to the right.

Physiological development of hydrochloric acid, intrinsic factor, pepsinogen, mucus, and gastric secretion occur throughout gestation. Around 9 weeks of gestation, glandular pits develop in the stomach and true parietal cells (acid-secreting) are identifiable by 11 weeks. Intestinal-type epithelium is found in the stomach during development but is usually replaced by characteristic gastric epithelium by term. Parietal cells, concentrated in the body and pyloric regions of the stomach, are capable of acid secretion at birth. Even the premature infant can secrete acid, suggesting that functional acid production is present early in gestation and awaits appropriate environmental and hormonal stimuli [5].

Pepsins, which are secreted by chief cells, have been of interest because of their role in the digestion of proteins. By 16 weeks of gestation, peptic activity is present in the stomach and increases as the fetus grows. Despite this activity, pepsinogen granules have not been shown in the chief cells. The reason for this discrepancy has not been explained.

At 11 weeks of gestation, intrinsic factor (IF), which is necessary for vitamin B_{12} absorption, is present. The function in utero of IF is unknown. Ingested vitamin B_{12} is bound to R factor in the stomach and then split from it by proteolytic enzymes in the proximal small intestine. The free B_{12} is rapidly bound to the IF secreted by the stomach. This B_{12}-IF complex is then recognized by specific receptors and transported across the epithelium where, upon exit from the cell, it is bound to transcobalamin II for transport in the blood.

Gastrin is detectable as early as 11 weeks of gestation in the duodenal mucosa, but its relationship to gastric acid secretion and parietal cell development is unclear. The observations that newborn gastrin levels are 2 to 3 times higher than maternal levels and that newborn umbilical cord venous samples are similar to umbilical cord arterial samples suggest that gastrin is synthesized by the fetus during gestation. There is some evidence in dogs that an elevated gastrin level in the final month of pregnancy leads to pyloric muscular hypertrophy. This has led to speculation that an analogous situation may occur in humans, but there is little supportive data.

During the first weeks of gestation, the small intestine grows in length at such a rapid rate that it loops into the umbilical cord. Following rotation around the superior mesenteric artery, the jejunum, ileum, cecum, ascending colon, and transverse colon elongate inside the cord. At 10 weeks the true abdominal cavity is large enough to reaccept the intestine. The jejunum reenters on the left side followed by the ileum on the right. The cecum becomes fixed in the left lower quadrant, and the ascending and transverse colon enter the abdominal cavity last.

During the elongation of the intestine, differentiation of the absorptive surface also takes place. Villi, which provide the surface area for absorption and whose cells contain brush border enzymes, begin to appear in the duodenum at 7 to 8 weeks. By 12 to 14 weeks, villi line the small intestine from the duodenum to the ileum. Crypts, whose cells provide the regenerative zone to replace sloughed epithelial cells, are present by 12 weeks. Peristaltic activity begins about this time. Lymphoid aggregates and Peyer's patches are present by 20 weeks.

The absorptive function of the fetal intestine has been studied extensively, but the significance of the data is undetermined. Using changes in potential difference, Koldovsky and colleagues [16] have shown that the fetal jejunum transports glucose at a greater rate than the ileum. Little is known about amino acid transport. Although the human fetus obtains IgG via the placenta, the intestine is capable of absorbing IgG as well as bovine serum albumin.

Disaccharidases of the small intestine provide the initial step in the absorption of dietary sucrose and lactose. Lactase, which is required for the absorption of the sugar found in milk, is detectable by 24 weeks of gestation and increases rapidly prior to birth. By term, the lactase level is 2 to 4 times greater than that of infants between 2 and 11 months of age. The cause for this rise in enzyme activity at birth is not known. Lactase activity in the fetus, as well as in the child and the adult, is greatest in the proximal intestine.

The colon develops and rotates with the small intestine. The rectum is derived from the cloaca and fuses with the sigmoid colon by 8 weeks. Failure of this union to occur results in imperforate anus, which is frequently associated with a fistula to the bladder or vagina. Colonic peristalsis can be noted as early as 8 weeks but the caudal migration of neuroblasts occurs near 12 weeks of gestation. At 24 weeks the fetus has ganglion cells present in the distal colon except 1 cm above the rectal sphincter, where there is a zone of normal hypoganglionosis. Hirschsprung's disease, or the absence of ganglion cells, is rare in the premature infant.

During fetal development, the colon as well as the small intestine serves as a reservoir for meconium. Meconium is a tenacious substance formed from intestinal secretions, cellular debris, serum proteins, and enzymes. Meconium is of little diagnostic value in reflecting in utero intestinal dysfunction although the meconium of infants with cystic fibrosis has an increased level of albumin.

The pancreas, which plays a central role in the digestion of protein and lipid, develops from the entoderm near the duodenum. Two primordial buds, one from the bile duct and the other from the duodenum, elongate to form the two ducts of the pancreas. They eventually fuse to form the main pancreatic duct (duct of Wirsung), which drains the body and tail of the pancreas, and a smaller accessory duct (duct of Santorini), which drains part of the head of the pancreas. Failure of fusion results in a pancreas divisum, which is the most common anatomical congenital pancreatic anomaly.

Pancreatic exocrine function is detectable in the second trimester of gestation. Lipase activity can be found by 16 weeks of gestation, and term levels are reached between 28 and 34 weeks [23, 28]. Amylase can be detected by 22 weeks [14], and trypsin may be present as early as 16 weeks of gestation.

Endocrine pancreatic function develops earlier than exocrine function, but the purpose of endocrine hormones in intestinal development remains unclear. Because maternal insulin does not cross the placenta, any insulin in the fetus is endogenously produced. Insulin is detected between 10 and 14 weeks of gestation and remains at a relatively constant level throughout gestation. Glucagon and somatostatin are found somewhat earlier (8 to 10 weeks and 11 weeks, respectively). The level of glucagon increases with fetal maturation [6].

EXTRAUTERINE DEVELOPMENT

Development of the gastrointestinal tract does not cease with birth. The nutritional needs of infants will be discussed in Chapter 5, but

Table 4-1. Dental Development

Teeth	Age of Eruption		Age of Shedding	
	Maxillary	Mandibular	Maxillary	Mandibular
Primary				
Central incisor	7½ mo	6 mo	7½ yr	6 yr
Lateral incisor	9 mo	7 mo	8 yr	7 yr
Cuspid	18 mo	16 mo	11½ yr	9½ yr
First molar	14 mo	12 mo	10½ yr	10 yr
Second molar	24 mo	20 mo	10½ yr	11 yr
Secondary				
Central incisor	7–8 yr	6–7 yr		
Lateral incisor	8–9 yr	7–8 yr		
Cuspid	11–12 yr	9–10 yr		
First bicuspid	10–11 yr	10–12 yr		
Second bicuspid	10–12 yr	11–12 yr		
First molar	6–7 yr	6–7 yr		
Second molar	12–13 yr	11–13 yr		
Third molar	17–21 yr	17–21		

Data from Howell, T. H. and Howard, R. B. Nutrition and Dental Health. In R. B. Howard and N. H. Herbold (Eds.), *Nutrition in Clinical Care* (2nd ed.). New York: McGraw-Hill, 1982.

the physiological basis for the extrauterine maturation of the gastrointestinal tract will be presented here.

The eruption of teeth portends the era of solid food. The neonate without dentition is limited to liquids or a soft bill of fare. As primary teeth are cut, the consistency of food can become more varied. Table 4-1 lists the expected time course of tooth eruption.

Swallowing is an obligatory function for the survival of the neonate. The sucking and swallowing reflex is so primitive that even infants with anencephaly are capable of nursing. Both the premature and the newborn infant occasionally have poorly coordinated swallows that may persist in a minority of children until the age of 2 years [11]. This is of more clinical significance in premature infants weighing less than 2,000 g who may have a number of uncoordinated attempts at deglutition.

The competency of the gastroesophageal function to prevent reflux of gastric contents is dependent upon the pressure of the lower esophageal sphincter and the angle between the stomach and the distal esophagus (angle of His) (see Chap. 11). As the cardia grows, the angle of His creates a valvelike mechanism to prevent reflux when the stomach is distended. There is controversy about whether or not the lower esophageal sphincter pressure rises or falls as the infant matures. In either situation, it is common for healthy infants under 15 months of age to regurgitate after a feeding. By 2 years of age, esophageal function should be as fully mature as that found in the adult.

Motility of the stomach is a continuation of esophageal peristalsis until 2 years of age. After this, gastric activity is regulated intrinsically. The pH of the stomach at birth is 6.0, and it rapidly falls to below 3.0 by 6 hours of age. The highest acid concentration occurs within 10 days after birth but is of little clinical relevance. Gastric acid output, which correlates with functional parietal cell mass, is low in the newborn, but approximates adult levels by the age of 3 months. In the premature infant over 32 weeks of gestation, gastric acid should be present; but in approximately one-third of premature babies, gastric acid was absent. Nevertheless, when stimulated even premature babies produce acid [4].

Intrinsic factor (IF) secreted by the parietal cell can be detected on the first day of life and, by 2 weeks of age, is half of the adult level. By 3 months of age, the neonate is producing an amount of IF comparable to that found in the adult [3]. The concentration of vitamin B_{12} in the umbilical cord blood of term and premature infants is approximately twice that found in the maternal serum. The level falls to a nadir by 1 month of age and then rises to the normal adult level by 4 months of age [17, 20].

The small intestine is the site for absorption of carbohydrate, fat, and protein. In term infants under 1 year of age, absorption of glucose is somewhat limited when compared with that of adults [27]. This might explain the occasional small amount of carbohydrate in the stool of healthy neonates. The premature infant is more vulnerable to this limitation, but the presence of small amounts of sugar in the stool is not by itself an indication to change formula.

Amylase cleaves starches to polymers of glucose and, like other pancreatic enzymes, has a reduced level in infants under 1 year of age [15]. However, following stimulation, the amylase activity increases, and intolerance of starch is rarely of clinical significance in either the premature or full-term infant. In the premature infant, some investigators believe that pancreatic function may depend upon the type of formula ingested [18]. The clinical relevance of this observation remains obscure, as clinical well-being and growth were not affected.

Cleavage of lactose to glucose and galactose by the brush border enzyme lactase is theoretically possible after 24 weeks of gestation; the lactase level begins to rise after 30 weeks of gestation. Thus, infants of less than 32 weeks' gestation may be lactose intolerant. By 28 weeks of gestation, the other disaccharidases—sucrase, maltase, and isomaltase—are at levels equivalent to those found in full-term infants. Consequently, even markedly premature infants should be able to tolerate properly selected formulas. The absorption of fat and protein is influenced by the integrity of the small intestinal mucosa but is more dependent on hepatic and pancreatic function.

Full-term infants do not absorb fat as efficiently as adults. The infant fed cow's milk–derived formula will continue to excrete between 5 and 20 percent of dietary fat until approximately 1 year of age [26]. In contrast, breast-fed babies will excrete less than 7 percent of ingested fat. Although the composition of dietary lipid is an important factor in determining absorption, there is also a physiological decrease in pancreatic lipase secretion as well as bile acid pool size. The bile acid pool size and synthetic rate are approximately half the adult value [24]. These deficits are accentuated in the premature infant, who excretes more dietary fat than the full-term baby. Premature infants fed cow's milk formula will excrete up to 40 percent of ingested fat; those fed human milk will excrete about 25 percent [22]. Again, dietary lipid composition is a factor in the difference, but premature infants have diminished lipase and bile salt secretion. They also have intraluminal bile salt concentrations less than those of term infants and below the necessary critical micellar concentration. In addition, bile acid synthetic rates are even less than those found in full-term infants [25].

Protein digestion in both full-term and premature infants appears to be intact [7], despite decreased secretion of trypsin following stimulation. Although premature infants may become hypoalbuminemic, it is not possible to determine whether this is related to nutritional deficiencies or poor absorption of protein. The absorption of amino acids in infants has not been adequately studied to determine if any deficit exists in premature or full-term infants.

Colonic function in full-term infants depends on diet. The frequency and consistency of stool is different in breast-fed versus formula-fed infants (see Chap. 5). The physiological factors contributing to these phenomena are unclear. In the premature infant, colonic function may be delayed, especially if the infant is sick.

The efficiency of digestion increases as the infant develops. Many of the mechanisms by which this occurs have been presented in this chapter. The practical application of these principles will be discussed in subsequent chapters.

REFERENCES

1. Abramovich, D. R. Fetal factors influencing amniotic fluid volume and composition of liquor amnii. *J. Obstet. Gynecol.* 77:865, 1970.
2. Abramovich, D. R. The volume of amniotic fluid and factors affecting or regulating this. In D. V. I. Fairweather, and T. K. A. B. Eskea (eds.)., *Amniotic Fluid.* Amsterdam: Excepta Medica, 1973. Pp. 29–51.
3. Agunod, M., et al. Correlative study of hydrochloric acid, pepsin, and intrinsic factor secretion in newborns and infants. *Am. J. Dis. Child.* 14:400, 1969.
4. Ahn, C. I., et al. Acidity and volume of gastric contents in the first week of life. *J. Korean Med. Assoc.* 6:948, 1963.

5. Ames, M. D. Gastric acidity in the first ten days of life in the prematurely born baby. *Am J. Dis. Child.* 100:123, 1960.
6. Assan, R. Pancreatic glucagon and glucagon-like material in tissues and plasma from human fetuses 6–26 weeks old. *Pathol. Biol.* 21:149, 1973.
7. Borgstrom, B., et al. Enzyme concentration and absorption of protein and glucose in duodenum of premature infants. *Am. J. Dis. Child.* 99:338, 1960.
8. Bryant, M. G., et al. Development of intestinal regulatory peptides in the human fetus. *Gastroenterology* 83:47, 1982.
9. Feldman, W. M. *The Principles of Ante-Natal and Post-Natal Child Physiology Pure and Applied.* London: Logmans, Green and Co., 1920.
10. Grand, R. J., et al. Development of the human gastrointestinal tract. *Gastroenterology* 70:790, 1976.
11. Gryboski, J. D. The swallowing mechanism of the neonate: 1. Esophageal and gastric motility. *Pediatrics* 35:445, 1965.
12. Gryboski, J. D., et al. Esophageal motility in infants and children. *Pediatrics* 31:382, 1963.
13. Hamosh, M., et al. Fat digestion in the stomach of premature infants. I. Characteristics of lipase activity. *J. Pediatr.* 93:674, 1978.
14. Keene, M. F. L., et al. Digestive enzymes of the human fetus. *Lancet* 1:767, 1929.
15. Klumpp, T. G., and Neale, A. V. The gastric and duodenal contents of normal infants and children. *Am. J. Dis. Child.* 40:1215, 1930.
16. Koldovsky, O., et al. Transport of glucose against a concentration gradient in everted sacs of jejunum and ileum of human fetuses. *Gastroenterology* 48:185, 1965.
17. Kumento, A. Studies on the serum binding of vitamin B_{12} in the newborn human infant. *Acta. Pediatr. Scand.* [Suppl.] 194:12, 1969.
18. Lebenthal, E., et al. The development of pancreatic function in premature infants after milk-based and soy-based formulas. *Pediatr. Res.* 15:1240, 1981.
19. Lebenthal, E., et al. Review article. Interactions of determinants in the ontogeny of the gastrointestinal tract: A unified concept. *Pediatr. Res.* 17:19, 1983.
20. Pathak, A., et al. Vitamin B_{12} and folic acid values in premature infants. *Pediatrics* 50:584, 1972.
21. Pritchard, J. A. Fetal swallowing and amniotic fluid volume. *Obstet. Gynecol.* 28:606, 1966.
22. Signer, E., et al. Role of bile salts in fat malabsorption of premature infants. *Arch. Dis. Child.* 49:174, 1974.
23. Tachibana, T. Physiological investigation of fetus. 1. Lipase in pancreas. *Jap. J. Obstet. Gynecol.* 11:92, 1928.
24. Watkins, J. B., et al. Bile salt metabolism in the newborn. *N. Engl. J. Med.* 288:431, 1973.
25. Watkins, J. B., et al. Bile salt metabolism in the human premature infant. *Gastroenterology* 69:706, 1975.
26. Weijers, A. A., et al. Analysis and interpretation of the fat-absorption coefficient. *Acta. Paediatr.* 49:615, 1960.
27. Younoszai, M. D. Jejunal absorption of hexose in infants and adults. *J. Pediatr.* 85:446, 1974.
28. Zoppi, G., et al. Exocrine pancreas function in premature and full-term neonates. *Pediatr. Res.* 6:880, 1972.

5. Feeding Throughout the First Year of Life

Frances J. Rohr and Judith A. Lothian

Infant feeding methods have come almost full circle during this century. Prior to the 1900s, practically all infants were breast-fed. Scientific advances in the processing of cow's milk, along with sociological influences such as industrialization and women's emancipation, led to greater use of formula. By the 1960s, the use of infant formula had spread to all socioeconomic groups and from industrialized to third world nations.

In the United States, the trend in infant feeding is changing again. The incidence and length of time that women are breast-feeding is increasing [61] (Fig. 5-1). Although primaparous mothers with some college education are most likely to breast-feed, breast-feeding is becoming more prevalent among women of all income and educational levels. In fact, a better understanding of the nutritional and immunological aspects of breast milk has led organizations such as the World Health Organization (WHO), the American Academy of Pediatrics, and the Canadian Pediatric Society to promote and support breast-feeding [4, 10, 83].

Although the incidence of breast-feeding is increasing in developed countries, it continues to decline in third world nations. This trend persists despite the fact that water supplies, storage facilities, and education are often inadequate for successful formula-feeding. Also, in third world nations where disease is often rampant, formula-fed infants do not receive the added protection of the immunological components of breast milk, rendering them less resistant to infection. Therefore, the sale of infant formulas in third world nations has caused an ethical controversy leading the WHO to issue a statement against the marketing of infant formulas in these nations [84].

While the environment in third world nations often makes formula-feeding inappropriate, the higher standards of living in developed countries give parents a choice about infant feeding: they may choose to breast-feed or bottle-feed. Because their choices may be shaped by medical, cultural, and personal influences, a variety of feeding practices exist. Despite these differences in feeding philosophies, most infants grow and appear to be well-nourished. However, we are learning that early feeding practices may exert subtle influences on health and that the control of dietary risk factors (i.e., fat, salt, and sugar [see Chap. 6]) begins in infancy. Therefore, the establishment of optimal nutrition should be an integral part of pediatric practice.

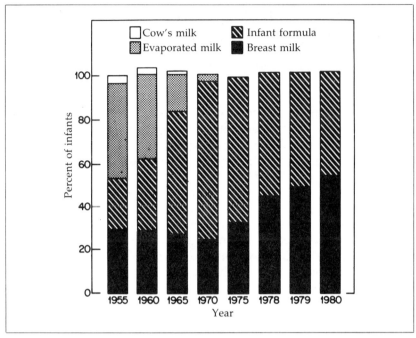

Figure 5-1. Trends in feeding infants (age 1 week) from 1955 to 1980. Breast-feeding incidence has nearly doubled since 1970, and the use of cow's milk and evaporated milk has virtually disappeared. The total may be greater than 100 percent because supplemental feedings (i.e., formulas in addition to breast milk) are included. Feedings representing less than 1 percent are not included. (Data from Martinez, G. A., Dodd, D. A., and Samartgedes, J. A. Milk feeding patterns during the first 12 months of life. Pediatrics 68:863, 1981.)

NUTRITIONAL NEEDS

Infancy is a period of great nutritional vulnerability because growth occurs rapidly during the first year. Birth weight usually triples or quadruples during the first year, and brain weight doubles. Thus, nutrient requirements are the greatest during the first year and especially during the first 6 months of life.

There are over 50 known nutrients that are essential to human life, but requirements have been set for fewer than half of them. A guide to the major nutrients in the infant's diet is found in Table 5-1. The Recommended Dietary Allowances (RDA) (see Appendix 1) are the standards most often used in the United States to determine dietary adequacy [38]. The Food and Nutrition Board of the National Academy of Sciences (NRCNAS) establishes the RDAs. These standards are updated about every 4 years and are based on current biochemical and clinical evidence from both animal and human studies. The RDAs are intended as guidelines in evaluating the dietary adequacy of populations, not individuals. They are set to meet the needs of specific age

Table 5-1. Nutrition in Infancy: Functions, Requirements, and Sources

Nutrient	Function	Daily Amount Recommended[a]	Good Sources in Infancy
PROTEIN	Synthesis of body proteins (tissues, enzymes, hormones, antibodies) and other nitrogen-containing compounds Energy source (4 kcal/gm)	8% total kcal 0.0–0.5 yr, 2.2 gm/kg 0.5–1.0 yr, 2.0 gm/kg	Breast milk, infant formula, cow's milk[b], infant foods: meat, fish, poultry, cheese, legumes, cereal, milk products
CARBOHYDRATE	Energy source (4 kcal/gm) Protein sparing Antiketogenic Synthesis of body compounds (ribose, deoxyribose)	Minimum requirement unknown 40–50% total kcal	Breast milk, infant formula, cow's milk[b], infant foods: cereal, juices, fruits, vegetables, grains
FAT	Energy source (9 kcal/gm) Provides fat-soluble vitamins Cushions vessels, nerves, and organs Structural component in cell and nucleus membranes Provides essential fatty acids necessary for growth and nerve myelinization Functions in association with phospholipid and cholesterol metabolism	40–50% total kcal (3% of total kcal as essential fatty acids)	Breast milk, infant formula, cow's milk[b], infant foods: poultry, meats, cheese, egg yolk

68

Table 5-1 (Continued)

Nutrient	Function	Daily Amount Recommended[a]	Good Sources in Infancy
FAT-SOLUBLE VITAMINS			
Vitamin A	Component of photosensitive pigment in eye Maintains integrity of epithelial membranes Aids in bone and tooth development	0.0–0.5 yr, 420 RE 0.5–1.0 yr, 2,000 IU (400 RE)	Breast milk, infant formula, infant foods: dark green or yellow fruits and vegetables
Vitamin D	Maintains calcium homeostasis and skeletal integrity Aids in absorption and utilization of calcium and phosphorus Regulates serum alkaline phosphatase	400 IU (10 μg cholecalciferol)	Breast milk, infant formula, cow's milk[b], exposure to UV light
Vitamin E	Antioxidant that stabilizes lipid portion of cell membrane, preventing oxidization	0.0–0.5 yr, 3 mg tocopherol 0.5–1.0 yr, 4 mg tocopherol	Breast milk, infant formulas
Vitamin K	Catalyzes synthesis of prothrombin in liver	No recommendations set 1 mg given to all newborns at birth	After newborn period, synthesized in gut Infant foods: widespread in foods, especially green leafy vegetables
WATER-SOLUBLE VITAMINS			
Ascorbic acid	Aids formation and maintenance of bone matrix, cartilage, dentin, collagen, and connective tissue	35 mg	Breast milk, infant formula, infant foods: fruits, vegetables, fortified infant juice

Vitamin	Function	Amount	Sources
	Enhances iron absorption Facilitates action of folic acid Related to metabolism of phenylalanine, tyrosine, and tryptophan	35 mg	Breast milk, infant formula, infant foods: fruits, vegetables, fortified infant juice
Thiamin	Energy production from carbohydrates, protein, fat Nerve impulse conduction Conversion of tryptophan niacin	0.0–0.5 yr, 0.4 mg 0.5–1.0 yr, 0.4 mg	Breast milk, infant formulas, infant foods: enriched cereal, grain products, whole grains
Riboflavin	Part of coenzymes FAD and FMN in hydrogen transfer reactions and deamination reactions	0.0–0.5 yr, 0.3 mg 0.5–1.0 yr, 0.5 mg	Breast milk, infant formula, infant foods: enriched cereals and grains, cheese, yogurt
Niacin	As part of NAD, NADP is involved in: Energy production (TCA and glycolytic pathways) Fatty acid metabolism Electron transport Pentose monophosphate shunt	0.0–0.5 yr, 6 mg 0.5–1.0 yr, 8 mg	Breast milk, infant formula, infant foods: enriched grains, meat, poultry, fish
Vitamin B_6	As part of coenzyme pyridoxal, phosphate is important in protein and amino acid metabolism in: Transamination Deamination Decarboxylation Desulfuration Involved in formation of heme precursor	0.0–0.5 yr, 0.3 mg 0.5–1.0 yr, 0.6 mg	Breast milk, infant formula, infant foods: pork, wheat germ, bananas, whole grains

Table 5-1 (Continued)

Nutrient	Function	Daily Amount Recommended[a]	Good Sources in Infancy
Folic acid	Coenzyme in formation of: Purines, pyrimidines Heme synthesis	0-0.5 yr, 30 µg 0.5-1.0 yr, 45 µg	Breast milk, infant formula, infant foods: green leafy vegetables, meat, poultry, legumes, whole grains
Vitamin B_{12}	Synthesis of nucleic acid and cell proteins Maturation of red blood cells in bone marrow Metabolism of nerve tissue	0.0-0.5 yr, 0.5 µg 0.5-1.0 yr, 1.5 µg	Breast milk, infant formula, infant foods: meat, fish, poultry, dairy products, vegetable sources: fortified soy milk, yeast grown on B_{12} enriched media
MINERALS Calcium	Bone and teeth formation Blood coagulation Nerve impulses Muscle contraction and relaxation (including cardiac)	0.0-0.5 yr, 360 mg 0.5-1.0 yr, 540 mg	Breast milk, infant formula, cow's milk[b], infant foods: cheese, yogurt, green leafy vegetables, legumes, whole grains
Phosphorus	Component of RNA and DNA Component of phospholipids Part of ATP, ADP-related to storage and release of energy	0.0-0.5 yr, 240 mg 0.5-1.0 yr, 360 mg	Breast milk, infant formula, cow's milk[b], infant foods: milk products, cereals, legumes, meat, fish, poultry
Magnesium	Mobilization of calcium from bone Cofactor in many phosphorylation reactions Involved in protein synthesis	0.0-0.5 yr, 50 mg 0.5-1.0 yr, 70 mg	Breast milk, infant formula, infant foods: vegetables, whole grains

Iron	Constituent of hemoglobin and myoglobin involved in O_2 and CO_2 transport	0.0–0.5 yr, 10 mg 0.5–1.0 yr, 15 mg	Breast milk (supplement after 4 mo), iron fortified formula, infant foods: fortified cereal, meat, poultry
Zinc	Constituent of many metalloenzymes Component of insulin Taste/olfactory activity Required for protein synthesis and sexual maturation	0.0–0.5 yr, 3 mg 0.5–1.0 yr, 5 mg	Breast milk, infant formula, infant foods: red meats, whole grains, chicken, fish
Iodine	Component of thyroid hormones	0.0–0.5 yr, 40 µg 0.5–1.0 yr, 50 µg	Breast milk, infant formula, infant food: widespread in small amounts in many foods
Fluoride	Structural component of bones and teeth		Fluoridated water, fluoride supplements
WATER	Contributes to structure and form of body through tissue turgor Provides aqueous environment necessary for cell metabolism Solvent for transport of nutrients and metabolic waste products Aids in maintaining body temperature	130–150 ml/kg	Breast milk, infant formula, infant foods: juices, water content of food (fruits and vegetables are highest)

[a]*Food and Nutrition Board: Recommended Dietary Allowances* (9th ed.). Washington D.C.: National Academy of Science National Research Council, 1980.
[b]Cow's milk may be added to infant's diet at the end of the first year.
Adapted from Getchell, E., and Howard, R. Nutrition in Development. In G. M. Scipien, et al. (Eds.), *Comprehensive Pediatric Nursing.* New York: McGraw-Hill, 1979.

groups of healthy people in the United States; variations in nutrient needs due to illness or other stress are not considered. The RDAs are based on the average nutrient need plus a 30 to 50 percent margin of safety. Thus, if two-thirds of the RDA for a nutrient is met, the intake is considered to be in the adequate range. For certain nutrients the NRCNAS has established "Safe and Adequate Dietary Intakes of Selected Vitamins and Minerals" (see Appendix 1). These are ranges of adequate subtoxic intakes, not recommended dietary intakes.

ENERGY

Energy requirements are based on longitudinal studies of the median energy intakes of thriving infants [38]. Ranges of energy intakes for infants growing at the tenth and ninetieth percentiles are listed in Appendix 1. For healthy infants, individual requirements are based on appetite, activity, and rate of weight gain. Infants gain an average of 25 to 39 gm per day during the first 3 months of life and 15 to 21 gm per day during the second 3 months [37]. Because this is the most rapid weight gain of any period in life, high energy intakes are required. To promote desirable growth in the first 6 months, an average of 115 kcal per kilogram is needed. By the end of the first year, the requirement decreases to approximately 105 kcal/kg [38]. Stress imposed by illness increases energy requirements.

The energy-yielding nutrients found in the infant's diet are carbohydrate (4 kcal per gram), protein (4 kcal per gram), and fat (9 kcal per gram). Although the RDAs give energy requirements, they do not provide guidelines on the percentage of energy to be derived from carbohydrate, protein, and fat. Fomon recommends a distribution of 35 to 65 percent carbohydrate, 7 to 16 percent protein, and 30 to 55 percent fat [36]. Infant formulas are regulated to this composition by the Food and Drug Administration.

Breast milk or formula is the major source of energy in the infant's diet, especially during the first 6 months of life. Breast milk and most infant formulas contain approximately 20 kcal per ounce (67 kcal/100 ml) with an energy distribution of about 40 to 50 percent carbohydrate, 6 to 15 percent protein, and 50 to 55 percent fat. Low fat milk (15 kcal per ounce) and skim milk (10 kcal per ounce) are not calorically dense enough to meet infants' energy demands. The reason for this is that infants are not able to drink sufficient volume to get the calories they require [37]. Although whole milk contains about 20 kcal per ounce, it is unacceptable for infant feeding because of its relatively high protein and low carbohydrate concentrations.

Infant formulas may be modified for increased energy needs due to illness, "catch up" needs, or fluid restrictions. Calorically dense formulas should be used only when the infant is treated by a medical provider. Sources of fat (MCT oil or corn oil) or carbohydrate (Polycose) may be added to increase calories, as shown in Table 5-2. Formulas

Table 5-2. Commonly Used Supplements in the Infant's Diet

Supplement	Description	kcal/ tbsp	Considerations for Use
CARBOHYDRATES			
Karo syrup	Glucose, maltose, dextrins	57	Very sweet taste, medium osmolarity, requires amylase for digestion
Polycose	Glucose polymer (hydrolyzed cornstarch—80% amylose, 20% amylopectin)	30	Tasteless, requires little or no amylase for digestion; low osmolarity powder and liquid forms
FAT			
Corn oil	Corn oil	126	Good source of linoleic acid; requires normal fat digestion and transport
MCT oil	Medium chain triglycerides; contains fatty acids with 8–12 carbons	115	Does not require bile salts or lipases for digestion
Lipomul	Polysorbate 60; glyceride phosphate, sodium saccharin	91	Perfume-like taste; combines with many foods
PROTEIN			Protein content should not exceed 15% of total calories
Casec	Calcium caseinate	17	Contains 75 mg Ca^{2+} per tbsp, 4 gm protein per tbsp

Note: Amount to be added to one quart of formula (20 kcal/oz) to make 25 kcal/oz concentration:
Karo syrup = 3.0 tbsp
Polycose = 6.0 tbsp
MCT oil = 1.5 tbsp
Corn oil = 1.5 tbsp
Adapted from Mikkola, M. L. The Cardiovascular System. In R. B. Howard, and N. H. Herbold, (Eds.), *Nutrition in Clinical Care*. New York: McGraw-Hill, 1982, and Getchell, E. (Ed.). *Handbook for Nutrition Services of the Dietary Department*. Boston: Children's Hospital Medical Center, 1982. P. 45.

Table 5-3. Breast Milk, Cow's Milk, and Infant
Formula Composition and Considerations for Use

Milk and Formula	Nutrient Source			Energy (kcal/oz)	Nutrients (gm/100 ml)		
	Protein	CHO	Fat		PRO	CHO	FAT
Breast milk	Lactalbumin casein	Lactose	Human milk fat	22	1.1	6.8	4.5
Cow's milk	Lactalbumin casein	Lactose	Butter fat	20	3.5	4.9	3.7
WELL INFANT FORMULAS							
Similac (Ross)	Nonfat cow's milk	Lactose	Soy oil, coconut oil	20	1.5	7.3	3.6
Enfamil (MJ)	Nonfat cow's milk	Lactose	Soy oil, coconut oil	20	1.5	7.0	3.7
PREMATURE							
Similac Low Birth Weight (Ross)	Nonfat cow's milk	Lactose, polycose	Soy oil, coconut oil, MCT oil	24	2.2	8.5	4.5
Enfamil Premature (MJ)	Demineralized whey, nonfat cow's milk	Glucose polymers, lactose	Corn oil, MCT oil, coconut oil	24	2.4	8.9	4.1
Special Care (Ross)	Nonfat cow's milk, demineralized whey	Lactose, corn syrup solids	Corn oil, coconut oil, MCT oil	24	2.2	8.6	4.4
INCREASED ENERGY/OZ.							
Similac 24 with Iron (Ross)	Nonfat cow's milk	Lactose	Soy oil, coconut oil	24	2.2	8.5	4.3
Similac 27 (Ross)	Cow's milk	Lactose	Coconut oil, soy oil	27	2.5	9.5	4.8
Enfamil 24 with Iron (MJ)	Nonfat cow's milk	Lactose	Soy oil, coconut oil	24	1.8	8.3	4.5
DECREASED ENERGY/OZ							
Similac 13 with Iron (Ross)	Cow's milk	Lactose	Coconut oil, soy oil	13.2	1.1	4.6	2.3
Enfamil 13 (MJ)	Nonfat cow's milk	Lactose	Soy oil, coconut oil	13.2	1.0	4.5	2.4

	Minerals					Osmolality (mOsm/kg H_2O)	Renal Solute Load (mOsm/liter)	
Iron (mg/100 ml)	mEq/Liter							Considerations
	Ca^{2+}	P^{2+}	Na^+	K^+	Cl^-			
0.1–0.15	17	8	7	13	11	280	75	Recommended for infant feeding whenever possible
0.05	59	60	22	35	28	288	230	Unmodified cow's milk not recommended for infant feeding. Avoid skim milk in first year. Evaporated cow's milk acceptable
With iron, 1.2	26	23	11	20	15	290	108	Formulas for normal, full-term infants. Breast milk substitute.
With iron, 1.2	28	27	12	18	15	290	110	Iron-fortified formulas recommended. Available in ready to use, concentrated liquid, and powder forms
0.3	36	33	16	26	24	290	154	Formulas used for infants with a limited intake or infants recovering from illness with in-
0.12	48	28	14	23	19	300	220	creased energy needs or illness-induced malnutrition. Available in ready to use form
0.3	70	46	15	26	18	300	147	
0.15	36	33	14	27	21	360	150	Formulas modified to meet the increased growth needs of the
trace	40	36	17	32	22	420	171	premature infant. Available in ready to use form
1.52	33	33	15	21	18	355	130	
0.7	20	18	10	15	12	190	84	Formulas used with infants who have not been fed enterally for
0.10	18	18	8	12	10	182	70	several days or weeks. Also used when a conservative initial formula is needed for newborns during first 24–48 hour period. Available in ready to use form

Table 5-3 (Continued)

Milk and Formula	Nutrient Source			Energy (kcal/oz)	Nutrients (gm/100 ml)		
	Protein	CHO	Fat		PRO	CHO	FAT
ELECTRODIALYZED							
SMA (Wyeth)	Nonfat cow's milk, demineralized whey	Lactose	Oleo, coconut oil	20	1.5	7.2	3.6
PM 60/40 (Ross)	Nonfat cow's milk, demineralized whey	Lactose	Safflower oil, soybean oil	20	1.6	7.6	3.5
SOY PROTEIN-LACTOSE FREE							
Isomil (Ross)	Soy protein isolate	Corn syrup, sucrose	Coconut oil, soy oil	20	2.0	6.8	3.6
Prosobee (MJ)	Soy protein isolate, supplement with L-methionine	Corn syrup solids	Soy oil, coconut oil	20	2.0	6.9	3.6
Hydrolyzed protein Nutramigen (MJ)	Casein hydrolysate	Sucrose, modified tapioca starch	Corn oil	20	2.2	8.8	2.6
Pregestimil (MJ)	Casein hydrolysate, L-tryptophan, L-cystine, L-tyrosine	Corn syrup solids, modified tapioca starch	Corn oil, MCT oil	20	1.9	9.1	2.7
ALTERED FAT-LACTOSE FREE							
Portagen (MJ)	Sodium caseinate	Corn syrup solids, sucrose	MCT oil (88%), corn oil (12%)	20	2.4	7.8	3.2

	Minerals							
		mEq/Liter				Osmolality (mOsm/kg H$_2$O)	Renal Solute Load (mOsm/liter)	
Iron (mg/100 ml)	Ca^{2+}	P^{2+}	Na$^+$	K$^+$	Cl$^-$			Considerations
1.26	22	20	6.5	14.4	10.4	300	91	Formulas provide a lower renal solute load and lower amounts
0.26	20	12	7	15	7	260	92	of sodium and potassium. (Whey is demineralized by electrophoresis.) Protein and mineral content is comparable to breast milk. Formulas are used with infants who have impaired renal or cardiovascular function and infants with diabetes insipidus. Have casein-whey ratios that resemble human milk. Available in ready to use, concentrated liquid, and powder forms
1.2	35	24	13	18	15	250	126	Formulas used for infants with milk protein hypersensitivity,
1.3	32	32	18.7	18	16	160	127	lactose or sucrose intolerance, galactosemia, and vegetarian diets. Available in powder form Other soy-based formulas including Neomulsoy (Syntex) and Soyalac (Loma Linda). Available in ready to use and concentrated liquid forms
1.27	32	28	14	17	13	443	130	Formulas used for infants sensitive to intact protein and infants recovering from pro-
1.27	32	25	14	18	16	338	125	longed diarrhea. These formulas avoid possible GI absorption of intact protein because the protein is hydrolyzed. The formulas contain a high percentage of free amino acids, and the remainder of the protein is in the peptide form. Available in powder form
1.88	32	28	14	22	16	236	150	Formula high in MCT oil, which is more readily hydrolyzed and absorbed, is used with infants who have a defect in the hydrolysis of fat (cystic fibrosis, pancreatic insufficiency, chronic liver disease, biliary atresia or obstruction), a defect in absorption (sprue, idiopathic steatorrhea, resection of intestine, blind-loop syndrome), a defective lipoproteinlipase system (hyperchylomicronemia), faulty chylomicron formation (β-lipoproteinemia), or defects in fat transportation (intestinal lymphatic obstruction, lymphangiectasia chylothorax, chyluria, chylous ascites, exudative enteropathy). Available in powder form

Table 5-3 (Continued)

Milk and Formula	Nutrient Source			Energy (kcal/oz)	Nutrients (gm/100 ml)		
	Protein	CHO	Fat		PRO	CHO	FAT
INBORN ERRORS OF METABOLISM							
Lofenalac (MJ)	Casein hydrolysate (most phenylalanine removed, fortified tyrosine, tryptophan, histidine, methionine)	Corn syrup solids, modified tapioca starch	Corn oil	20	2.2	8.8	2.7
Phenyl Free (MJ)	L-amino acids	Sucrose, corn syrup solids, modified tapioca starch	Corn oil	25	3.8	6.2	6.4
CARBOHYDRATE-FREE							
RCF (Ross)	Soy protein isolate		Soy oil, coconut oil	Varies with CHO added	2.0		3.6
TRANSITION FORMULA							
Advance (Ross)	Cow milk, soy protein	Corn syrup, lactose	Soy oil, corn oil	20	2.0	5.5	2.7
WATER/ELECTROLYTE MAINTENANCE							
Pedialyte (Ross)	—	Glucose	—	6	—	5.0	—
Lytren (MJ)	—	Corn syrup solids, glucose	—	9	—	7.6	—
5% glucose	—	Glucose	—	6	—	5.0	—
10% glucose	—	Glucose	—	12	—	10.0	—

may be prepared to contain higher energy concentrations by diluting the powder or liquid with less water. For example, adding 8 ounces of water to a 13-ounce can of concentrated liquid formula raises the caloric density from 20 to 25 kcal per ounce. Also, for special medical conditions, proprietary formulas with increased caloric concentrations are available (i.e., Enfamil Premature [Mead Johnson], Similac Low Birth Weight [Ross], and SMA 27 [Wyeth]). Table 5-3 gives information on formula compositions and indications for use.

When infant foods are introduced, they begin to replace breast milk or infant formula as the major source of energy. The caloric density of infant foods varies, as seen in Table 5-15. By the time most infants reach 9 months of age, about half of their total energy requirements is met by solid foods.

Iron (mg/100 ml)	Minerals					Osmolality (mOsm/kg H₂O)	Renal Solute Load (mOsm/liter)	Considerations
	mEq/Liter							
	Ca²⁺	P²⁺	Na⁺	K⁺	Cl⁻			
1.3	32	28	13.9	17.4	13.3	454	130	Formula used for infants and children with phenylketonuria. Initially to meet phenylalanine needs, whole milk or formula is added. Available in powder form
2.3	57	55.2	20.7	34.1	26.8	920	170	Formula used for older children with phenylketonuria. Contains no phenylalanine. Available in powder form
—	35	32.2	12	18.2	14.9	Varies with CHO added	126	Formula used for infants with carbohydrate intolerances. Carbohydrate of choice can be added (i.e., polycose, dextrose) slowly to provide 6.4% of total energy. Available in powder form
1.2	26	23	13	22	16	210	131	Formula used as transition between infant formula and cow's milk. Available in ready to use form
—	4	—	30	20	30	405	—	Formulas used for mild to moderate diarrhea (water and electrolyte maintenance or replacement). Initial oral feeding after NPO. Available in ready to use form
—	4	5	30	25	25	290	—	
—	—	—	—	—	—	276	—	IV solutions for acute illness.
—	—	—	—	—	—	552	—	

MJ = Mead Johnson, Evansville, Indiana; Ross = Ross Laboratories, Columbus, Ohio
Note: The nutrient composition of formulas changes frequently. For the most current information, contact the manufacturer.
Adapted from Howard, R. B. Growth and Nutrition. In R. B. Howard and N. H. Herbold (Eds.), *Nutrition in Clinical Care* (2nd ed.). New York: McGraw-Hill, 1982.

PROTEIN

Protein requirements depend both on body size and growth rate. In infancy, and especially during the first 6 months, protein requirements are greatest due to the rapid synthesis of protein into tissues, enzymes, and hormones. The RDA for protein during the first 6 months of life is 2.5 gm/kg per day, which is nearly three times the adult requirement. Protein utilization changes with age. Fomon demonstrates that infants use about 60 to 70 percent of their protein requirement for growth, whereas toddlers use only 10 to 15 percent for growth [35]. If caloric intake is inadequate, protein is used to provide energy. Because of the interrelationships between protein and energy metabolism, protein requirements are often expressed as gm/100 kcal. Current recommendations set by the Food and Drug Administration suggest that the minimum protein intake for normal infants should be about 1.8 gm protein per 100 kcal [1].

The American Academy of Pediatrics recognizes that up to 4.5 gm of protein per kilogram may be required in infancy, depending on the quality of protein in the infant's diet [2]. The quality of protein can be determined objectively by calculating the protein efficiency ratio (PER). The PER has been derived experimentally by feeding rats various proteins and measuring their growth [35]. The PER is defined as the weight gain in grams divided by the grams of protein consumed. Casein is the protein used as the standard to which other proteins are compared. If a protein used in a formula has a PER of less than 100 percent of the PER for casein, then the total amount of protein must be increased to compensate for the lower protein quality. An example of this is soy protein, which has a lower PER; therefore, soy formulas have greater total protein concentrations than milk-based formulas (see Table 5-3). Proteins that have a PER of less than 70 percent of casein cannot be used in infant formulas [1].

Although both human and cow's milk contain casein, their protein contents differ both qualitatively and quantitatively. The compositional differences between cow's milk and human milk protein, as well as the modifications of cow's milk for infant use, are shown in Table 5-4. Breast milk contains less total protein (1.6 gm/100 kcal) than cow's milk, but has a higher whey-casein ratio and more alpha-lactalbumin. In addition, the non-protein nitrogen content of human milk is higher, a factor that may be beneficial in promoting growth [57]. Demineralized whey is added to some infant formulas to approximate the higher whey-casein ratio in breast milk. The demineralization process causes electrolyte loss; therefore, these formulas have lower sodium and chloride concentrations, as seen in Table 5-3.

When breast-feeding is not possible and cow's milk formulas are not tolerated, soy formulas are most commonly used (i.e., Prosobee [Mead Johnson], Isomil [Ross]). The decreased PER of soy protein is due to the relatively low amounts of the amino acid methionine; therefore, some soy formulas have added methionine. One of the most common reasons for using a soy formula is cow's milk hypersensitivity. The suspected incidence of cow's milk hypersensitivity ranges from 0.1 to 8 percent of infants [31], but because there are no objective diagnostic criteria, the condition is often overdiagnosed. Infants may also be allergic to soy protein; approximately 30 percent of children with milk enteropathy are also intolerant of soy protein (see Chap.

Table 5-4. Comparison of Human and Cow's Milk Protein

Protein Component	Human Milk	Cow's Milk	Significance for Infant Feeding
Total protein content (gm/100 ml)	1.2	3.3	Unmodified cow's milk is not recommended because protein content is too high. Infant formulas based on cow's milk contain 1.5–1.8 gm/dl (which is acceptable)
Casein-whey ratio	40 : 60	20 : 80	Cow's milk is more allergenic. Some formulas are modified to provide the same casein-whey ratio as human milk
α-Lactalbumin (mg/100 ml)	150	90	Part of enzyme lactose synthetase. Parallels lactose content of milk
β-Lactoglobulin (mg/100 ml)	—	300	Chief protein in cow's milk, believed to be related to milk hypersensitivity
Nonprotein nitrogen (percent of total nitrogen)	25	5	Higher nonprotein nitrogen in human milk is believed to promote growth
Amino acids pattern: methionine-cysteine ratio	1	7	Newborn and preterm infants cannot efficiently metabolize methionine
Total aromatic amino acid content (mg/100 ml)	126	363	Newborns have low levels of enzymes required to metabolize aromatic amino acids

Data from Mata, L. Breast-feeding: Main promoter of infant health. *Am. J. Clin. Nutr.* 31: 2058, 1978, American Academy of Pediatrics Committee on Nutrition and the Nutrition Committee of the Canadian Pediatric Society. Breast-feeding, a commentary in celebration of the International Year of the Child, 1979. *Pediatrics* 62:591, 1978, and Lawrence, R. A. *Breast-feeding: A Guide for the Medical Profession.* St. Louis: Mosby, 1980.

8). If the infant is hypersensitive to both cow's milk and soy formula, formulas that contain meat as the protein source may be tried. MBF (Gerber) is a meat-based formula that is available for hypersensitive infants.

For infants who cannot utilize intact protein, casein hydrolysates are used as the protein source in other proprietary formulas, such as Nutramigen and Pregestimil (Mead Johnson). These formulas may be used in prolonged diarrheal illnesses because they contain peptides that are more easily digested and absorbed than intact proteins [63]. Formulas containing casein hydrolysates sometimes are supplemented with amino acids that may be lost in the hydrolysis process [56].

Specific free amino acids are used as the nitrogen source in formulas designed for children with inborn errors of amino acid metabolism (i.e., Phenyl Free, MSUD Powder [Mead Johnson]; PKU-1 [Milupa]). Because these formulas are devoid of essential amino acids, they are not suitable for general use and should be used with strict medical supervision.

LIPIDS

Lipids serve a variety of functions in the infant diet. They supply a major source of energy (9 kcal/gm), fat-soluble vitamins A, D, E, and K, as well as essential fatty acids. Lipids are also a component of phospholipids (the structural components of cell membranes) and prostaglandins and leukotrienes (potent regulators of cellular function).

The NRCNAS has not established an RDA for lipid. The American Academy of Pediatrics recommends that infant formulas provide between 30 and 54 percent of total calories as fat [1]. Lower amounts of dietary fat may cause caloric inadequacy or essential fatty acid deficiency. A diet too high in fat can cause ketosis and/or acidosis in the normal infant.

Lipids account for approximately half the calories in human milk. The lipid content of human milk is the most variable. When the maternal diet is deficient in calories, the total fat content of breast milk is reduced [48]. Caloric supplementation of the maternal diet increases the lipid concentration in breast milk. In addition, there are diurnal and within-feeding variations in breast milk lipid content [45]. The lipid concentration of breast milk is the lowest in the morning and increases during the day. During a feeding, the lipid content also rises. Both the total lipid content and the fatty acid composition of breast milk are influenced by diet. For example, the essential fatty acid, linoleic acid, is found in higher concentrations in the breast milk of women who consume diets high in vegetable oils and other unsaturated fats.

Essential Fatty Acids

Linoleic acid (C 18 : 2)* is the principal essential fatty acid. A deficiency of linoleic acid may result in growth failure and skin lesions. Human milk contains between 8 and 10 percent of its fat calories as linoleic acid. The Food and Drug Administration requires that infant formulas contain a minimum of 2 percent of total calories as essential fatty acids; the American Academy of Pediatrics recommends that formulas contain 300 mg of linoleic acid per 100 calories (approximately 2.7 percent

---

*Formula represents the length of carbon chain and number of double bonds.

of total calories) [1]. No upper limit for linoleic acid content in commercial preparations has been established. The linoleic acid content of most infant formulas is about 4 percent of total calories. Soy, corn, cottonseed, sunflower, sesame, and safflower oils are rich in linoleic acid [49]. Most infant formulas contain one or more of these oils in order to provide sufficient essential fatty acids.

When linoleic acid or other polyunsaturated acids are prevalent in the infant's diet, there is an increased need for vitamin E, an antioxidant that prevents the oxidation of double bonds. Formulas with high concentrations of polyunsaturated fatty acids (PUFA) are not recommended for preterm infants who are born with low vitamin E stores and may not absorb vitamin E well [18]. For these reasons, premature infants are supplemented with vitamin E and are given special formulas that contain acceptable amounts of PUFA (i.e., Enfamil Premature [Mead Johnson], Similac Low Birth Weight [Ross]).

Triglycerides

Triglycerides are composed of three fatty acids arranged on a backbone of glycerol. The type of fatty acid and the configuration of the fatty acids on the glycerol molecule affects absorption. Fatty acids range in size from 4 to 24 carbon atoms. They also range in degree of hydrogen saturation, which is determined by the number of single bonds (saturated) or double bonds (unsaturated) in the molecule. Animal fats contain saturated fats, whereas vegetable fats contain unsaturated fats, with the exception of palm and coconut oils that have a high proportion of lauric acid (C 14 : 0). The fatty acid composition of various milks and infant formulas are presented in Table 5-5.

Short-chain triglycerides contain fatty acids with 4 to 8 carbons. They provide fewer calories (5.3 kcal/gm) than do other fats. Because of their instability, they are not an important contributor to the infant's diet [35]. Medium-chain triglycerides (MCT) contain fatty acids with 10 to 14 carbons and provide 8.3 kcal/gm. These triglycerides are easily absorbed into the portal vein because they do not require micellar formation and lymphatic transport. Pregestimil and Portagen (Mead Johnson) are formulas that contain added MCT (C 8 : 0 to C 12 : 0) and are indicated in diseases with steatorrhea (e.g., cystic fibrosis). MCT also may be used as an energy source for infants or children with increased caloric needs and/or volume restrictions.

Long-chain triglycerides (greater than 14 carbon atoms) provide 9 kcal/gm and are the predominant source of fat in standard formula-fed and breast-fed infants' diets. Unsaturated fats are more readily absorbed than saturated fats, and the position of the fatty acid on the glycerol molecule also appears to affect absorption (see Table 5-5). The abundant unsaturated fatty acid, oleic acid (C 18 : 1), found in

Table 5-5. Fatty Acid Composition of Various Milks and Formulas

Type of Feeding	Fat Source	Fatty Acid Composition Weight (%)										
		4:0–8:0	10:0	Lauric 12:0	Myristic 14:0	Palmitic 16:0	Palmitoleic 16:1	Stearic 18:0	Oleic 18:1	Linoleic 18:2	Linolenic 18:3	Other
Breast	Human	—	1.3	3.1	5.1	20.2	5.7	5.9	46.4	13.0	1.4	0.4
Cow	Cow	6.2	3.0	3.1	14.2	42.9	3.7	5.7	16.7	1.6	1.8	1.3
Goat	Goat	8.2	8.4	3.3	10.3	24.6	2.2	12.5	28.5	2.2	—	—
Enfamil (Mead Johnson)	Soy, coconut	1.9	1.1	10.0	4.1	11.1	—	3.8	21.1	41.1	5.9	—
Similac (ready to feed) (Ross)	Soy, coconut	4.2	3.6	29.7	11.7	9.5	—	2.8	13.6	21.3	3.6	—
SMA (Wyeth)	Oleo, coconut, safflower, soy	2.0	1.4	14.5	6.0	12.8	—	7.4	38.9	13.1	1.1	2.8
Portagen (Mead Johnson)	MCT, corn	68.0	20.0	1.0	—	1.4	—	—	3.2	6.8	—	—
MBF (Gerber)	Beef, sesame	—	—	—	0.7	14.4	—	7.3	43.0	32.7	0.7	1.2

Data from Jensen, R. G., Hagerty, M. M., and McMahon, K. E. Lipids of human milk and infant formulas: A review. *Am. J. Clin. Nutr.* 31:990, 1978, and Fomon, S. J. *Infant Nutrition* (2nd ed.) Philadelphia: Saunders, 1974.

breast milk and safflower oil is easily absorbed by infants. Arachidonic acid (C 20:1) is another unsaturated fatty acid that is an important precursor to prostaglandins and leukotrienes.

Among the saturated fats found mainly in human and animal milks and to a lesser degree in infant formulas, stearic acid (C 18:0) is absorbed poorly [46]. Palmitic acid (C 16:0) possibly is more easily absorbed if it is the second fatty acid on the triglyceride as compared with either terminal position on the molecule [35]. This may be the reason for the efficient absorption of palmitic acid in human milk [49]. Too high a concentration of either palmitic or stearic acid is not desirable because both are believed to interfere with the absorption of calcium by binding calcium in the lumen of the gut. The effect of saturated and unsaturated fatty acid intake on serum cholesterol levels is a pediatric concern.

Cholesterol

Because the atherosclerotic process leading to cardiovascular disease begins during the pediatric years, it has been postulated that lowering serum cholesterol in infancy may help prevent atherosclerosis. However, because cholesterol levels are affected by both dietary intake and endogenous synthesis of cholesterol and because human milk contains higher amounts of cholesterol and more saturated fat than infant formulas, there may be a biological need for cholesterol. Some speculate that cholesterol may be important for central nervous system development as well as for bile salt synthesis [35, 49]. This is supported by the evidence that if mothers are given low-cholesterol, high-PUFA diets, their breast milk cholesterol content does not change significantly [49].

Many infants in the United States are fed cholesterol-free formulas from birth, which has caused some to question the safety of these diets. A three-year study of infants who were fed low-saturated fat, low-cholesterol diets showed that they did not differ from controls in growth and development or any biochemical measurement with the exception of serum cholesterol [40]. At present, no restriction of cholesterol or dietary fat is recommended during the first year of life. However, as infants move into the toddler years, it is prudent to monitor the total fat and cholesterol content of their diets (see Chap. 6).

CARBOHYDRATE

Carbohydrates supply the infant both with energy (4 kcal/gm) and the structural components of biological compounds (see Table 5-2). The simplest form of carbohydrates called monosaccharides include hexoses and pentoses. The hexoses (six-carbon sugars) including glucose, fructose, galactose, and mannose are the most important nutritionally. The body uses glucose as its energy source. The central nervous system is especially dependent on glucose for energy, although in prolonged starvation the brain utilizes ketones. Pentoses (five-carbon sugars) can be synthesized via the pentose monophosphate shunt and are incorporated into compounds such as riboflavin, certain coenzymes, and nucleoproteins. Disaccharides (i.e., lactose, maltose) and more complex carbohydrates are a major source of glucose, but they require luminal digestion in order to be absorbed.

Lactose, a disaccharide containing glucose and galactose, is the most important (and in some cases the only) carbohydrate in the infant's diet. It comprises about 38 percent of the total calories in breast milk [4] and is uniform in its concentration despite maternal diet [48]. In standard infant formulas, between 40 and 59 percent of calories are provided by carbohydrate, principally lactose.

Lactase, a brush border enzyme necessary for the breakdown of lactose to glucose and galactose, is rarely congenitally deficient in infants of more than 30 weeks' gestation [57]. In contrast, in adults lactase deficiency is common, especially among black, Oriental, and Jewish populations. Although plentiful in infancy, lactase activity declines in these groups during childhood. Secondary lactase deficiency may result following any mucosal injury to the small intestine but is reversible when the causative agent is removed [43].

Alternatives to commercial infant formulas that contain lactose are needed for infants who have primary or secondary lactase deficiency, milk protein allergy, or galactosemia (an inborn error of carbohydrate metabolism). For these infants, formulas are required that contain other carbohydrate sources such as sucrose, maltose, corn syrup solids, and Polycose. Formulas with sucrose or maltose have sweeter tastes than those containing lactose. Sucrose, composed of fructose and glucose, is usually well tolerated. Primary sucrase deficiency is rare, and secondary deficiency is found in severe intestinal injury. In the intestine healing from villous injury, sucrase activity returns before lactase activity.

Maltose may be found in the infant's diet in the form of corn syrup and corn syrup solids [56]. These hydrolysates of corn starch require amylase for digestion; maltase then cleaves the resulting disaccharide into two glucose monomers. Maltase is a plentiful brush border enzyme and is less likely to be deficient than either sucrase or lactase [43]. Hence, corn syrup and corn syrup solids are often used as carbohydrate sources in formulas intended for children with mucosal injury. Also, because glucose polymers (e.g., Polycose [Mead Johnson]) are readily absorbed, they are frequently added to formulas for premature infants such as Enfamil Premature (Mead Johnson) and Similac Low Birth Weight (Ross). Because digestive enzymes in the premature infant do not function optimally, these infants are especially vulnerable to carbohydrate malabsorption.

Malabsorbed carbohydrate is metabolized by colonic bacteria producing hydrogen gas, which is subsequently expired and may be detected in the breath. The hydrogen breath test is a noninvasive test used to detect lactose or other carbohydrate malabsorption [65]. In addition, colonic bacteria convert nonabsorbed carbohydrate to volatile fatty acids that may be absorbed in the colon and used as an energy source [56].

As long as the infant is breast- or formula-fed, sources of carbohydrate in the diet are limited. Other disaccharides, such as fructose and sucrose, and polysaccharides, such as starch and fiber, become increasingly more important in the diet as other foods are introduced (see Chap. 6).

WATER

Water is a physiologically important nutrient in infancy. Under normal conditions, the water requirement in infancy is the sum of the water that is lost via the skin, stool, urine, and respiratory system plus the small amount that is needed for growth [35]. In febrile conditions, approximately 10 percent more water is lost through the skin than normally; in diarrhea, 5 to 6 times the amount of water is lost in the stool.

The NRCNAS has not established a requirement for fluid; however, a healthy infant should receive about 130 to 155 ml of fluid per kilogram per day [15]. This is equivalent to about 30 ounces of breast milk or formula for a 6-kg infant. Because the amount of fluid necessary per kilogram decreases with age, at the end of the first year of life, about 120 to 135 ml/kg is needed [15]. Barring unusual circumstances such as extreme heat, increased temperature, or exceptional fluid loss, fluid requirements are met by breast milk or infant formulas of standard dilution fed to meet caloric needs. When special formulas with high renal solute loads are used, the infant requires more fluid; this usually is not an issue unless the infant receives concentrated formula.

VITAMINS AND MINERALS

The need for vitamin and mineral supplementation depends on nutrient stores at birth and the bioavailability of nutrients in the diet. Table 5-6 gives supplementation guidelines. Dietary requirements in the first 6 months of life can be met by breast milk or infant formulas with appropriate supplementation. The following section will focus on the vitamins and minerals with questionable adequacy in the infant's diet. (Functions and sources of other vitamins and minerals are found in Table 5-1.)

Table 5-6. Vitamin and Mineral Supplementation Guide for Normal Infants

	Nutrient (dose)[a]			
Type of Feeding	Vitamin D (400 IU)	Vitamin C (35 mg)	Iron (1 mg/kg/day up to 15 mg)	Fluoride (see table 5-9)
Breast	±[b]		+	±[c]
Iron-fortified formula				±[c]
Non-iron fortified formula			+	±[c]
Home-prepared evaporated milk formula	±[d]	+	+	±[c]

Note: ± indicates supplement should be given under the conditions specified in footnotes.
[a]Supplements should start shortly after birth; iron supplements to be started no later than 4 months of age.
[b]If maternal diet is low in vitamin D or mother and infant are not exposed to sunlight.
[c]Where the fluoride content of local water is less than 0.03 ppm.
[d]If milk used in preparation is not fortified.
Adapted from American Academy of Pediatrics Committee on Nutrition. Vitamin and mineral supplementation needs in normal children in the United States. *Pediatrics* 66: 1015, 1980, and Fomon, S. J., et al. Recommendations for feeding normal infants. *Pediatrics* 63:52, 1979.

Vitamin D

Vitamin D is sometimes called the "sunshine" vitamin because it can be synthesized in skin that has been exposed to ultraviolet light. Vitamin D is found in breast milk, formulas, fortified cow's milk, and fish oils.

Vitamin D is a steroid that acts as a hormone to regulate calcium and phosphorus homeostasis. (A detailed review of vitamin D metabolism is provided by DeLuca [29].) A deficiency of vitamin D causes osteomalacia in adults and rickets in children. In rachitic states, the diminished deposition of calcium and phosphorus results in malformation of primarily the long bones. The amount of vitamin D required from dietary sources is dependent on the amount of sun exposure and may vary seasonally. The current recommendation for vitamin D in infancy is 400 International Units (IU) or the equivalent, 10 units of cholecalciferol [38].

Most formula-fed infants receive sufficient vitamin D. Infants fed home-prepared formulas need supplementation only if the milk used in preparation is not vitamin D fortified. Vitamin D supplementation is controversial for breast-fed infants. Rickets have been reported to occur in breast-fed infants, but most often in association with strict vegetarian maternal diets [32]. Rickets is uncommon among breast-fed infants despite the fact that human milk contains small amounts of vitamin D (approximately 22 IU/liter [4]. It has been proposed that vitamin D in breast milk is easily absorbed as a water-soluble sulfate analogue [55]. However, studies have demonstrated that this component has little antirachitic activity [58]. Most evidence suggests that unconjugated forms of vitamin D, especially 25-hydroxyvitamin D, are the main antirachitic metabolites in human milk, but the total amount of these metabolites appears to be less than the amount required for normal skeletal development [80]. In a study of unsupplemented breast-fed infants without clinical manifestations of rickets, serum 25-hydroxyvitamin D levels were similar to levels found in infants with rickets [44]. At 12 weeks of age, the bone mineral concentration of unsupplemented breast-fed infants in this study was significantly less than that of supplemented infants given similar calcium and phosphorus intakes. By age 1 year, there was no difference between the groups in any biochemical measurements [44]. Thus the physiological value of vitamin D supplementation in breast-fed infants is still questionable; nevertheless, supplementation is recommended.

It is likely that the need for vitamin D supplementation depends on the infant's stores at birth. Children of women who had inadequate vitamin D intakes during their pregnancies are at the highest risk for being deficient. If the infant does not receive adequate sunlight exposure or if maternal diet is low in vitamin D, then the American Academy of Pediatrics recommends that breast-fed infants receive supplemental vitamin D [6]. It is essential for the health provider to take a dietary history of a breast-feeding mother, beginning with the prenatal diet (see Chap. 7). The recommended supplementation level of 400 IU of vitamin D can be given as vitamin drops or cod-liver oil. Table 5-7 provides information on commercially available vitamin preparations.

Vitamin C

Vitamin C is essential for the development of normal collagen. It also enhances iron absorption and is required for the metabolism of certain amino acids. Although adequate amounts of vitamin C are present in formulas and breast milk, formulas made from evaporated cow's milk require vitamin C supplementation [6]. Vitamin C is included in nearly all infant vitamin preparations, often in conjunction with vitamins A and D. Because of the abundant availability of vitamin C, deficiencies are rare (see Table 7-18). Vitamin C is water soluble; therefore, toxicity is only a concern with megadosages. In adults, chronic high dose administration acidifies the urine and may predispose to renal stones.

Table 5-7. Common Vitamin/Mineral Supplements for Infants and Toddlers

Supplement	Recommended Dose	Vitamin A (IU)	Vitamin D (IU)	Vitamin E (IU)	Vitamin C (mg)	Thiamin (mg)	Riboflavin (mg)	Niacin (mg)	Pyridoxin (µg)	Vitamin B12 (µg)	Folic Acid (µg)	Pantothenic Acid (µg)	Biotin (µg)	Fluoride* (mg)	Iron (mg)
Tri-Vi-Sol[a]															
Drops	1 ml	1500	400	—	35	—	—	—	—	—	—	—	—	—	+
Tablets	1	2500	400	—	50	—	—	—	—	—	—	—	—	—	—
Tri-Vi-Flor[a]															
Drops	1 ml	1500	400	—	35	—	—	—	—	—	—	—	—	0.25	+
Drops	1 ml	1500	400	—	35	—	—	—	—	—	—	—	—	0.50	—
Tablets	1	2500	400	—	60	—	—	—	—	—	—	—	—	1.0	—
Poly-Vi-Sol[a]															
Drops	1 ml	1500	400	5	35	0.5	0.6	8.0	0.4	2	—	—	—	—	+
Tablets	1	2500	400	15	60	1.05	1.2	13.5	1.05	4.5	0.3	—	—	—	‡
Poly-Vi-Flor[a]															
Drops	1 ml	1500	400	5	35	0.5	0.6	8.0	0.4	2	—	—	—	0.25	—
Drops	1 ml	1500	400	5	35	0.5	0.6	8.0	0.4	2	—	—	—	0.50	+
Tablets	1	2500	400	15	60	1.05	1.2	13.5	1.05	4.5	0.3	—	—	0.50	—
Tablets	1	2500	400	15	60	1.05	1.2	13.5	1.05	4.5	0.3	—	—	1.0	‡

Vi-Penta Multi-vitamin Drops[b]	0.6 ml	5000	400	2	50	1.0	1.0	1.0	1.0	—	—	10	30.0	—
Chocks-Bugs Bunny Multivitamin tablets[c]	1	2500	400	15	60	1.05	1.2	13.5	1.05	4.5	300	—	—	‡
Pals multi-vitamin tablets[d]	1	3500	400	—	60	0.8	1.3	14.0	1.0	2.5	50	5	—	‡
One-A-Day Vitamin tablets[c]	1	5000	400	15	60	1.5	1.7	20.0	2.0	6	400	—	—	‡

[a]Mead Johnson, Evansville, In.
[b]Roche Laboratories, Nutley, N.J.
[c]Miles Laboratories, Inc., Elkhart, In.
[d]Bristol-Myers, New York, N.Y.
*Fluoride drops without vitamins are available when only fluoride is needed. (See Fluoride Supplementation Schedule, Table 5-9).
†Available with iron (10 mg) or without iron.
‡Available with iron (12 mg) or without iron.
Data from *Physicians' Reference for Nonprescription Drugs*. Oradell, N.J.: Medical Economics Company, 1980. *Physicians' Desk Reference* (36th ed.). Oradell, N.J.: Medical Economics Company, 1982.

B Vitamins

The functions of the B vitamins are presented in Table 5-1. Vitamin B complex deficiencies are rare in breast-fed infants; however, deficiencies may occur in breast-fed infants whose mothers follow restricted diets [8]. Vitamin B_{12} deficiency has been reported in breast-fed infants whose mothers follow strict vegan (no animal products) diets [28, 85]. For this reason, vitamin B_{12} supplements are recommended for vegetarian women. There are no naturally occurring non-animal sources of vitamin B_{12}; however, synthetic vitamin B_{12} preparations are available for the mother or the infant [28]. The requirement for vitamin B_{12} in infancy is 0.5 to 1.5 μg per day; for breast-feeding mothers the requirement is 4 μg per day [38].

Iron

Iron deficiency is a common problem in infancy and childhood. The Center for Disease Control Coordinated Nutrition Surveillance Program estimates the prevalence of anemia (defined as hemoglobin less than 11 mg/100 ml) in infants aged 6 to 11 months to be between 23 and 34 percent depending on the ethnic population [22]. About 6 to 9 percent of these infants have hemoglobin levels of less than 10 mg/100 ml. Iron deficiency anemia is more prevalent among infants and children from lower socioeconomic groups. It places these at-risk children at further risk because iron deficiency may impair learning by disrupting cerebral oxidative metabolism, neurotransmitter synthesis, or brain cell mitosis [70]. In addition, resistance to infection is lower in the iron-deficient child [3]. An excellent review of iron deficiency in infancy and childhood has been written by Dallman [27]. Deficiency states and the need for supplementation can be related to iron stores at birth.

Full-term healthy infants are born with iron stores of about 75 mg/per kg, which they receive transplacentally in the form of red blood cells. An inadequate placental transfusion of red blood cells at birth may be the initiating factor in the development of inadequate iron stores. As newborn erythrocytes reach senescence (lifespan of about 120 days), hemoglobin levels decline, and most of the iron from these senescent red blood cells is transported to the bone marrow where it forms the infant's iron stores. As iron reserves increase, absorption of dietary iron decreases. By the age of 2 months, hemoglobin levels reach their lowest point. This is followed by erythropoiesis and the utilization of iron stores. By the age of 4 months, there is an increased reliance on dietary iron to replenish low iron stores because of rapid growth. This is the time when term infants are most responsive to dietary iron supplements. In the preterm infant or the infant who for any reason is anemic at birth, iron stores may be exhausted more quickly, and iron supplementation may be required at the age of 2 to

3 months [27]. The adequacy of iron stores can be assessed by serum ferritin, which will reflect iron deficiency prior to abnormalities in red cell hemoglobin or red cell number.

To ensure adequate iron stores and to prevent anemia, the RDA for iron is 10 mg per day until the age of 6 months and 15 mg per day between 6 months and 3 years [38]. The American Academy of Pediatrics recommends that full-term infants receive 1 mg/kg per day of iron and preterm infants receive 2 mg/kg per day, not to exceed 15 mg of iron per day [2]. Both breast and cow's milk are poor iron sources, however, breast milk iron appears to be better absorbed and iron deficiency anemia is rare in purely breast-fed infants [64]. Lactoferrin, ascorbic acid, lactose, and phosphorus may enhance the absorption of iron from breast milk [64]. Lactoferrin, which must be unsaturated with iron in order to be effective [20], has an important bacteriostatic action in the breast-fed infant. Theoretically, oral iron supplementation could interfere with this action, but the American Academy of Pediatrics Committee on Nutrition has reviewed the available evidence on the relationship between iron status and the incidence of infection and concluded that iron supplementation is beneficial [3]. With respect to infant formulas, those that are iron fortified provide sufficient iron. However, unmodified cow's milk is low in iron and may also cause occult intestinal blood loss [31]. Thus, whole milk should not be given during the first year of life. Table 5-8 compares the iron content and absorption of breast milk and infant formulas.

Certain food components have been found to either inhibit or enhance iron bioavailability. Heme (flesh) iron and ascorbic acid promote iron uptake, whereas phytates (present in whole grains and legumes) and tannins (in tea) interfere with iron absorption [27]. The addition of solid food to breast-fed infants' diets diminishes iron absorption and necessitates the use of iron supplementation. The form of iron used in supplementation or food fortification also affects utilization

Table 5-8. The Iron Content and Percent Absorption of Iron in Infant Milk Feedings

Type of Feeding	Approximate mg Fe/liter	Absorption %	Iron Absorbed per Liter (mg)
Breast milk	0.5–1.0	49	0.25–0.5
Iron-fortified infant formula	12	4	0.5
Non-iron fortified infant formula	2.0	10	0.2

Data from Dallman, P. R., Siimes, M. A., and Stekel, A. Iron deficiency in infancy and childhood. *Am. J. Clin. Nutr.* 33:86, 1980.

[2]. Iron is poorly absorbed from iron pyrophosphate, ferric ortho-phosphate, and reduced iron of large particle size. Absorption is good from ferrous sulfate and from reduced iron of small particle size. This is the type currently used in iron-fortified infant cereals.

Usually by the age of 4 months, supplementation is needed in breast-fed infants. A number of infant vitamin preparations are available with iron (see Table 5-7). Preparations that also provide vitamin D are best suited for the breast-fed infant. Iron-fortified cereals, introduced between 4 and 6 months of age, may be adequate if iron-supplemented formula has been used. Although iron supplementation has been as-sociated with gastrointestinal distress, colic, and constipation in young infants, the direct effect of iron has not been established [36].

Fluoride

Fluoride helps to prevent dental caries later in life by changing the structure of tooth enamel. In the presence of fluoride, a fluoroapatite or a mixed hydroxyfluoroapatite crystal is formed in the tooth enamel instead of hydroxyapatite [66]. The fluoroapatite crystal is larger, more perfectly shaped, and more stable than hydroxyapatite, causing teeth to be less acid soluble and more resistant to caries. In addition, fluoride may interfere with the metabolism of oral bacteria and improve tooth morphology by creating smoother occlusal surfaces that are less re-tentive to food [35].

The optimum amount of fluoride in an infant's diet is between 0.05 and 0.07 mg per kilogram of body weight [74]. This level cannot be achieved without supplementation. However, excessive fluoride dep-osition in infancy may cause a mottling of teeth, known as fluorosis, which has caused much debate in medical and dental communities regarding the correct level of fluoride supplementation. In 1979, the American Academy of Pediatrics Committee on Nutrition revised their fluoride supplementation schedule (Table 5-9) to optimize fluoride in-take and prevent fluorosis [5]. This supplementation schedule is based on the child's age and the fluoride content of the local water. Because fluoride does not pass readily into breast milk and breast-fed infants consume little additional water, some feel that breast-fed infants re-quire fluoride supplementation regardless of the local water fluoride content [5]. Because formula manufacturers use nonfluoridated water in their preparations, the same argument may be made for infants who receive ready-to-use formulas. Nevertheless, current guidelines for fluoride supplementation in both breast-fed and formula-fed infants depend on the local water supply.

The time to add fluoride to an infant's diet is not definite. Although mineralization of deciduous teeth begins early in infancy, supple-mentation with fluoride as late as age 6 months seems to reduce the incidence of dental caries. The American Academy of Pediatrics rec-

Table 5-9. Fluoride Supplementation Dosage Schedule (mg/day)

Age	Local Water Fluoride Concentration (ppm)		
	0.3	0.3–0.7	0.7
2 wk–2 yr	0.25	—	—
2 yr–3 yr	0.50	0.25	—
3 yr–16 yr	1.0	0.50	—

Note: 2.2 mg sodium fluoride contains 1 mg fluoride
Source: American Academy of Pediatrics Committee on Nutrition. Fluoride supplementation: Revised dosage schedule. *Pediatrics* 63:150, 1979.

ommends that fluoride supplementation, when necessary, should begin shortly after birth [5, 6]. Table 5-7 lists infant vitamin preparations that contain fluoride. Fluoride drops may be given separately when it is not necessary to give additional vitamins or minerals.

THE IMMUNOLOGY OF BREAST-FEEDING

Human milk with appropriate supplements or iron-fortified formulas meet infants' nutritional requirements. Although iron-fortified formula is the best substitute for breast milk, it cannot provide the immunological factors that are contained in breast milk.

Infants are born with stores of maternal IgG because it is actively transported across the placenta. However, newborns are susceptible to infection because of their immature immunological systems. Through colostrum and breast milk, infants receive additional immunoglobulins. Breast-feeding has been reported to be protective against many infantile illnesses [23, 34] including gastroenteritis, respiratory illnesses [79], meningitis, and salmonella [39] and botulinum [14] infections. Because there are inherent problems in comparing breast- and bottle-fed children, the protective effect of breast-feeding is viewed with occasional skepticism. Epidemiological studies on breast-feeding are often challenged because breast-feeding mothers as a group tend to have more education and better health, factors that would, in themselves, lead to lower infant mortality [23]. However, the health advantage to breast-feeding has been demonstrated even when socioeconomic status is controlled as an experimental variable [25, 26].

A number of factors have been identified in breast-milk that help to explain its immunoprotective value. Breast-milk contains both cellular and humoral components that provide protection against infection. Some of these factors protect against specific antigens while others nonspecifically inhibit bacterial growth. Table 5-10 provides a summary of these factors.

Secretory IgA is the most abundant immunoglobulin in human milk.

Table 5-10. Factors in Colostrum and Human Milk that Confer Immunity to Infants

Factor	Description	Effect on Host Resistance
Immunoglobulins (IgA, IgM, IgG)	IgA is the predominant immunoglobulin in human milk. All immunoglobulins are found in specific B lymphocytes	Confers passive mucosal protection of GI tract against penetration of intestinal organisms and antigens
Lactoferrin	Iron-binding protein	Inhibits E. coli and staphylococci by competing for available iron
Lysozyme	Heat- and acid-stable enzyme. 300 times more abundant in human than cow's milk	Bacteriostatic agent against Enterobacteriaceae and gram-positive microorganisms. Aids in lysis by IgA antibodies
Bifidus Factor	Nitrogen containing carbohydrate without an amino group	Promotes growth of L. bifidus, predominant flora in breast-fed infants' guts, which creates low stool pH and inhibits pathogens
Leukocytes Macrophages	Large complex phagocytes; making up 90% of leukocytes found in colostrum	Phagocytosis of microorganisms. Produce complement, lysozyme, and lactoferrin
Lymphocytes	Comprise 10% of leukocytes found in colostrum. Both B cells and T cells are present	B cells: Produce IgA antibody. T cells: Believed to transfer delayed hypersensitivity from mother to infant

Data from Lawrence, R. A. Breast-Feeding, A Guide for the Medical Profession. St. Louis: Mosby, 1980. Pp. 73–91, American Academy of Pediatrics Committee on Nutrition and the Nutrition Committee of the Canadian Pediatric Society. Breast-feeding, a commentary in celebration of the International Year of the Child, 1979. Pediatrics 62:591, 1978, and Chandra, R. K. Immunological aspects of human milk. Nutr. Rev. 36:265, 1978.

Evidence suggests that IgA is transported through the intestinal epithelial cell where the secretory piece is attached. This complex binds
to the luminal surface of the epithelial cell and the IgA is then available
to bind antigens such as bacteria. The immobilization of the antigen
makes it accessible to proteolytic digestion by intraluminal pancreatic
enzymes. The mechanism may be important in eradicating entero-
viruses and agglutinating bacteria. Because the secretory IgA concentration of colostrum is higher than that of mature milk, colostrum is
immunologically important in the early neonatal period. Secretory IgA
concentration decreases during the first 3 months of lactation but is
maintained at about the same level from the age of 3 months to 1 year
[42, 67].

Other soluble factors, lactoferrin and lysozymes, also found in breast
milk, play a role in protecting the infant from infection. Lactoferrin,
an iron-binding protein competes with bacteria (e.g., E. coli and
Staphylococcus) for available iron [19]. Only lactoferrin that is unsaturated with iron is bacteriostatic, leading some to hypothesize that
iron supplementation could interfere with its effectiveness. Maternal
iron supplementation does not reduce the function of lactoferrin;
however, heating breast milk reduces the iron-binding capacity.
Therefore, infant formulas and heated breast milk lack this bacteriostatic factor [4].

Lysozymes are enzymes that are found in greater concentrations
in human milk than in cow's milk. They aid in lysis of bacteria and
are effective against Enterobacteriaceae and gram-positive bacteria [2].
Lysozyme levels vary with the phase of lactation; the highest levels
are present in colostrum. The concentration declines during the first
month and rises thereafter, remaining at the highest concentration
throughout the first year of lactation [42].

Another characteristic of breast milk that is believed to confer immunological protection is the bifidus factor, a nitrogen-containing
polysaccharide that is more abundant in human milk and colostrum
than in cow's milk [23, 57]. In the gut of the breast-fed infant, the
bifidus factor promotes the growth of the microorganism, Lactobacillus
bifidus (L. bifidus). This bacteria metabolizes lactose, which produces
lactic and acetic acids and results in a lower stool pH. The acidic environment inhibits the growth of many gram-negative organisms and
selects for nonpathogenic colonic flora [57]. Formula fed-infants have
mixed floras with some L. bifidus but with a predominance of gram-
negative anaerobic bacteria such as Bacteroides, Clostridium, and Proteus.

Other resistance factors are present in breast milk but are not well
defined. These include an antistaphylococcus factor (a fatty acid–like
compound that protects against staphylococcal infections), lactoper-
oxidase (present in both cow's and human milk and which retards

bacterial growth in vitro), and interferon (an antiviral glycoprotein produced by human milk leukocytes) [23, 62].

In addition to the soluble factors, cellular constituents of human milk, including macrophages and lymphocytes, are also of immunological significance in the breast-fed infant. About 90 percent of the viable leukocytes in human milk are phagocytic macrophages. They are capable of ingesting bacteria and immune complexes. In addition, they produce the bacteriologically active substances lactoferrin, lysozyme, and complement [4]. Lymphocytes, including both T cells and B cells, are also present in human milk. Lymphocytes, sensitized in the mother's gut to a specific antigen, are believed to migrate through the lymphatic system to the mammary gland where they produce antigen-specific antibodies. The term *enteromammary system* is used to describe this synergistic process of breast milk immunity. The mother, when exposed to her infant's bacteria, produces antibodies to those specific strains of intestinal bacteria; the infant receives both antibody and sensitized lymphocytes via the breast. Evidence exists for a similar system that links the respiratory system and the mammary gland [42].

Whether or not breast-feeding protects against allergies is less clear. Although the protein in breast milk is believed to be less allergenic than that in cow's milk (see Chap. 8), epidemiological evidence regarding the effect of breast-feeding on allergies has been inconclusive. For example, some claim that breast-feeding and the delayed introduction of solid food decreases the incidence of atopic eczema [24], while others find no difference in the incidence of eczema between formula-fed and breast-fed infants studied prospectively [54].

The infant is believed to be most susceptible to allergies during the first 6 weeks of life when the digestive tract is immature both anatomically and immunologically [57]. Theoretically, the antibodies in breast milk may protect the infant from absorbing antigenic proteins across the intestinal mucosa. Families with a history of food sensitivity, asthma, or atopic symptoms should be encouraged to breast-feed and delay the introduction of solid foods [57].

Some infants appear to be allergic to substances in breast milk, but this is rare. The allergic reactions, often manifested by colic or vomiting, may be caused by a maternally ingested protein that appears in breast milk [41]. Cow's milk protein is suspect. Some mothers report that colic disappears when they exclude milk from their diets and substitute processed dairy products such as yogurt or cheese. Other maternally ingested foods have been reported to be poorly tolerated by breast-fed infants. These are not allergic reactions, and the reasons for difficulty is unknown. "Gassy" vegetables such as garlic, onion, cabbage, turnip, and broccoli may cause colic in infants [57]. Large amounts of fruit in mothers' diets sometimes cause diarrhea in infants.

Although most mothers do not need to restrict the types of foods they eat, infants react differently to mothers' diets. If a mother suspects that a food is causing problems, she should either temporarily avoid that food or observe the infant for 24 hours after she has ingested the suspect agent [57]. Breast-milk allergy is rarely a contraindication to breast-feeding; however, there are certain conditions in which breast-feeding is not advised.

CONTRAINDICATIONS TO BREAST-FEEDING

Although most women are capable of breast-feeding, some choose not to or cannot breast-feed. Commonly, personal, not medical, reasons influence women's decisions regarding breast-feeding. However, there are some medical reasons that preclude breast-feeding [19] (Table 5-11).

Infants with galactosemia should never breast-feed because they are unable to metabolize the galactose component of lactose in milk. Breast milk jaundice may be a reason to discontinue breast-feeding temporarily; however, the incidence of breast milk jaundice is less than 1 in 200 births [57]. Breast-feeding usually does not have to be terminated, but enough formula should be given to keep the infant's bilirubin below 12 mg/100 ml [57]. Other reasons for not breast-feeding include maternal breast cancer or the infectious diseases hepatitis, cytomegalovirus, and type B streptococcal disease. Some feel that cytomegalovirus is not a contraindication to breast-feeding because the risk of infection is small compared to the benefits obtained by breast-feeding [75].

The bottom section of Table 5-11 indicates special circumstances in which breast-feeding may be successful. Success depends on the severity of the infant's medical condition, the mother's commitment to breast-feeding, and the available support. Specialized techniques for managing breast-feeding in the problem infant have been described in detail by Lawrence [57].

MATERNAL DIET

The RDAs for lactation reflect the nutrient demands of breast-feeding (see Appendix 1). Most women in the United States consume conventional diets and produce breast milk that is adequate in quantity and composition. Table 5-12 shows an adequate daily dietary guide for a breast-feeding woman. Well-nourished, well-hydrated women produce an average of 700 ml of breast milk per day [48]. Two to three quarts of liquid are needed daily to produce sufficient quantities of breast milk. If insufficient fluid is consumed, compensation occurs by a decrease in maternal urine volume and an increase in its concentration. With chronic underhydration, breast milk volume is compromised. Adequate protein and energy intakes are also needed to pro-

Table 5-11. Breast-feeding Considerations

Factors	Comment
BREAST-FEEDING CONTRAINDICATED	
Maternal	
Informed personal decision against breast-feeding	Most common reason for not breast-feeding
Breast cancer	Priority is cancer treatment
Infectious disease (hepatitis, cytomegalovirus, β-streptococcus)	May transmit disease to infant
Infant	
Galactosemia	Inability to metabolize galactose found in human milk
BREAST-FEEDING POSSIBLE	
Maternal	
Nipple problems (engorgement, cracked nipples, mastitis)	See text for treatment
Medications	Medication that least affects infant can be prescribed and timed to minimize risk to infant (see Appendix 7)
Exposure to pollutants	Depends on extent of exposure
Mental illness	Depends on the severity of disorder and type and amount of medication used. Mothers taking Lithium should not breast-feed
Infant	
Low birth weight, small-for-gestational age Down syndrome Congenital anomalies	Depends on the severity of problem and infant's ability to suck. Mother may temporarily need to express milk until any medical problems are resolved and infant is able to breast-feed or special feeding techniques are instituted
Phenylketonuria	Infants are given a combination of breast milk and formula low in phenylalanine, and blood phenylalanine levels are monitored
Breast milk–induced jaundice	Rarely a serious problem. If prolonged and severe may require a temporary discontinuation of breast-feeding. Resolves as infant's ability to conjugate and excrete bile matures

Adapted from Berger, L. R. When one should discourage breast-feeding. *Pediatrics* 67:300, 1981.

Table 5-12. Daily Dietary Guide for a Lactating Woman

Food Group	Major Nutrients Provided	Minimum No. of Servings per Day	Serving Size
PROTEIN Animal (meat, fish, poultry, egg)	Protein, iron, vitamin B_{12}, thiamin, vitamin B_6, zinc, iodine	2	3 oz or equivalent
Vegetable (nuts, legumes)	Protein, iron, folic acid, vitamin B_6, vitamin E, magnesium, zinc, fiber	2	Depends on type of vegetable. Nutritionists should plan to ensure protein complementation.
MILK AND MILK PRODUCTS	Protein, calcium, vitamin D, vitamin A, riboflavin, vitamin B_6	4–5	8 oz or equivalent (i.e., 1 oz cheese, 8 oz yogurt)
GRAINS (whole grain or enriched)	Thiamin, niacin, iron, phosphorus (if whole grain, zinc, magnesium, fiber)	4	1 slice bread, ½ cup pasta or rice, ¾ cup cereal, or ½ cup cooked cereal
FRUITS AND VEGETABLES		4 total	
Vitamin C-rich	Vitamin C, fiber	1	½ cup fruit or juice, ¾ cup vegetable
Leafy greens	Folate, vitamins A, E, K, B_6, iron, magnesium, fiber	2	1 cup raw or ¾ cup cooked
OTHER (e.g., beans, squash, carrots, pears, apples)	Varies with fruit or vegetable (vitamin A if dark green or yellow)	1	½ cup fruit, ¾ cup vegetable
FLUID		8–10	8 oz

Note: Guidelines for total energy content of diet not included. Caloric requirement varies depending on age and activity (an average of 500 kcal should be added to RDA for age group).

Adapted from Herbold, N. H. Nutrition in Pregnancy, Lactation, Middle and Later Years. In R. B. Howard and N. H. Herbold (Eds.), *Nutrition in Clinical Care* (2nd ed.). New York: McGraw-Hill, 1982. P. 319.

duce sufficient milk. Some energy for lactation is supplied from fat stores that are formed during pregnancy; in fact, about one-third of prenatal weight gain consists of lactation stores [48].

If a woman consumes an adequate diet during lactation, she does not require vitamin and mineral supplementation with the exception of iron. Because iron stores are often depleted during pregnancy and delivery, iron supplementation started during pregnancy should continue for several months post partum. In well-nourished women, vitamin supplementations do not significantly increase the vitamin levels in breast milk [76].

In undernourished women, the volume of breast milk is compromised before the composition is altered. Fat composition, vitamin A, and B complex vitamins are the most diet-dependent components of breast milk and therefore are the most likely to be suboptimal in the breast milk of poorly nourished women [48]. Women who follow unconventional diets may acquire specific deficiencies in breast milk, such as inadequate vitamin B_{12} in the milk of women on very restrictive vegan diets [28, 85]. Also, because of the difficulty in maintaining an adequate intake, dieting usually is not recommended during lactation. Taking a careful nutritional history and evaluating the adequacy of a lactating woman's diet should be an integral part of infant care.

Drugs in Breast Milk

Most ingested substances appear in breast milk to some degree. The extent to which a substance passes into breast milk depends on how it is administered, absorbed, metabolized, and excreted. The question of exactly when a substance becomes harmful to the infant depends on several factors. For example, tetracycline may be passed to the infant in breast milk and result in the discoloration of the baby's teeth. If medication is needed, the effects of the drugs on the infant can be minimized by choosing a drug that passes into the milk in the smallest quantity. Also, taking medications right after breast-feeding usually minimizes the amount that appears in the milk at the next feeding. Appendix 7 contains an extensive list of medications and their effects on breast-fed infants.

Some over-the-counter medications and certain foods in the maternal diet contain stimulants that may cause irritability and poor sleep patterns in a breast-fed infant. Methylxanthines, including theobromines (chocolate) [71], theophyllines (teas), and caffeine (coffee, cola, teas, cocoa) are all common stimulants that can pass into breast milk [77]. The infant's ability to metabolize caffeine does not mature until about age 3 to 4 months; therefore, caffeine may accumulate and cause symptoms [12] such as irritability. The stimulatory effect of caffeine may be accentuated by maternal nicotine. Alcohol, if consumed in small quantities, may promote the let-down reflex, but larger amounts

(2 to 3 ounces) will cause lethargy in infants [57]. Thus, during lactation, mothers should be encouraged to avoid smoking and caffeine, to control alcohol consumption, and to check with their physicians about using nonprescription drugs.

POLLUTANTS

Most pollutants are not present in sufficient quantities in breast milk to be of concern. Contaminants that appear in breast milk in the highest concentrations are those that are lipid soluble, metabolically stable, and abundant in the environment [72]. Two compounds, polychlorinated biphenyls (PCB) and dichlorodiphenyltrichloroethane (DDT), will be briefly discussed here.

Polychlorinated biphenyls are a group of synthetic organic compounds that have been widely used in industry and have leaked or been disposed of into waters and landfills [82]. Fish from contaminated water may contain high levels of PCB. Women who are exposed to PCB either by diet or occupation store the fat-soluble compound in adipose tissues and excrete large amounts of PCB during lactation. Although the long-term effect of PCB on infants is not known, lactating women are advised (1) to eliminate eating fish from contaminated waters, (2) to avoid quick weight loss that will mobilize fat stores, and (3) to test their breast milk for PCB content if they suspect excessive exposure [82].

Dichlorodiphenyltrichloroethane (DDT), also fat soluble, is likewise readily excreted during lactation. DDT is poisonous and may cause central nervous system dysfunction (tremors, seizures, convulsions) and abnormal liver function in adults consuming 16 to 286 mg/kg of DDT per day [72]. Effects on infants have not been studied; however, caution is warranted. Where exposure is suspect, each case must be considered individually, and the benefits of breast-feeding must be weighed against the potential risk of contamination.

THE PRACTICAL ASPECTS OF BREAST-FEEDING

While much attention is given to the content of breast milk, another area of equal concern is the actual techniques of breast-feeding. Frustrated parents often search for practical information that will ensure a successful breast-feeding experience for mother, infant, and family. Once viewed as a natural, instinctive method of feeding, breast-feeding now is considered an art requiring special preparation and support to be successful. Preparation for breast-feeding should begin during pregnancy and include a discussion of the advantages and disadvantages of breast-feeding. There needs to be an opportunity to dispel myths and address individual concerns. A session discussing breast function, potential difficulties, and available resources (i.e., support groups, breast pumps) is useful. The role of a maternal-child health professional is to educate women regarding their choices about infant feeding and to support their decisions with educational and practical information.

PREPARATION FOR BREAST-FEEDING

Western women rarely expose their breasts to air. Because they tend to protect their breasts with bras and layers of clothing, nipples are often "shocked" by the infant's vigorous sucking. To toughen nipples beforehand, the following measures may be beneficial:

1. Removing the bra for a few hours each day (the friction of clothes rubbing against the breast toughens the nipples).
2. Washing breasts with plain water only, because soaps and lotions soften the nipples.
3. Gently stimulating the nipple. With one hand supporting the breast from underneath, the nipple is gently grasped with the other hand and pulled forward. Alternatively, the nipple can be rolled between two fingers, rotating the fingers around the nipple.

Inverted or flat nipples are difficult for the infant to grasp adequately. When this condition is identified during pregnancy, the use of Woolrich Shields helps the nipples to protrude. These shields may be obtained from local pharmacies or the Le Leche League.

THE FIRST ENCOUNTER

Women are often anxious about their first nursing experience with an infant who is also thrust into a new learning experience (Fig. 5-2). In a relaxed supportive environment, the mother's confidence, which is the key to successful breast-feeding [51], increases. Immediately after delivery, infants are usually more alert than they will be for the next several days. This is an excellent time to initiate breast-feeding. This early interaction fosters bonding [53] and, when continued at frequent intervals, is the most significant variable in preventing sore, cracked nipples [59]. As breast-feeding commences, mothers should be encouraged to wash their hands; however, breasts do not need to be washed prior to feeding.

POSITIONING

The relaxed mother, given time, will be comfortable breast-feeding in a variety of positions. Initially, breast-feeding may be easiest when lying down. A mother can lie on her side with one or two pillows placed behind her back and one under her head.

When a mother sits in bed to breast-feed, the infant can be placed on a pillow on the mother's lap. She can then pull her legs up to bring the infant closer and lean forward to get the nipple closer. When sitting in a chair or in bed, the mother places the infant in the crook of her

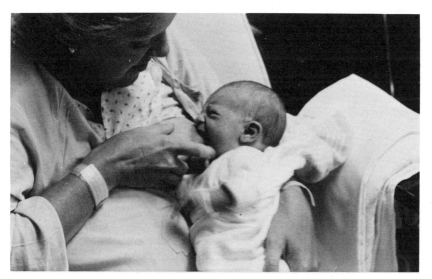

A

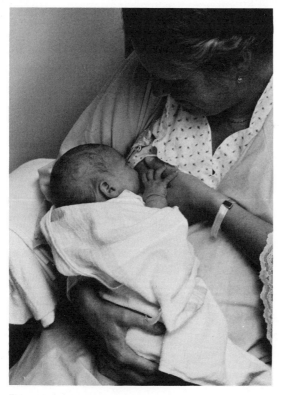

B

Figure 5-2. A and B. The first encounter. With confidence and support, mother and infant adjust to the new feeding experience.

arm. In this position, the other hand is available to help place the nipple in the infant's mouth.

Once positioned, infants should be encouraged to grasp the entire areola, because grasping only the nipple will contribute to soreness. The up and down pressure on the areola releases milk from the ducts. Mothers can help their infants to get hold of the areola by compressing the breast with two fingers or a finger and thumb. When infants take the nipple only, they should be removed from the breast by gently inserting a finger in the side of the infants' mouth and breaking the suction. Then the breast may be offered again. If mothers lightly stroke their infants' lips with the nipple, infants eventually will open their mouths wide enough to accommodate both the nipple and the areola.

If the breasts are large or engorged, the mother needs to press a finger on the breast to keep it away from the infant's nose. Expressing milk by hand from the engorged breast before feeding will make it easier for the infant to latch onto the nipple.

For the first 2 to 3 days, the breasts produce colostrum. The milk, which is a thin bluish liquid, comes in around the third day. Because the milk supply increases rapidly if the infant is nursed frequently, every effort should be made to allow the mother to nurse (either in her room or in the nursery) when the infant is willing. Breast-feeding mothers are encouraged to nurse during the night feeding as well to ensure production of an adequate supply of milk for the infant. Both breasts are used at each feeding to stimulate rapid increases in supply and prevent "lopsided" breasts. Alternating the first breast offered to the infant at each feeding ensures fairly equal stimulation of both breasts.

COMMON PROBLEMS AND INTERVENTIONS

Most women experience some difficulties when they breast-feed for the first time. Because the mother's confidence is important for successful breast-feeding, exploring all difficulties and offering encouragement and a variety of solutions is of more value than offering rigid advice.

Uterine Cramps

Nursing and the subsequent release of oxytocin stimulates uterine contractions that prevent postpartum hemorrhage. Cramping is usually a problem for the first 48 to 72 hours and medication (e.g., acetaminophen) may be taken one-half hour before nursing to relieve the pain.

Leaking

Leaking of breast milk is a common problem, especially when the supply is being established. It is an indication of a good let-down reflex. Nursing pads without plastic liners or small cotton handkerchiefs slipped inside the bra are useful in absorbing leakage. These should be changed frequently to prevent sore, cracked nipples.

When the let-down reflex is anticipated by a tingling, warm, or full sensation in the breast, pushing firmly against the breast with the palm of the hand until the tingling stops may impede leaking. As the let-down reflex becomes more efficient and the milk supply is well-established, leaking is not as frequent.

Failure of the Let-Down Reflex

Fatigue and tension inhibit the let-down reflex. If let-down is a problem, exploring family routines and emotional climate usually provides clues leading to specific solutions.

Mothers should be encouraged to let the infant suck until the let-down reflex occurs. Most infants will wait as long as 5 minutes for this reflex. When the infant is frustrated or impatient, a pump or hand massage can be used until let-down occurs, and then the infant can be put to the breast. Mothers also may want to try conscious relaxation techniques such as Lamaze breathing, yoga, transcendental meditation, or listening to soft music. To enhance let-down, a glass of wine or beer may be taken prior to feeding. Applying heat to the breasts also may help if let-down fails to occur. If having other people around produces tension, mothers should be encouraged to isolate themselves.

Inadequate Milk Supply

The more an infant feeds, the more milk is produced. Frequent feeding ensures an adequate milk supply and is not an indication that the mother is not producing sufficient quantities of milk. Giving supplementary bottles of formula or small amounts of cereal restricts sucking time and breast stimulation. Mothers need to be reassured that unrestricted feedings are the best way to enhance milk production. Inadequate fluid consumption can lead to inadequate milk supplies. Breast size is not related to the ability to nurse or to the amount of milk produced.

Sore Nipples

Some soreness in the nipples is usual in the first week of breast-feeding. If soreness persists, it must be determined if the infant is grasping only the nipple instead of the areola or if suction is being broken prior to removing the infant from the breast. Once the milk lets down, the soreness usually eases. Milk can be expressed by pump or hand until let-down occurs; then the infant can be put to the breast.

There are other suggestions to alleviate sore nipples. Nipples should be exposed to air (i.e., by keeping bra flaps down). Nursing pads should be changed frequently, and those with plastic liners should be avoided because they trap moisture. Warm compresses or ice packs can be applied. Nursing should begin on the breast with the least discomfort because the infant's sucking is less vigorous on the second breast. Nipple shields can be used for a few feedings but may prevent the breast from emptying evenly or completely, which may result in clogged ducts and affect milk production. Vitamin E oil may help soften nipples and can be applied by breaking open a vitamin capsule and spreading the contents on the areola and around the nipple. If used sparingly, oil does not need to be washed off prior to feeding. With appropriate therapy, soreness usually begins to ease by 5 to 7 days post partum.

Cracked Nipples

Tender, sore nipples can progress to cracking of the areola or nipple, often with bleeding. The mother needs reassurance that a small amount of blood in the milk will not harm her infant. The suggestions discussed for sore nipples also can be used for cracked nipples. In addition, using a shield or not using the affected breast for several feedings may be warranted. If the breast is not used, hand massage (under warm water) or using a pump stimulates the let-down reflex and maintains milk supply until the infant sucks again.

Engorgement

Engorgement should not be a problem if the infant is allowed to nurse frequently. When engorgement does occur, the infant may have trouble grasping the nipple and areola. Hand-expressing milk or using a small hand pump before the infant is put to the breast may soften the breast and reduce some fullness.

Using warm water (taking a shower or leaning over the sink and pouring warm water over the breasts) or applying ice packs to the breast also may provide relief. Mothers should be encouraged to drink fluids and to nurse frequently. Tight bras or binders cause clogged ducts and exacerbate the problem.

Mastitis

If the breast is not emptying evenly or completely, a duct can become blocked and infection may develop. The causes of a clogged duct are tight bras, sleeping or feeding positions that cause focal pressure on the breast, or incomplete let-down reflex. The symptoms of a blocked duct are a sore area of the breast, a red hot patch of skin, achy flu-like symptoms, and fever.

Treatment is started immediately. Frequent nursing initiated on the affected breast allows the duct to reopen. Also, guidelines for let-down problems should be followed (see p. 107). It may take 24 hours before symptoms resolve. Sometimes antibiotics are administered to the mother, but this is usually not necessary unless an abscess has developed.

Breast Abscess

A breast abscess may develop if a clogged duct is not treated adequately and breast-feeding is stopped. Signs and symptoms include a high fever and a tender, hot, swollen area on the breast. Abscesses are treated with antibiotics and the infant should be seen by the pediatrician for the possibility of sepsis. Breast-feeding does not need to be terminated, but the infant should not nurse on the affected side until the infection has cleared. Milk should be pumped or hand-expressed from the affected side and discarded. Once the infection resolves, normal breast-feeding can be resumed.

Colicky Infant

Most infants have periods of crying and fussing. Mothers may offer the breast for comfort as well as nourishment and accept short periods of crying and fussing as normal. The true "colicky" infant is often uncomfortable and inconsolable, and an organic cause for the discomfort is often sought through medical evaluations. Environmental factors such as maternal stress and diet may be etiological agents. For example, one report links maternal ingestion of cow's milk with infant colic (see Chap. 8). Although the etiology of colic remains undetermined, it usually is resolved by the age of 3 to 4 months.

BIRTH CONTROL AND BREAST-FEEDING

As long as the infant breast-feeds exclusively, the level of the hormone prolactin remains elevated and can prevent ovulation. Nevertheless, breast-feeding is not a reliable method of birth control, and ovulation can occur. Even after menstruation returns, the ovulatory cycle is often irregular throughout breast-feeding. Oral contraceptives should be used with caution during lactation because they may reduce milk supply [60]. (See Appendix 7 for further explanation.)

BREAST-FEEDING UNDER SPECIAL CONDITIONS

CESAREAN SECTION

A mother who has had a cesarean section can breast-feed if both she and the infant are able. However, following surgery, infants often are lethargic from the anesthesia and mothers may require pain medication. Unless the medication is excessive, it will not affect the infant initially. However, if maternal medication is required beyond 48 hours after birth, it should be given immediately after breast-feeding so that the least amount of the drug appears in the breast-milk.

PREMATURE INFANT

The degree of prematurity and the general health of the infant dictate the efficacy of breast-feeding. Until the infant is strong enough to suck at the breast, the mother should hand-express milk or use a pump to maintain her milk supply. This milk can be stored until the infant is ready to feed or given to the infant via gavage feedings. Breast milk from mothers of premature infants is 30 percent higher in protein than the milk produced by mothers of full-term infants. Thus, the milk may be particularly suited to the premature infant's nutrient needs (see Chap. 8).

TWINS

Twins can be breast-fed successfully. Some women find that they can nurse both infants at once—one on each breast. Positioning is the key and, with mother either sitting or lying, infants can be supported by pillows on the mother's abdomen. Some women prefer to nurse the infants one at a time, and others find that nursing only one infant at each feeding and bottle-feeding the other is best. Being flexible and allowing the infants' personalities and needs to shape caregiving are even more essential with twins than with one infant.

ILLNESSES

Common maternal illnesses such as colds or gastrointestinal upsets generally are not an indication to stop breast-feeding. In fact, the mother's antibodies transmitted in her breast milk help confer immunity to the infant. Likewise, if the infant is ill, the mother may produce antibodies to the infant's infective agent and then pass them back through the breast milk (see p. 95). In addition, suckling at the breast is usually comforting to the sick infant.

STORING BREAST MILK

In instances where mother or infant temporarily are unable to breast-feed, mother may need to express breast milk either by hand or pump and store the milk for later use. The technique should be as sterile as possible to avoid contamination. Mothers are encouraged to wash their hands well; however, breasts do not need washing. Expressed milk should be placed in sterile bottles, refrigerated, and used within 24 hours after collection. If the milk must be transported from home to the hospital, it should be kept on ice.

Breast milk that will not be used within 1 day should be frozen immediately, although this will destroy the cellular constituents (see p. 95). The safe storage time depends on the type of freezer used. In chest-type deep freezers, milk can be frozen at 0°F for up to a year. In frost-free freezers, the temperature fluctuates because of the freeze and thaw cycles; therefore, breast milk is only safe for about 4 months.

SUPPORT FOR THE BREAST-FEEDING MOTHER

Rest is important for the breast-feeding mother. Family support is needed to ensure that the mother's energies are focused on caring for herself and her infant. For the first few weeks, the physical demands of around the clock breast-feeding leave little energy for homemaking chores or professional activities. Ideally, preparation (e.g., cooking and freezing meals before delivery and arranging for help with cleaning) helps ease the stress. Because fatigue and tension adversely affect the let-down reflex and milk production, having extra help and simplifying life is a necessity. Successful breast-feeding demands that the mother be paced by her infant. If rushed and harried, this is impossible; once milk production is well established, the infant's schedule will follow fairly predictable patterns. The transition to motherhood and breast-feeding can be further complicated by postpartum depression. It is important that mother and family not connect the "blues" with breast-feeding, but recognize the phenomenon as normal for most mothers in this period of changing roles.

Another adjustment for both mothers and fathers is the reestablishment of interpersonal relationships. Breast-feeding should not interfere. However, there is a need for partners to communicate their feelings and preferences, especially when they resume sexual relations. Some women find pressure on their full breasts painful, and others complain of dry vaginal lining. Whatever the issues, open discussions will enhance relationships and facilitate problem solving.

THE PRACTICAL ASPECTS OF FORMULA-FEEDING

Successful formula-feeding does not end with choosing an appropriate infant formula. Attention to a few practical considerations may prevent problems in the formula-fed infant.

PREPARING INFANT FORMULAS

Most infant formulas are available in concentrated liquid or ready-to-use forms. Table 5-3 lists the availability of various infant formulas. Convenience and cost are factors determining the type of formula used. Ready-to-use formulas generally cost about 30 percent more than their concentrated equivalents, but eliminate preparation and the chance of errors. Families preparing formulas from evaporated milk should use 1 part evaporated milk to 2 parts water plus 5 percent corn syrup. In one survey, over 60 percent of mothers questioned claimed that they do not prepare formulas exactly according to manufacturers' directions [50].

Both concentrated liquid and powder-type formulas require dilution, and although gross errors are uncommon, they can be serious. In attempt to stretch limited food budgets, a dilute formula may be prepared. Feeding overly diluted formula can result in failure to thrive. Also, water intoxication resulting in seizure disorders has been reported in infants fed large amounts of overly diluted formula or excessive free water [68].

Concentrated formulas may cause osmotic diarrhea. Mammalian milk has an osmolarity of about 300 mOsm per liter, as do most infant formulas when diluted according to recommendations (see Table 5-3). Tolerance to more concentrated formulas varies widely from infant to infant; however, the American Academy of Pediatrics recommends that formulas having osmolarities over 400 mOsm per liter should bear warning statements on their labels [1]. Special formulas for metabolic disorders (i.e., Phenyl Free [Mead Johnson]) may be hyperosmolar even at normal dilutions because they contain osmotically active free amino acids.

STERILIZATION

In households supplied with chlorinated water, sterilization is usually not necessary if good sanitary procedures are used in formula preparation. Bottles, nipples, and utensils should be washed carefully in hot, soapy water and rinsed well before filling. Prepared formula should be stored below 40°F for no longer than 24 hours.

Where sanitary conditions are substandard (i.e., contaminated water supplies or inadequate refrigeration), the risk of bacterial contamination and consequent infection is higher, and sterilization is recommended. Common sterilization methods are *terminal* sterilization and *aseptic* sterilization. In the terminal method, bottles containing formula are sterilized in boiling water for 25 minutes, allowed to cool, and then refrigerated. With the aseptic method, all equipment (bottles, nipples, and utensils) is boiled for 5 minutes. The formula is then prepared in a clean environment and poured into bottles and refrigerated. The terminal method may be easiest to carry out in most homes [73]. By about age 3 months, the infant's digestive tract is well colonized with bacteria, and sterilization is not necessary.

NIPPLES AND BOTTLES

There are a number of commercially available nipples and bottles. Because infants' needs vary, no one bottle or nipple is recommended for all. Some nipples are designed to mimic the human nipple (i.e., Nuk nipple) and may be more readily accepted by infants who are both bottle- and breast-fed. Long or soft nipples often are used for premature infants or infants with poor suck reflexes because these nipples promote easier sucking. Nipples with enlarged holes may facilitate formula flow; however, they can cause infants to choke or thrust their tongues forward to stop the flow, which encourages a pattern of tongue thrusting. If the nipple hole is too small, the infant may swallow large amounts of air, which can lead to regurgitation or colic. Formula should flow from an inverted bottle in a rapid succession of drops but not a continuous stream [78]. Observing the feeding habits of the infant will provide a clue as to the adequacy of the flow.

POSITIONING

An infant should be held in an upright position with the head supported. The infant's head should be slightly forward, not tilted back. If the infant's head is back or the infant is lying with the bottle propped up, there is a chance of choking or regurgitating the formula into the eustachian tubes [17]. The upright position enhances esophageal clearance. The infant can be held properly either in the lap or the arms of the feeder. Facing the parent during feeding optimizes one-to-one interaction. The bottle should be tilted so that the neck of the bottle is always filled with formula. This will prevent excessive air swallowing and allow a more consistent milk flow.

BURPING

Whether breast- or bottle-fed, infants need to be burped periodically throughout the feeding. The infant should be burped after every few ounces during feeding or between breasts if breast-fed. Burping is accomplished by holding the infant forward in the parent's lap or up against the parent's shoulder and gently patting or rubbing the infant's back. After feeding, the infant should be kept upright or placed on the right side to promote gastric emptying.

AMOUNT TO FEED

The timing of feedings and the amount of formula an infant takes is highly variable. Most infants require 6 to 8 feedings per day for the first few weeks of life. A normal full-term infant needs about 150 ml of formula per kilogram of body weight at the age of 1 week. During the first 5 months of life, a rule of thumb regarding the number of ounces of formula an infant needs is the infant's age in months plus 3 ounces per feeding. Thus, an infant of 4 months would require about 7 ounces each feeding.

OVERFEEDING OR UNDERFEEDING

A common question parents have, regardless of the feeding method, is when to stop feeding. Parents should be encouraged to recognize their infant's signs of hunger and satiety and to discontinue feeding when the infant first shows signs of fullness. Signs of overfeeding are excessive weight gain, regurgitation, vomiting, diarrhea, or frequent large stools. Signs of underfeeding are inadequate weight gain, irritability, and constipation [47]. The infant's appetite is a good indicator of needs and will vary according to the infant's growth rate. With bottle-feeding, parents may push the last ounce into the infant so no formula is wasted. Breast-fed infants also can be overfed if they are offered the breast frequently or for too long. Whether or not obesity in infancy is a predictor of later weight problems remains unclear [30].

Nevertheless, obesity is a major health problem in the United States and prevention is important (see Chap. 10).

INFANT FOODS

READINESS

Infants are ready for beikost (foods other than breast milk or formula) at about 5 to 6 months of age. There is no advantage to earlier beikost introduction. The common claim that feeding solids causes an infant to sleep through the night is unfounded [36]. Solid foods do, however, provide supplemental nutrients to breast milk or formula that are often necessary during the second 6 months of life.

Physiologically, infants show readiness for beikost at about 4 to 6 months of age. By this time, infants' kidneys can tolerate the increased solute loads of protein and electrolytes. Production of pancreatic amylase is mature, and the intestine is less permeable to foreign proteins. Neuromuscularly, infants are ready to eat solid food by the age of 6 months. The suck-swallow reflex wanes, facilitating the swallowing of nonliquid foods. Head and neck control, hand-to-mouth motion, and unassisted sitting all develop at about 6 months, allowing the infant to become more involved in feeding (see Table 2-2). Trying to feed beikost to an infant who is not developmentally ready may result in an unnecessary struggle. Conversely, if solids are introduced much later than about 6 months, the infant is accustomed to being nourished via the breast or bottle and may be more reluctant to accept food from a spoon.

FOOD INTRODUCTIONS

Guidelines for introducing beikost are presented in Table 5-13. These suggestions should be individualized according to parent's preferences and lifestyles. Cultural beliefs may influence what feeding advice parents accept; even if a family is mostly acculturated, certain food beliefs and symbolism may persist. For example, Puerto Rican families may delay weaning or Vietnamese families may refuse cow's milk and prefer sweetened condensed milk. Table 5-14 highlights some cultural feeding practices that may be helpful to understand when individualizing suggestions regarding the introduction of new foods.

CEREAL

The first solid food an infant receives should be an iron-fortified single grain infant cereal [7]. These cereals are usually well tolerated and are a good source of energy and iron. Commercially prepared infant cereals contain bioavailable reduced iron of small particle size [2]. Packaged combinations of fruit and cereal have lower nutrient densities and cost more than plain infant cereal. Ensuring iron adequacy in the second 6 months of life is important because iron deficiency anemia

Table 5-13. Solid Food Introductions During the First Year

Food	0–2	2–4	4–6	6–8†	8–10†	10–12†
Breast milk or iron-fortified formula	5–9 feedings (16–32 oz)	4–7 feedings (20–36 oz)	4–6 feedings (24–40 oz)	3–4 feedings (24–32 oz)	3–4 feedings (16–32 oz)	3–4 feedings (16–32 oz)
Grains			Infant cereal,* single grain (i.e., rice, barley, oatmeal)	Infant cereal, all varieties	Infant cereals, plain hot cereal (adult type), plain crackers, toast	Infant cereal, cooked cereal, bread products, rice, pasta
Vegetables				Strained or mashed vegetables (plain)	Cooked, mashed table vegetables	Cooked vegetable pieces, raw vegetables (finger foods)
Fruit			Fruit juice (from cup)	Strained fruit, applesauce, mashed bananas, fruit juice (from cup)	Soft peeled fruit (i.e., banana, pear, apple, peach), fruit juice (from cup)	Fresh fruits (peeled), canned fruits (packed in own juice), fruit juice (from cup)
Protein foods				Plain yogurt, strained meats, egg yolk, tofu, cottage cheese	Strained meats, egg yolk, tofu, cottage cheese, legumes (sieved)	Small pieces of chicken or meat (tender), whole egg, cooked dry beans (mashed), peanut butter

Age (mo)

*Iron-fortified dry, boxed cereals are better sources of iron and protein than jarred cereals mixed with fruit.
†This is a time when the sodium content of the infant's diet can increase greatly; highly processed, canned, and salted foods should be avoided.

frequently presents at this time. For infants who are breast-fed beyond 6 months of age, iron-fortified cereal is recommended for supplying supplemental iron. Otherwise, adequate iron can be provided by iron-fortified formula or medicinal iron.

Cereals should always be spoon-fed. Feeding cereal and formula through a bottle or an infant-feeder does not promote proper oral-motor development because infants continue to suck instead of learning to move their tongues laterally and swallow solid food. In addition, diluted solids fed by bottle may lead to overfeeding and obesity.

Table 5-14. Infant Feeding Practices in Selected Cultures

Culture	Common Feeding Practices
American Indian (Fomon and Anderson)	Breast-feeding varies with degree of acculturation (least common in working mothers and where other milk supplies are available). Canned evaporated milk formula is most frequently used. Goat's milk may be used when available. Soft drinks, powdered fruit-flavored drinks, coffee, and tea are fed by bottle. Bottle-feeding often continues beyond 2 yr. Food introductions reported to occur either early (within 1st week) or later (several months of age).
Chinese (Ho)	Breast-feed to 1 yr. Foods introduced between 3 and 8 mo, including rice and rice products such as gruel, soup, rice flour paste, minced fish, pork, and occasionally eggs. Fruit or vegetable purees generally not given.
Mexican (Fomon and Anderson)	Breast-feed beginning at third day when milk lets down; colostrum considered unfit for infant. Herb teas (e.g., yerba buena, manzanilla, cinnamon, oregano, rosa de castilla, anise, lemon, and orange leaves) are given during this period. Teas considered medicinal, and human milk and teas comprise basic neonatal diet. Breast-feed until 3–9 mo. Food introduced by age 6 mo, including mainly fruits (banana, orange, and apple), bean soup (caldo de frijol), and tortillas. Other foods used are gruel (atoles), bread, crackers, cookies, a watery noodle soup (sopa aguada), cocoa, coffee with milk, eggs, and Jell-O. Cow's milk is usually boiled. By 2 yr, children share in family meals. Foods prohibited during illness include fruit, avocado, beans (frijoles), and pork.

Table 5-14 (Continued)

Culture	Common Feeding Practices
Puerto Rican* (Fomon and Anderson)	Breast-feeding practiced by only 3% of mothers, most often by recent immigrants. Bottles given on demand by age 3 weeks. Cereal added to milk in bottle. Foods introduced at 2–3 mo, including egg yolk, juice (especially orange), and strained homemade soup. Ripe banana and egg yolk may be added to the bottle. Cereal rarely fed after 1 yr. Bottle-feeding may continue until age 6 yr. Soft drinks become main beverage during toddler years.
Vietnamese (Eichelberger and Miller)	Breast-feeding common, but many change to bottle. Sweetened condensed milk used. Cereal added to bottle. Wean from bottle during second year. Foods introduced at about 6 mo, including rice water gruel with bits of vegetable or meat. Juices diluted and sugar added. Fruit-flavored beverage powders used. Children often refuse cow's milk.

Note: This table is meant only to sensitize the practitioner to the nuances of cultural feeding practices. Over time and with acculturation into the American lifestyle, feeding practices change, and not always for the better. Many new refugees enter into urban poverty where bottle-feeding continues to prevail.
*Based on feeding practices of Puerto Rican families living in the Philadelphia metropolitan area.
Data from Fomon, S. J., and Anderson, T. A. (Eds.). Practice of Low Income Families in Feeding Infants and Small Children with Particular Attention to Cultural Subgroups. Proceedings of a National Workshop, March 17–18, 1971. U.S. Dept. of Health, Education, and Welfare. DHEW Publication No. (HSA) 75-5605, Ho, Z. Breast feeding in XinHui district in South China. *Food and Nutrition Bulletin* 2:43, 1981, and Eichelberger, B. J., and Miller, L. *Dietary habits and Nutritional Problems of Vietnamese Refugees*. WIC Notes, Mead Johnson, 4th Quarter, 1981.

OTHER FOODS

When cereals are well accepted, strained vegetables, tofu, fruits, and meats can be added to the infant's diet. The order of introduction does not seem to be important in determining which foods a child will accept. Parents should be encouraged to wait 4 to 5 days after adding new foods to check for skin rashes or changes in bowel habits. Eggs are considered potentially allergenic and should not be offered before 1 year of age [7]. However, the egg yolk is not as allergenic as the egg white and may be introduced earlier.

From a nutritional standpoint, offering a variety of foods promotes a balanced diet and sound eating habits. The breast-fed infant requires good sources of protein (i.e., cereals with milk or formula, meats) to complement the relatively low protein content of breast milk. As more solid foods are ingested, the infant's intake of breast milk or formula will decrease. However, a minimum of about 16 ounces of milk (breast, cow's, or formula) is needed to supply adequate amounts of calcium [7]. If a source of milk is not acceptable, yogurt, cheese, and tofu (which has been processed using calcium) are other calcium sources that can be added to the infant's diet.

JUICES

Juices, a source of vitamin C, can be offered when the infant is able to drink from a cup, usually at about the age of 5 to 6 months. There is no nutritional need for juice if adequate breast milk or formula is given because both supply adequate amounts of vitamin C. Feeding juice from a bottle may promote nursing bottle caries, especially if the bottle is given at bedtime or frequently throughout the day. Sweetened beverages (i.e., soft drinks, fruit drinks, and "ades") provide little besides empty calories.

COW'S MILK

Infant formula or breast milk is the best choice for milk-feeding throughout the first year of life. Ingestion of cow's milk protein can cause insidious intestinal blood loss that may contribute to anemia. However, many infants receive whole cow's milk during the latter part of their first year of life without any untoward effects. Fomon believes that cow's milk is acceptable for older infants consuming 200 gm of solid food (1½ jars of infant food) [36], but the American Academy of Pediatrics recommends that cow's milk be given after 1 year of age. Low fat or skim milk is not recommended during infancy largely because infants fed milk with reduced fat contents are unlikely to consume enough to meet their caloric needs [36].

WATER

Water is not needed by infants who are totally breast- or formula-fed, except possibly in very hot weather. Once foods with high renal solute loads are introduced, such as meats and egg yolk, water should be offered.

COMMERCIAL INFANT FOODS

As public interest in good nutrition increases, more families are preparing their own infant foods. However, most infants still receive commercial infant foods, and one study showed that infants receive an average of 300 baby food preparations in their first year [33]. Commercial infant foods have improved within the last decade. Additives and preservatives, such as monosodium glutamate and certain modified food starches, were previously used to make infant foods taste or look more acceptable to parents. The use of many additives was discontinued in the 1970s after questions about their safety were raised. More recently, commercial infant food companies have discontinued using salt and sugar in many of their products. Food manufacturers also screen ingredients to determine if levels of pesticides, aflatoxins, and other contaminants are within acceptable limits set by the U.S. Department of Agriculture.

READING THE LABEL

By learning to read labels, nutritious baby foods can be selected. Ingredient lists on baby food labels are mandatory. Ingredients are listed on the label in decreasing order by weight (i.e., the first ingredient listed on the label is most abundant, and so on) (Fig. 5-3). A food that has water listed as the main ingredient is just that, mostly water. Water is added to many infant fruits and vegetables to facilitate processing and achieve a desired consistency. The ingredient list also shows whether fillers or sweeteners have been added to the product. Many food manufacturers now draw special attention to the fact that additives or preservatives have not been added to their products.

Although not mandatory, nutrition labeling may also show the caloric content and the number of grams of protein, carbohydrate, and fat provided per serving. The "Percent U.S. RDA" of key nutrients are sometimes listed and can be used to compare products for their nutrient quality. Because nutrition labeling is left to the discretion of the manufacturers, it is sometimes difficult to make a fair comparison. Table 5-15 provides examples of the protein and energy contents of a few infant foods. "High-protein" meat and vegetable combinations contain more protein and calories than vegetables but less than meats. "Desserts" tend to have higher carbohydrate and energy contents but lower nutrient densities than fruits. These desserts are sometimes recommended for infants who are not gaining weight. Commercially

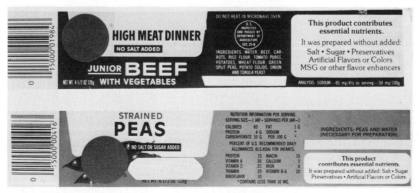

Figure 5-3. Learn about the ingredients and nutritional quality of different infant foods from the label.

Table 5-15. Energy and Protein Content of Selected Infant Foods

Food	Protein (gm/tbsp)	Energy (kcal/tbsp)
Rice cereal (dry)	0.2	15
Oatmeal	0.5	15
Beef, strained	1.9	13
Chicken, strained	2.1	20
Beef with vegetables (high meat dinner)	0.9	12
Squash, strained	0.1	4
Creamed corn, strained	0.3	9
Pears, strained	Trace*	7
Peach cobbler dessert, strained	Trace	13

*Contains less than 0.1 gm protein/tbsp
Data from Nutrient Values, Gerber Baby Foods, Gerber Products Company, Fremont, Michigan, 1981.

prepared infant fruits, vegetables, and meats closely resemble home-prepared infant foods.

HOMEMADE INFANT FOODS

Some parents prefer to make their own baby foods in order to control what their infants receive. Being "homemade" carries the connotation of being nutritious and wholesome; however, the nutritional value of infant foods depends on preparation. Cooking and preparation techniques that maximize the nutritional value of adult foods also apply to infant foods. This includes selecting food that is fresh and in season whenever possible, avoiding overcooking (steaming vegetables only until they are soft enough to be pureed), avoiding frying, and using minimal amounts of water for cooking and pureeing [21].

Certain items should not be added to infant foods such as salt, sugar, spices, and fat. Studies have shown that the sodium content of homemade infant food sometimes exceeds that of commercial infant foods [52]. This may occur when parents either add salt or use canned foods in the preparation of infant foods. Canned vegetables are higher in sodium than fresh or frozen vegetables. For example, the sodium content of various forms of peas (per 100 gm) is: fresh, 2 mg; strained commercial infant peas, 100 mg; frozen peas, 115 mg; and canned peas, 236 mg [69]. Canned foods also should be avoided because unless the can was specifically designed to contain infant foods, it may have a high lead content [36]. Acidic foods, especially, tend to leach lead from cans. Canned infant foods are specially packaged to avoid lead contamination.

Sugar or other sweeteners do not need to be added to homemade infant foods because they contribute little besides calories. Spices, especially pepper and mustard, should not be used in infancy because they can irritate the gastrointestinal tract. Fats, which are a potent caloric source, do not need to be added unless there are special conditions demanding higher than normal energy intakes.

Fancy equipment and a lot of time are not required for the proper preparation of infant foods, but proper sanitation and planning are critical in preventing food-borne illnesses. Working surfaces and equipment should be cleaned with regular soap and water and rinsed well. Household chlorine bleach (prepared according to directions on the package) may be used to sanitize surfaces and utensils.

Infant foods are microbiologically safe if they are refrigerated below 40°F for less than 24 hours. Foods that will not be used in that time period should be frozen. Leftovers should be reheated to 140°F before feeding and should not be allowed to remain at room temperature for long periods of time. More complete information on preparing and storing infant foods can be found in some cookbooks [21].

SERVING TIPS FOR INFANT FOODS

Infant foods can be fed at room temperature or slightly warmed. Infant foods should be spoon-fed and never given from a bottle. When feeding, the amount of food that the infant usually eats should be removed from the container and the rest refrigerated. If the infant is fed directly from the jar, salivary enzymes are introduced and may break down the remaining food. Leftovers should be used within 24 hours.

Heating jarred commercial infant foods in a microwave oven is generally not recommended because the food may heat unevenly and could explode. Some infant foods specifically have the warning "Do Not Heat in Microwave Oven" on the label. Other foods may be heated in a microwave oven if the metal caps are removed.

Many parents ask how much infant food they should feed. The amount of food an infant takes varies considerably depending on the infant's sex, size, and the amount of breast milk or formula consumed. Parents should be advised to let the infant's appetite dictate the amount given, as long as the infant is growing well. Initially, most infants take about 1 or 2 tablespoons of dry cereal mixed with either formula or breast milk. When commercial infant foods are used, the jar often becomes the unit of measure; however, this amount does not necessarily represent the ideal amount to feed. As a guideline, a 6-month-old male growing at the fiftieth percentile and consuming 4 to 5 breast or formula feedings (approximately 28 ounces) would take about 5 tablespoons of infant foods at each of three meals [47].

ADVANCING TEXTURE

At about age 7 to 9 months, infants can tolerate some textured foods. Strained foods decrease in importance in the diets as infants learn to move their tongues laterally, munch, and chew. Although first teeth

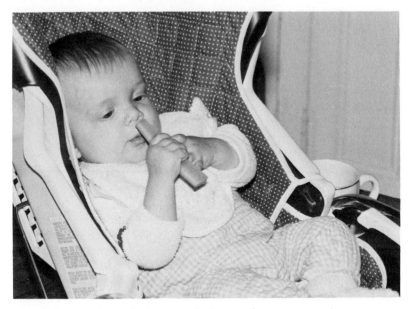

Figure 5-4. First finger foods—a perplexing.puzzle—a new experience.

usually appear between ages 7 and 9 months, the acceptance of textured foods varies widely. Soft or mashed table foods can be mixed with strained foods initially; then texture can be increased gradually. Table 5-13 gives guidelines for advancing texture in the normal infant's diet (see also Table 2-2).

When children sit alone and develop eye-hand coordination, they can be offered soft finger foods such as zwieback or toast. Whole grain bread products have lower sugar contents and are less cariogenic than teething biscuits and cookies. By about age 9 to 10 months, infants develop pincer grasps and finger-feed quite well (Fig. 5-4). Soft finger foods (e.g., peeled pieces of fruit and vegetables, tender meat, cheese, and tofu) can be managed, but fibrous or stringy foods, nuts, raisins, and popcorn should not be offered because they may cause choking. With the introduction of finger foods, the sodium content of the diet can increase greatly unless careful attention is paid to the types of foods offered. Surveys show that table foods contribute nearly two-thirds of the sodium content of the infant's diet at age 10½ months [9]. (Table 6-10 shows the sodium content of foods that are commonly included in the infant's diet).

WEANING

WEANING THE BREAST-FED INFANT

When to wean the infant from the breast is an individual decision. As solid food or supplementary bottles are introduced and the infant takes less milk at the breast, the milk supply naturally decreases. If this is a gradual process, there should be no breast engorgement or discomfort. The small amount of milk present in the breasts after the last breast-feeding is reabsorbed by the body.

Gradual weaning can be accomplished at any time. By substituting formula for every other breast-feeding, complete weaning can be accomplished over a period of a few days to a week. If breast-feeding must be terminated abruptly, wearing a bra, reducing fluid intake, and applying ice to the breasts helps to relieve the discomfort.

Although there are individual differences, weaning naturally starts at about age 6 to 9 months when infants are ready and eager for solid food. Some infants are ready to discontinue nursing at 9 to 12 months of age. When infants begin playing and socializing during feedings, refuse to nurse, or nurse for increasingly shorter periods of time, they may be ready to stop breast-feeding. Nursing sessions should gradually shorten and be eliminated. Some infants enjoy the breast-feeding relationship and continue to nurse beyond 12 to 18 months of age. Some mothers may be content to breast-feed for 2 to 3 years. If a mother is having a difficult time ending the nursing relationship, counseling may be beneficial. Discussing specific strategies may be helpful (i.e., postponing nursing or suggesting alternate activities when the child wants to nurse). Assisting the mother in identifying whether she is satisfying the infant's needs or her own needs can encourage a resolution (see Chap. 3).

WEANING THE FORMULA-FED INFANT

By the end of the first year of life, an infant can drink from a cup and is ready to be weaned from the bottle. Weaning may be more easily accomplished at this stage when the infant is developmentally ready than if bottle-feeding is prolonged and becomes a habit. Prolonged bottle-feeding and/or breast-feeding can contribute to nursing bottle caries (see Fig. 6-2). Many infants remain on the bottle well into their second or third years of life because the bottle may also represent a source of comfort that the child is reluctant to give up. Weaning age is culturally determined as well. Weaning is most easily accomplished by gradually increasing the amount of liquid that is offered from a cup while decreasing bottle feedings. The nighttime bottle often is the last to go; this will not be a problem if the infant has never taken a bottle to bed.

NUTRITIONAL CONCERNS AND THE PRUDENT DIET IN INFANCY

Much remains to be learned about the influence of nutrition in the first year on later health and eating habits. Nevertheless, it appears that some moderation is warranted in the infant's diet. Diet is recognized as a risk factor in cardiovascular disease, hypertension, cancer, and dental disease. Although controversial, questions now arise about prevention through early nutritional control of sodium, sugars, fat, and food additives (see Chap. 10).

Sodium

Infants can tolerate a wide range of sodium intakes (see Appendix 1). For example, breast milk contains from 3 to 19 mEq of sodium per liter with a mean of about 7.5 mEq per liter, while most infant formulas contain approximately 15 mEq per liter. The amount of sodium contributed by infant foods has changed in recent years. Whereas commercial infant foods used to be a large source of sodium in the infant's diet, presently, the greatest sodium sources are cow's milk and table foods that are added during the weaning period [9].

The long-term effects of high sodium diets in infancy are not known. Epidemiological and animal studies suggest that excessive dietary sodium contributes to the development of hypertension . However, the amount of salt in the infant's diet does not appear to be related to childhood hypertension. A study of black infants fed either high sodium (about 9 mEq NaCl/100 kcal) or low sodium (about 2 mEq NaCl/100 kcal) diets from age 3 to 8 months showed no difference in blood pressure at ages 1 and 8 years [81]. Preference for salt at age 8 years did not appear to be related to sodium content of the diet in infancy, suggesting that imprinting of a taste for salty foods did not occur. At present, the American Academy of Pediatrics does not recommend further sodium restriction in products intended for infant use (see Chap. 6).

Sugars

While preference for sweets is evident in newborns and even premature infants, recent longitudinal studies indicate that postnatal feeding experience may influence responses to sweets [16]. Preference for sweets may be modified somewhat by frequency, type, and amount of exposure. Presently, it appears that there is significant exposure to sweets during the first year. Even though infant food manufacturers have discontinued adding sugar to many of their products, Andrew and associates found sugar to be a noticeable part of infants' diets [11]. Of children age 5 to 12 months, 32 percent received a sweet snack on 24 hour recall that, in this age group, implies parental consent.

Lactose in milk and fructose in fruit should provide the simple sugars in the infant's diet. Additional sugar (i.e., sweetened beverages or table sugars) provides no nutritional value other than calories. Honey is not recommended for infants because it can potentially contain the bacteria C. botulinum, and honey-induced botulism has been reported [13]. Because infants are especially susceptible to the botulinum toxin, honey should not be offered prior to age 1. Nutritionally, honey is similar to sucrose; it provides mainly calories (honey contains 61 kcal per tablespoon; sugar contains 46 kcal per tablespoon) [69].

FOOD ADDITIVES AND PRESERVATIVES

Food manufacturers have discontinued using potentially harmful additives in infant foods [33]. As the infant's diet advances and table foods make up a greater proportion of the diet, the potential for introducing foods containing additives increases. In many cases, the relationship between food additives and cancer or hyperactivity is unclear. In general, because food additives do not benefit the infant, it seems wisest to avoid or at least limit their use (see Appendix 5). Nitrates are a particular concern, not only because of their possible relationship to cancer, but because they may cause methemoglobinemia in young infants. Methemoglobinemia is formed by the oxidation of hemoglobin in the presence of nitrates. Because methemoglobin cannot bind oxygen, high concentrations may lead to cyanosis.

CONCLUSION

Until more is learned about the early influences of diet on later health status, encouraging an adequate diet that is not excessive in sodium, sugar, or fat is the prudent approach. At this point, even if specific disease states cannot be linked to the infant's diet, there is enough information to warrant moderation because eating habits in infancy establish the basis for lifetime eating habits. Breast-feeding, the delayed introduction of solid foods, and the use of table foods that are consistent with the U.S. Dietary Guidelines (see Chap. 6) provide optimum infant nutrition.

REFERENCES

1. American Academy of Pediatrics Committee on Nutrition. Commentary on breast-feeding and infant formulas, including proposed standards for infant formulas. *Pediatrics* 57:278, 1976.
2. American Academy of Pediatrics Committee on Nutrition. Iron supplementation for infants. *Pediatrics* 58:756, 1976.
3. American Academy of Pediatrics Committee on Nutrition. Relationship between iron status and incidence of infection in infancy. *Pediatrics* 62:246, 1978.
4. American Academy of Pediatrics Committee on Nutrition and the Nutrition Committee of the Canadian Pediatric Society. Breast-feeding, a commentary in celebration of the International Year of the Child, 1979. *Pediatrics* 62:591, 1978.
5. American Academy of Pediatrics Committee on Nutrition. Fluoride supplementation: Revised dosage schedule. *Pediatrics* 63:150, 1979.
6. American Academy of Pediatrics Committee on Nutrition. Vitamin and mineral supplement needs in normal children in the United States. *Pediatrics* 66:1015, 1980.

7. American Academy of Pediatrics Committee on Nutrition. On the feeding of supplemental foods to infants. *Pediatrics* 65:1178, 1980.
8. American Academy of Pediatrics Committee on Nutrition. Nutrition and lactation. *Pediatrics* 68:435, 1981.
9. American Academy of Pediatrics Committee on Nutrition. Sodium intakes of infants in the United States. *Pediatrics* 68:444, 1981.
10. American Academy of Pediatrics Policy Statement based on Task Force Report. The promotion of breast-feeding. *Pediatrics* 69:654, 1982.
11. Andrew, E., et al. Infant feeding practices of families belonging to a pre-paid group practice health care plan. *Pediatrics* 65:978, 1980.
12. Aranda, J. V., et al. Maturation of caffeine elimination in infancy. *Arch. Dis. Child.* 54:946, 1979.
13. Arnon, S. S., et al. Honey and other environmental risk factors for infant botulism. *J. Pediatr.* 94:331, 1979.
14. Arnon, S. S., et al. Protective role of human milk against sudden infant botulism. *J. Pediatr.* 100:568, 1982.
15. Barness, L. A. Nutrition and Nutritional Disorders. In W. E. Nelson, et al. (Eds.), *Textbook of Pediatrics* (11th ed.). Philadelphia: Saunders, 1979.
16. Beauchamp, G. K., and Maller, O. The Development of Flavor Preferences in Humans: A Review. In M. R. Kare and O. Maller (Eds.), *The Chemical Senses and Nutrition*. New York: Academic Press, 1977. Pp. 292–315.
17. Beauregard, W. G. Positional otitis media. *J. Pediatr.* 79:294, 1971.
18. Bell, E. F., et al. Vitamin E absorption in small premature infants. *Pediatrics* 68:830, 1979.
19. Berger, L. R. When one should discourage breast-feeding. *Pediatrics* 67:300, 1981.
20. Brock, K. H. Lactoferrin in human milk: Its role in absorption and protection against enteric infections in the newborn. *Arch. Dis. Child.* 55:417, 1980.
21. Castle, S. *The Complete New Guide to Preparing Infant Foods*. New York: Doubleday, 1981.
22. Center for Disease Control. Nutrition surveillance—United States. *M.M.W.R.* 30:521, 1981.
23. Chandra, R. K. Immunological aspects of human milk. *Nutr. Rev.* 36:265, 1978.
24. Chandra, R. K. Prospective studies of the effects of breast-feeding on incidence of infection. *Acta. Paediatr. Scand.* 68:691, 1979.
25. Cunningham, A. S. Morbidity in breast-fed and artificially-fed infants. I. *J. Pediatr.* 90:726, 1977.
26. Cunningham, A. S. Morbidity in breast-fed and artificially-fed infants. II. *J. Pediatr.* 95:685, 1979.
27. Dallman, P. R., Siimes, M. A., and Stekel, A. Iron deficiency in infancy and childhood. *Am. J. Clin. Nutr.* 33:86, 1980.
28. Davis, J. R., Goldenring, J., and Lubin, B. H. Nutritional vitamin B_{12} deficiency in infants. *Am. J. Dis. Child.* 135:566, 1981.
29. DeLuca H. F. The vitamin D system in the regulation of calcium and phosphorus metabolism. *Nutr. Rev.* 37:161, 1979.
30. Dine, M. S., et al. Where do the heaviest children come from? A prospective study of white children from birth to five years. *Pediatrics* 63:1, 1979.
31. Eastham, E. J., and Walker, W. A. Adverse effects of milk formula ingestion on the gastrointestinal tract. *Gastroenterology* 76:365, 1979.
32. Edidin, D. V., et al. Resurgence of nutritional rickets associated with breast-feeding and special dietary practices. *Pediatrics* 65:232, 1980.

33. EPSGAN Committee on Nutrition. Guidelines on infant nutrition II. Recommendations for the composition of follow-up formula and beikost. *Acta. Paediatr. Scand.* 290[Supp.]:4, 1981.
34. Fallot, M. E., et al. Breast-feeding reduces incidence of hospital admissions for infections in infants. *Pediatrics* 65:1121, 1980.
35. Fomon, S. J. *Infant Nutrition* (2nd ed.). Philadelphia: Saunders, 1974.
36. Fomon, S. J., et al. Recommendations for feeding normal infants. *Pediatrics* 63:52, 1979.
37. Fomon, S. J., et al. Body composition of reference children from birth to age ten years. *Am. J. Clin. Nutr.* 35[Supp.]:1169, 1982.
38. Food and Nutrition Board: *Recommended Dietary Allowances* (9th ed.). National Academy of Science National Research Council: Washington, D.C., 1980.
39. France, G. L., Marmer, D. J., and Steele, R. W. Breast-feeding and salmonella infection. *Am. J. Dis. Child.* 134:147, 1980.
40. Friedman, G., and Goldberg, S. J. An evaluation of the safety of a low-saturated fat, low cholesterol diet beginning in infancy. *Pediatrics* 58:655, 1976.
41. Gerrard, I. W. Allergy in breast-fed babies to ingredients in breast milk. *Ann. Allergy.* 42:69, 1979.
42. Goldman, A. S., et al. Immunologic factors in human milk during the first year of lactation. *J. Pediatr.* 100:563, 1982.
43. Greene, H. L., McCabe, D. R., and Merenstein, G. B. Protracted diarrhea and malnutrition in infancy: Changes in intestinal morphology and disaccharidase activities during treatment with intravenous nutrition or oral elemental diets. *J. Pediatr.* 87:695, 1975.
44. Greer, F. R., et al. Bone mineral content and serum 25-hydroxyvitamin D concentrations in breast-fed infants with and without supplemental vitamin D: One year follow-up. *J. Pediatr.* 100:919, 1982.
45. Hall, B. Uniformity of human milk. *Am. J. Clin. Nutr.* 32:304, 1979.
46. Hanson, J. M., and Kinsella, J. E. Fatty acid composition of infant formulas and cereals. *J. Am. Diet. Assoc.* 78:250, 1981.
47. Howard, R. B. Growth and Nutrition. In R. B. Howard and N. H. Herbold (Eds.), *Nutrition in Clinical Care* (2nd ed.). New York: McGraw-Hill, 1982.
48. Jelliffe, D. B., and Jelliffe, E. F. The volume and composition of human milk in poorly nourished communities: A review. *Am. J. Clin. Nutr.* 31:492, 1978.
49. Jensen, R. G., Hagerty, M. M., and McMahon, K. E. Lipids of human milk and infant formulas: A review. *Am. J. Clin. Nutr.* 31:990, 1978.
50. Jones, R. A., and Belsey, E. M. Common mistakes in infant feeding: A survey from a London borough. *Br. Med. J.* [Clin. Res.] 2:112, 1978.
51. Kemberling, S. R. Supporting breast-feeding. *Pediatrics* 63:60, 1979.
52. Kerr, C. M., Reisinger, K. S., and Plankey, F. W. Sodium concentration of home made baby foods. *Pediatrics* 62:331, 1978.
53. Klaus, M., and Kennel, J. *Maternal Infant Bonding.* St. Louis: Mosby, 1976.
54. Kramer, M. S., and Moroz, B. Do breast-feeding and delayed introduction of solid foods protect against subsequent atopic eczema? *J. Pediatr.* 98:546, 1981.
55. Lakdawala, D. T., and Widdowson, E. M. Vitamin D in human milk. *Lancet* 1:167, 1977.
56. Lake, A. M., Kleinman, R. E., and Walker, W. A. Enteric alimentation in specialized gastrointestinal problems: An alternative to total parenteral nutrition. *Adv. Pediatr.* 28:319, 1981.

57. Lawrence, R. A. *Breast-feeding: A Guide for the Medical Profession*. St. Louis: Mosby, 1980.
58. Leerbeck, E., and Sondergaard, H. The total content of vitamin D in human milk and cow's milk. *Eur. J. Nutr.* 44:7, 1980.
59. L'Esperance, C. Pain or pleasure: The dilemma of early breast-feeding. *Birth and Family Journal* 7:21, 1980.
60. Lonnerdal, B., Forsum, E., and Hambraeus, L. Effect of oral contraceptives on composition and volume of breast milk. *Am. J. Clin. Nutr.* 33:816, 1980.
61. Martinez, G. A., Dodd, D. A., and Samartgedes, J. A. Milk feeding patterns during the first 12 months of life. *Pediatrics* 68:863, 1981.
62. Mata, L. Breast-feeding: Main promoter of infant health. *Am. J. Clin. Nutr.* 31:2058, 1978.
63. Matthews, D. M., and Adibi, S. A. Peptide absorption. *Gastroenterology* 71:151, 1976.
64. McMillian, J. A., Landaw, S. A., and Oski, F. A. Iron sufficiency in breast-fed infants and the availability of iron from human milk. *Pediatrics* 58:686, 1976.
65. Newcomer, A. D., et al. Prospective comparison of indirect methods for detecting lactase deficiency. *N. Engl. J. Med.* 293:1232, 1975.
66. Nizel, A. E. *Nutrition in Preventive Dentistry: Science and Practice*. Philadelphia: Saunders, 1972.
67. Ogra, S. S., and Ogra, P. L. Immunologic aspects of human milk. I. Distribution characteristics and concentrations of immunoglobins at different times after the onset of lactation. *J. Pediatr.* 92:546, 1978.
68. Partridge, J. C., et al. Water intoxication secondary to feeding mismanagement. *Am. J. Dis. Child.* 135:38, 1981.
69. Pennington, J. A., and Church, H. N. *Bowes and Church's Food Values of Portions Commonly Used* (13th ed.). Philadelphia: Lippincott, 1980.
70. Pollet, J., and Leibel, D. Iron deficiency and behavior. *J. Pediatr.* 88:372, 1976.
71. Resman, B. H., Blumenthal, H. P., and Jusko, W. J. Breast milk distribution of theobromine from chocolate. *J. Pediatr.* 91:477, 1977.
72. Rogan, W. J., Bagniewska, M. A., and Damstra, T. Pollutants in breast milk. *N. Engl. J. Med.* 302:1450, 1980.
73. Siegenthaler, E. J., Byrne, A. M., and Ekpenyong, I. An evaluation of the effectiveness of sterilization of infant formulas by thermal heating and an aseptic method. *Ecol. Food. Nutr.* 4:215, 1976.
74. Singer, L., and Ophang, R. Total fluoride intake of infants. *Pediatrics* 63:460, 1979.
75. Stagno, S., et al. Breast milk and the risk of cytomegalovirus infection. *N. Engl. J. Med.* 302:1073, 1980.
76. Thomas, M. R., et al. The effects of vitamin C, vitamin B_6, vitamin B_{12}, folic acid, riboflavin, and thiamin on breast milk and the maternal status of well nourished women at 6 months postpartum. *Am. J. Clin. Nutr.* 33:2151, 1980.
77. Tyrala, I. E., and Dodson, W. E. Caffeine secretion into breast milk. *Arch. Dis. Child.* 54:787, 1979.
78. Valman, H. B. Feeding and feeding problems. *Br. Med. J.* [Clin. Res.] 2:457, 1980.
79. Watkins, C. J., Leeder, S. R., and Corkhill, R. T. The relationship between breast and bottle feeding and respiratory illness in the first year of life. *J. Epidemiol. Community Health* 33:180, 1979.
80. Weisman, V., et al. Vitamin D metabolites in human milk. *J. Pediatr.* 100:745, 1982.

81. Whitten, C. F., and Stewart, R. A. The effect of dietary sodium in infancy on blood pressure and related factors. *Acta. Paediatr. Scand.* 279[Supp.]:3, 1980.
82. Wickizer, T. M., and Brilliant, L. B. Testing for polychlorinated biphenyls in human milk. *Pediatrics* 68:411, 1981.
83. *World Health Organization Twenty Seventh World Health Assembly, Part I: Infant Nutrition and Breast-feeding.* Official Records of the World Health Organization, 217:20, 1974.
84. *World Health Organization Code on Marketing of Breast Milk Substitutes.* Albany, New York: WHO Publications, 1981.
85. Zmora, E., Gorodischer, R., and Bar-Ziv, J. Multiple nutritional deficiencies in infants from a strict vegetarian community. *Am. J. Dis. Child.* 133:141, 1979.

6. Nutrition and Toddler Feeding

Rosanne B. Howard

Spilled food, sticky hands, and frustrated parents best describe mealtimes with children between the ages of 1 and 3 years. Toddlers use mealtime as a testing ground for autonomy. While eating, the toddler can exert control (e.g., refuse foods or spit out lumps). Food jags and finicky appetites dominate this developmental period. As toddlers vacillate between feelings of separation and security, regressions in feeding behavior are seen. Ambivalence, negativism, and independence abound at toddler mealtime.

It is in this milieu that food for growth is provided. During this period, lasting food habits are formed amid cultural and environmental influences—food habits that ultimately can influence health and longevity.

ENVIRONMENTAL INFLUENCES ON TODDLER FEEDING

Today's family, buffeted by changing parental roles, single parents, and working mothers, is in transition. These changes are reflected at family meals. Traditional family dinners are being relegated to special occasions with more individualized meals scheduled around work, day care, or leisure activities. Increasingly, there is a reliance on day care centers, restaurants, vending machines, and convenience and fast foods for meals. The time and energy once spent on food preparation is being used for other activities.

In 1979 the United States Department of Agriculture reported that 35 percent of food dollars was spent for meals outside the home [62] and fast foods sales increasingly account for more food dollars. Between 1963 and 1979 sales rose 83 percent in eating places and 300 percent in fast food places [61]. In one survey, nearly 94 percent of families ate out at least once in an eight-week period [50]. These families frequented all restaurants labelled "quick service" an average of 2.14 times per week [18]. Nutritional status is not significantly influenced in these families, but data do show that fast-food meals may be nutritionally inadequate and calorically excessive due to the nature of the menus in fast-food restaurants [57] (Table 6-1). The nutritional impact of fast foods on the toddler is unclear, but the exaltation of fast foods by the media has promoted hamburgers and french fries to be among the most accepted toddler fare; outings to fast-food restaurants are now considered special treats for children.

In addition to fast-food meals, mini meals or snacks are taking the place of three square meals per day in many households. With full schedules and less time to shop and prepare food, there is a growing

Table 6-1. Nutritional Analyses of Fast Food

	Wt (g)	Energy (kcal)	PRO (g)	CHO (g)	Fat (g)	Chol (mg)	Vitamins A (IU)	B₁ (mg)	B₂ (mg)	Nia. (mg)	B₆ (mg)	B₁₂ (μg)	C (mg)	D (IU)	Minerals Ca (mg)	Cu (mg)	Fe (mg)	K (mg)	Mg (mg)	P (mg)	Na (mg)	Zn (mg)	Mois-ture (g)	Crude fiber (g)
MCDONALD'S																								
Egg McMuffin®	138	327	19	31	15	229	97	0.47	0.44	3.8	0.21	0.75	<1.4	46	226	0.12	2.9	168	26	322	885	1.9	70.7	0.1
English muffin, buttered	63	186	5	30	5	13	164	0.28	0.49	2.6	0.04	0.02	0.8	14	117	0.69	1.5	71	13	74	318	0.5	21.7	0.1
Hotcakes w/butter & syrup	214	500	8	94	10	47	257	0.26	0.36	2.3	0.12	0.19	4.7	5	103	0.11	2.2	187	28	501	1070	0.7	97.8	0.2
Sausage (pork)	53	206	9	tr	19	43	<32	0.27	0.11	2.1	0.18	0.53	0.5	31	16	0.05	0.8	127	9	95	615	1.5	22.9	0.1
Scrambled eggs	98	180	13	3	13	349	652	0.08	0.47	0.2	0.19	0.93	1.2	65	61	0.06	2.5	135	13	264	205	1.7	68.1	<0.1
Hashbrown potatoes	55	125	2	14	7	7	<14	0.06	<0.01	0.8	0.13	0.01	4.1	<1	5	0.04	0.4	247	13	67	325	0.2	30.9	0.3
Big Mac®	204	563	26	41	33	86	530	0.39	0.37	6.5	0.27	1.8	2.2	33	157	0.18	4.0	237	38	314	1010	4.7	100.4	0.6
Cheeseburger	115	307	15	30	14	37	345	0.25	0.23	3.8	0.12	0.91	1.6	13	132	0.11	2.4	156	23	205	767	2.6	108.4	0.2
Hamburger	102	255	12	30	10	25	82	0.25	0.18	4.0	0.12	0.81	1.7	12	51	0.10	2.3	142	19	126	520	2.1	48.0	0.3
Quarter Pounder®	166	424	24	33	22	67	133	0.32	0.28	6.5	0.27	1.88	<1.7	23	63	0.17	4.1	322	37	249	735	5.1	83.7	0.7
Quarter Pounder® w/ch	194	524	30	32	31	96	660	0.31	0.37	7.4	0.23	2.15	2.7	25	219	0.18	4.3	341	41	382	1236	5.7	96.0	0.8
Filet-O-Fish®	139	432	14	37	25	47	42	0.26	0.20	2.6	0.10	0.82	<1.4	25	93	0.10	1.7	150	27	229	781	0.9	59.5	0.1
Regular fries	68	220	3	26	12	9	<17	0.12	0.02	2.3	0.22	<0.03	12.5	<1	9	0.03	0.6	564	27	101	109	0.3	25.4	0.5
Apple pie	85	253	2	29	14	12	<34	0.02	0.02	0.2	0.02	<0.04	<0.8	2	14	0.05	0.6	39	6	27	398	0.2	38.3	0.3
Cherry pie	88	260	2	32	14	13	114	0.03	0.02	0.4	0.02	<0.02	<0.8	<2	12	0.06	0.6	35	7	27	427	0.2	38.9	0.1
McDonaldland® cookies	67	308	4	49	11	10	<27	0.23	0.23	2.9	0.03	0.03	0.9	10	12	0.07	1.5	52	11	74	358	0.3	2.2	0.1
Chocolate shake	291	383	10	66	9	30	349	0.12	0.44	0.5	0.13	1.16	<2.9	44	320	0.19	0.8	580	49	335	300	1.4	203.0	0.3
Strawberry shake	290	362	9	62	9	32	377	0.12	0.44	0.4	0.14	1.16	4.1	32	322	0.07	0.2	423	31	313	207	1.2	207.9	<0.3
Vanilla shake	291	352	9	60	8	31	349	0.12	0.70	0.3	0.12	1.19	3.2	26	329	0.09	0.2	422	31	314	201	1.2	211.3	<0.3
Hot fudge sundae	164	310	7	46	11	18	230	0.07	0.31	1.1	0.13	0.7	2.5	16	215	0.13	0.6	410	35	236	175	1.0	97.9	0.2
Caramel sundae	165	328	7	53	10	26	279	0.07	0.31	1.0	0.05	0.6	3.6	14	200	0.09	0.2	338	30	230	195	0.9	93.2	<0.2
Strawberry sundae	164	289	7	46	9	20	230	0.07	0.30	1.0	0.05	0.6	2.8	16	174	0.11	0.4	290	28	80	96	0.8	101.0	0.2

Source: Reprinted with permission from Young, E. A., Brennan, E. H., and Irving, G. L.: Nutritional Analysis of Fast Foods. *Dietetic Currents* 8:5–12, 1981. Published by Ross Laboratories, Columbus, Ohio 43216.

feeling that meal patterns need to be more flexible in order to conform to faster-paced and less structured lifestyles. Between-meal eating is becoming a way of life, and snack foods laden with salt and fat are the most popular consumer items (see Table 6-9). Snack foods such as potato chips, pretzels, nuts, crackers, and spreads gross 9 billion dollars per year [60]. It is estimated that 18 percent of all shoppers buy such snack items and the number of these items purchased appears to increase with rising family income [14, 41]. The proportion increases substantially when either family groups or women with children do the buying [14]. Thus, it can be inferred that toddlers have access to these high caloric, low-nutrient snack foods.

In a study of environmental factors associated with preschool obesity, the typical pattern of children age 2 followed a trend of eating five meals or snacks daily [16]. Parents most frequently allow children of this age group to make their own snack and breakfast selection, therefore allowing them to determine possibly one-third or more of their daily nutrient intake. Snacking is not intrinsically antithetical to sound nutrition; however, attention needs to be given to the type of foods selected and the amount consumed according to each child's needs. Parents must be aware that because of the incidental nature of snacking, it can be used to fulfill unconscious emotional needs and to relieve boredom. Many parents comment that the refrigerator door is opened continually on rainy days or when the children complain that they have "nothing to do." Another observation is that snacking is often paired with television watching.

To what degree television affects toddlers' eating behavior is highly speculative. The food tastes of 4-year-old children have been found to be influenced by television advertising [16]. The most frequent request resulting from advertising was for presweetened dry cereals, many of dubious nutritional content and high in sugar (Table 6-2). It is estimated that children under 12 years of age who watch a moderate amount of television see 21,300 commercials per year [2]. Many of these commercials are devoted to snack foods, soft drinks, and breakfast cereals. A Federal Trade Commission report on television advertising for children emphasizes that many of the products advertised on television are sweets [28]. Mothers often report that children request products or brands of candy and snacks frequently. Not only can television influence food requests, but the passive process of watching keeps children from expending energy on physical activities. This is a concern with a population at risk for childhood obesity (see Chap. 10).

Besides the messages emanating from television, toddler's developing food repertoires are influenced by the messages of numerous caretakers. With more mothers of young children working (45.4 percent of all women with children under the age of 6) [68], infants and

Table 6-2. Sugar Content of Selected Breakfast Cereals

Cereal	Percent of Sucrose
Shredded Wheat (large biscuit)	1.3
Cheerios	2.0
Puffed Rice	2.4
Puffed Wheat	3.5
Corn Flakes (Kellogg)	7.8
Rice Krispies	10.0
Raisin Bran (Kellogg)	10.6
Sugar Frosted Corn Flakes	15.6
Alpha Bits	40.3
Cap'n Crunch	43.3
Kaboom	43.8
Franken Berry	44.0
Frosted Flakes	44.0
Count Chocula	44.2
Boo Berry	45.7
Froot Loops	47.4
King Vitamin	58.5
Super Orange Crisp	68.0

Data from: Shannon, Ira L. Sucrose and glucose in dry breakfast cereal. *J. Dent. Child.* 41:347, 1974.

toddlers are exposed to a variety of caretakers, each with their own habits and cultural attitudes toward food, causing interpretation of the same food practices to vary. "For example, eating everything on the plate in some cultures may mean that there is not enough to eat; in other cultures it may mean thrift or waste not, want not; in still other cultures it may mean that the person is selfish in not thinking ahead to take home food to share with the family" [40]. The subtle nuances of these food attitudes are transmitted from caretaker to the child during feeding as food is used to fill emotional as well as bio-logical needs (Table 6-3). For example, food is often used as a reward for good behavior. Eppright found 23 percent of preschool parents used food as a reward and 29 percent used food as a pacifier [27]. Some of the stress imposed by diet alterations (e.g., allergy diets) can be related to previous unconscious food meanings, especially when foods with "special meanings" such as milk or reward foods are taken away.

Another effect of multiple caretakers is that parents are no longer solely responsible for their children's intakes. In many cases, five food decisions are being left to babysitters and day care personnel who must provide meals and snacks that contribute up to 75 to 80 percent of children's nutrient intake [68]. These short-term caretakers may not have the same long-term interest in nutrition as parents. Again, the nutritional impact is hard to measure, but the implication is for

Table 6-3. Symbolic Meanings of Food

Food Symbol	Symbol Formation
Love, security, trust, gratification, sensory pleasure	Food from early feeding experiences imparts feelings of security, trust, love; the infant that suckles from breast or bottle is cuddled closely, is filled with warm milk, feels sensory pleasure
Reward, punishment	Food can be used as a method of discipline, withheld to enforce behavior (a tool to provoke fear or hunger) or given as a reward for good behavior
Self-fulfillment	Food, so paramount to the infant's development, can become the focus of the parent-child relationship and, as such, the means through which parents achieve self-fulfillment. For example, the act of feeding becomes the act of nurturing, and the fulfillment of parental esteem is heavily at stake in feeding the family

Religion
  foods that derive a separate meaning only from religious rites on feast days (e.g., matzo)
Prestige
  foods whose major value is to demonstrate an ability to pay (e.g., gourmet or exotic foods such as cavier or quality foods such as brand-name products)
Taboo
  foods proscribed for irrational and nonscientific reasons (e.g., Hindu prohibition of beef)
Socialization
  food and eating that carry the perceptible symbolic undertone of sociability (e.g., a wedding banquet, testimonial dinner, holiday feast, coffee klatch, cocktail party)
Health
  foods purported to have magical properties (e.g., used to cure ailments, ward off old age, or function as aphrodisiacs)
	Food customs are part of our cultural heritage. From the beginning, societies developed patterns around the conduct of food activities. These standardized practices are unique to each society, having evolved from different environmental factors and having been incorporated into the society to maintain the viability of the group

Table 6-3 (Continued)

Food Symbol		Symbol Formation
Language		Foods communicate meanings
meat, steak, potatoes	= masculinity, aggression	that justify the simile of a language
vegetables, fruits	= femininity	
fruits ("bearing fruit," fruition)	= love, affection, sexuality	
olives	= sophistication or adult taste	
peanut butter	= childhood	

Source: Howard, R. B., and Herbold, N. (Eds.). *Nutrition in Clinical Care* (2nd ed.). New York: McGraw-Hill, 1982.

communication between all parties involved in feeding in order to ensure nutritional adequacy.

Despite the myriad of influences on toddler feeding, it is still the parents who have the most authority, especially parents who agree about child-rearing practices. Wakefield and Merrow studied child-rearing beliefs of parents of 150 children [71] using the procedure of Centers and Centers [13]. They found that parents who agreed on child-rearing practices had average-weight children who consumed diets containing nutrients equal to more than 90 percent of the RDA. Children from families who disagreed about child-rearing practices had poor nutrient intakes and were relatively under- or overweight. It is important, therefore, for parents to understand their own food attitudes in order to give a consistent message at meals. Also, if parents or older siblings dislike foods, children are likely to do so. (Interestingly, food dislikes of children are found to be associated more closely with dislikes of fathers and older brothers than with the dislikes of mothers and older sisters [27]. Family influences seem to be strong determinants in developing food behavior.

The extent to which food faddism affects toddler eating is mostly impressionistic. Usual reasons for practicing fad diets include poverty, religious and philosophical beliefs, and misguidance. These fad diets can result in poor nutritional status. For the most part, food fads do not involve the feeding of young children except in certain cults. Edidin and colleagues found 10 cases of nutritional rickets associated with low calciferol intake due to unsupplemented breast-feeding, dietary manipulation, or fad diets [25].

People with similar beliefs sometimes form food cults, in which the health risks to children vary. For example, the extremism among the adherents of the Zen macrobiotic diet (who follow the teachings of

Zen Buddhist monks in a Yin and Yang food philosophy) places them in the high nutritional risk category. After ten increasingly restrictive stages, the diet consists of cereals and a minimum quantity of water. At the highest diet level, scurvy, anemia, hypoproteinemia, hypercalcemia, emaciation, loss of kidney function due to restricted fluid intake, and even death may result [58]. Fortunately, most followers adhere to lower levels of the diet that allow 25 to 30 percent of energy to be provided by food of animal origin. Energy, calcium, riboflavin, and iron (in women only) are the limiting nutrients [11]. Children in these macrobiotic families are at particular risk for malnutrition because they use a mixture of seeds, rice, beans, and water as a replacement for milk early in life. Kwashiorkor has been reported in infants fed macrobiotic diets [10, 43] (see p.158).

The rising cost of the food dollar poses another type of nutritional threat. Inflation is causing everybody, especially the poor, to cut back on food costs and unfortunately, in many instances, on food quality. The nutritional status of the nation's poor is further affected by rising unemployment and cutbacks in federally supported child food programs and food stamp programs. (see Appendix 9). Also, food shopping by the inner city's urban poor is often hampered by lack of competitive supermarkets. Unless they have transportation, they must depend on corner grocery stores that have a limited number of food items and higher costs.

Not only the poor economize on food bills. According to a nationwide poll, 72 percent of those surveyed (many of them from middle and upper-middle income families) said that they had been forced to economize because of inflation and recession [72]. Money, now more than ever, seems to dictate family meals. While almost three-quarters of those surveyed in 1978 reported that they had sought to improve nutritional quality, less than one-quarter of those surveyed in 1982 said the same thing.

With higher food costs, there is no room for impulse buying on weekly shopping trips. Items must be selected with cost and nutrition in mind. Reading food labels is important (see Fig. 5-3). However, interpreting labels can be a problem, especially for groups with limited education. Consumers must now decide among the 12,000 or so items that line the average supermarket while trying to interpret the nutritional value of a highly processed food or the significance of food additives. Professional guidance in these areas is needed.

The use of additives to preserve color and flavor or thicken food (see Appendix 5), as well as the concern about pesticide and fertilizer residues, has provoked consumer concern. This concern has prompted some consumers to seek *organic* foods. The term *organic* is somewhat of a misnomer because all foods actually are organic. The USDA defines organic food as food free from synthetic fertilizers, pesticides, growth regulators, and chemical additives. However, there are no guarantees that foods will be completely free of pesticide and fertilizer residues when organically grown. Some may contain pesticide residues because traces of such chemicals remain in the soil years after their use has stopped. Also, they may be present in dust, wind, and rainfall runoff from nearby farms. Researchers at the USDA found pesticide residues in 5 out of 6 heads of organic lettuce bought at health food stores [63]. The residue level of one head exceeded that of nonorganic lettuce bought at the supermarket. Thus, even when goods are bought at reputable markets where food is definitely organically grown, they may not be totally free from chemical residues. In these economically difficult times as families try to get the most from their food dollars, it is important to remember that organically grown foods are usually more expensive and have not proven to offer extra nutritional benefit.

The cumulative effects of many additives and chemical residues are unknown, and their relationships to allergies, cancer, birth defects, and interactions with drugs need to be investigated. The subtleties of intolerance to additives is just now being recognized. For example, the FDA estimates that 50,000 to 100,000 people are intolerant to tartrazine (food color yellow, no. 5), which pervades our food supply [59]. It is contained in aspirin, ice cream, sherbets, desserts, (gelatins and puddings), salad dressings, bakery products, candies as well as in orange, lime, and lemon flavored drinks to name but a few frequently consumed items. A list of additives generally recognized as safe (GRAS) has been compiled by the FDA. Health professionals should keep informed about the potential problems of additives and advise families to consume a varied diet in order to minimize exposure to any one additive. In children who appear to be sensitive to certain additives (e.g., salicylates, tartrazine), an additive-free diet can be devised (see Appendix 3). The relationship of certain food additives to hyperactivity is controversial; nevertheless, parents often claim improvement in their child's behavior when given additive-free diets. (It is difficult to assess whether behavior changes are due to the diet itself or a placebo effect.) There is no harm in trying such diets, as long as they are nutritionally sound. Parents should realize that additive-free diets may take extra time and planning to implement properly. They must also realize that additive-free diets should not be used universally in the treatment of childhood hyperactivity.

It is in the complex environment of additives, processed foods, fast-paced schedules, television commercials, and shrinking food dollars that toddlers' nutrient needs must be met. With so many stimuli and numerous caretakers, food decisions cannot be left to chance. Priority must be given to foods that supply nutrient needs.

NUTRIENT NEEDS AND CONCERNS

Unpredictable appetites, undeveloped feeding skills, and ritualistic behavior can sometimes make toddler meals a trial for even the most enlightened and patient parents (Fig. 6-1). As the rapid growth of infancy subsides and energy needs per kilogram of body weight decrease, appetites fluctuate, making toddlers nutritionally vulnerable. However, data found in three major surveys (the Ten State Nutrition Survey, 1968-1970 [66], the Preschool Nutrition Survey, 1968-1970 [51], and the Health and Nutrition Examination Survey [HANES], 1971-1972 [55]) indicates that United States preschoolers are relatively well-nourished. To date, only the HANES I survey sample of 1,500 children is considered representative of United States preschoolers [55]. (The HANES II data collected from 1976–1980 is being analyzed.) For the most part, poorer growth and substandard dietary intakes could be associated with lower socioeconomic status. The clinical signs of malnutrition were rarely found (0 to 2 percent for most deficiency signs) but iron deficiency was widespread. Almost 87 percent of preschoolers were found to have deficient iron intakes [51]. These findings were supported by the Nationwide Food Consumption Survey (1977–1978) [64]. It was found that food intakes of children age 1 to 2 years averaged only 55 percent of the RDA for iron, lower than for any other age group.

To meet the iron needs of children in this age group, 15 mg of iron is required daily [32]. Table 6-4 lists the amount of iron found in some foods (see also Appendix 4). With some creative planning, iron-rich foods can be incorporated into the diet of the child with even the most finicky appetite. For example, gravies can be made from strained baby meats. Infant cereals can be reinstituted as hot cereal for breakfast; or iron-fortified cereals such as Instant Cream of Wheat can be used. However, the use of adult fortified cereals to meet iron needs should be discouraged. Crawford and associates found some parents feeding cereals fortified with 14,080 IU of vitamin A and 3.52 to 4.2 mg of iron per 100 gm to their children [16]. These children ate one to two cups (30 to 40 gm per cup) of these cereals per day, either as a breakfast cereal or as between-meal snacks. In their study of diets of second and sixth grade pupils, Cook and Payne found eight children who were consuming a total daily average of over 10,000 IU of vitamin A [15]. Although cereals intended for adults can provide a source of iron, there could be a concern in certain children for excess vitamin A when taken with other food sources and vitamin supplements, as shown in both of these studies.

Although iron is a nutrient to be stressed in the diets of preschoolers, the developmental characteristics of this age group often conspire against the consumption of iron-containing foods. At the end of the

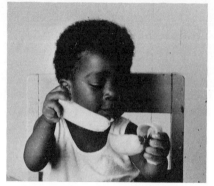

A

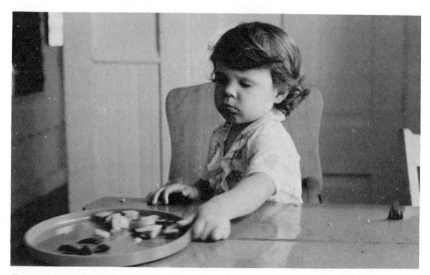

B

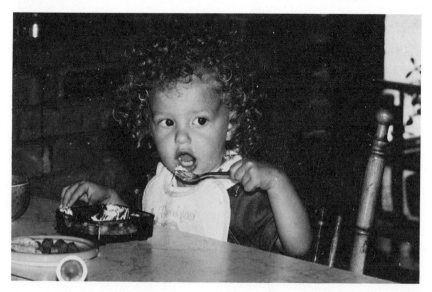

C

Table 6-4. Iron Content of Selected Foods

Sources of Iron	Amount	Iron (mg)
HEME		
Beef (hamburger)	1 oz	1.39
Chicken (light meat)	1 oz	0.37
Fish (haddock)	1 oz	0.14
Liver (calf)	1 oz	4.05
Lamb (leg, lean)	1 oz	0.88
Pork	1 oz	1.04
NONHEME		
Infant cereal (oatmeal)	6 tbsp	14.2
Fortified cereal (Cheerios)	1 cup	4.0
Cream of Wheat (cooked)	½ cup	7.8
Wheat germ	1 oz	2.6
Whole grain bread	1 slice	0.5
White enriched bread	1 slice	0.6
Rice (enriched, all varieties)	½ cup	0.6
Lentils (cooked)	⅓ cup	1.1
Egg	1 med	1.1
Raisins	1 tbsp	0.4
Prunes	4 med	1.5
Spinach (cooked)	¼ cup	1.5
Black strap molasses (unsulphured, Grandma's)	1 tbsp	0.4

Data from J. A. Pennington and H. H. Church, *Food Values of Portions Commonly Used* (13th ed.). Philadelphia: Lippincott, 1980.

first year, toddlers generally have been weaned from iron-containing breast milk or formula, and iron-fortified infant cereals usually have been discontinued. Many toddlers dislike meat—the best source of heme iron. Often this is due to their immature chewing skills (good rotary chewing does not develop until around age 2 ½ years). In fact, some toddlers will chew meat into a small bolus and spit it out. They must become accustomed to the texture of meat as well as the different taste from that of cereals, fruits, and vegetables. Toddlers' ritualistic behavior sometimes makes it difficult to incorporate new iron-containing foods into their diets, and their small, fluctuating appetites further complicate maintenance of adequate iron stores.

These developmental characteristics may also affect children's zinc status. Hambridge and colleagues found preschool and school-age children from low- and middle-income families to possibly be ingesting

Figure 6-1. A, B, and C. The many faces of toddler feeding. (Part C courtesy of William Epstein.)

inadequate amounts of zinc [38]. Forty percent of Denver Head Start children 3.5 to 6 years old with heights less than the third percentile had low concentrations of hair zinc and 69 percent had low plasma zinc concentrations. Zinc is found chiefly in red meats and seafood, particularly oysters, which are not part of the standard toddler fare. Cereals and legumes can be considered fair sources. Zinc is found in other foods such as milk, fruit, and vegetables, but in lesser amounts.

Calcium is another nutrient that may be below the RDA in the preschool group. In the HANES I survey, calcium intakes were the poorest in the 2- to 3-year-old age group [55] and lower in black children than in white children. Eppright and coworkers found that only children less than 1 year of age averaged a consumption of 3 or more cups of milk daily; thereafter, the mean daily intakes of milk approximated 2 ½ cups [27]. Crawford and associates found the decrease in calcium related to the decrease in milk consumption associated with the increase in consumption of solid foods at the ages of 1 and 2. Although calcium was the second most frequent nutrient deficiency (after iron), no mothers stressed calcium-containing foods in the diets of their preschoolers [16]. At 1- to 2-years old, children require 800 mg of calcium per day, which is mainly provided by milk or dairy foods. Certain foods such as spinach and kale contain calcium, but the fiber, phytate, and oxalate content decrease the bioavailability of calcium and make them less reliable sources.

The frequent spills that accompany weaning and some toddlers' reluctance to drink from the cup can further compromise calcium intake. Other calcium-containing foods such as cheese, tofu processed with calcium, and yogurt should be encouraged. Powdered or evaporated milk can be added to soups and puddings. To encourage milk drinking, the excessive use of other beverages (i.e., soda, fruit juices) may need to be curtailed (Table 6-5). In children who do not drink milk or milk substitutes and do not eat dairy foods, there is need for calcium supplementation. Table 6-6 provides a schedule of calcium supplementation for these children. Nondairy creamers cannot provide the calcium or protein that is needed. Parents must be aware that low milk consumption is also associated with low intakes of vitamin A and riboflavin [55].

Preschoolers from the lowest socioeconomic stratum (below the poverty level) were found to have the highest prevalence of low serum vitamin A [55]. Vitamin A nutriture is further reduced by the toddler's indifference to vegetables. Sixty percent of the mothers surveyed by Crawford and coworkers said that their children disliked vegetables the most [16]. Many mothers do not realize the desirability of including vitamin A and C–rich fruits and vegetables in their children's diets;

Table 6-5. Calcium Content of Selected Foods

Type	Amount	Calcium (mg)
Milk, whole (3.5% fat)	8 oz	288
Milk, lowfat (2% fat), protein fortified	8 oz	352
Evaporated, condensed milk	1 oz	81
Skim milk solids, instant	1 tbsp	48.5
Yogurt, whole	8 oz	275
Yogurt with nonfat milk solids	8 oz	415
Cheese: cheddar, American	1 oz	211
Cottage cheese	1 rounded tbsp	26
Ice cream (10% fat)	½ cup	88
Pudding, vanilla from mix (with whole milk)	½ cup	149
Tofu	1½ oz	64

Data from J. A. Pennington and H. H. Church, *Food Values of Portions Commonly Used* (13th ed.). Philadelphia: Lippincott, 1980.

Table 6-6. Schedule of Calcium Supplementation

Type	Calcium (mg)	Age	Amount/day
Neo Calglucon (calcium gluconate)	115 mg/tsp	1–6 mo	1 tsp × 3
		6 mo–3 yr	2 tsp × 3
Tums Tablets (calcium carbonate not completely absorbed)	500 mg per tablet	3 yr–5 yr	1 tablet × 3
		5 yr–10 yr	2 tablet × 3

Note: Supplementation is indicated for children on a milk-free diet not drinking milk substitute or child refusing milk and milk products for longer than 1 month. These supplements *do not* replace protein, vitamin D, calories, and other nutrients contained in milk, so careful consideration must be given to the total nutrient replacement.
Data from *Handbook for Nutrition Services of the Dietary Department*, The Children's Hospital, Boston, Ma., 1982.

the vitamin C content of preschoolers' diets was found to be well below standard in more than 20 percent of the population [64].

By the age of 3 years, many children have already developed a dislike of certain foods, especially vegetables. Thus, vegetables should be among the first foods introduced to infants before an aversion can develop. With preschoolers, the vegetable dilemma often can be solved by presenting raw vegetables as easy-to-pick-up snack foods. These raw vegetables can begin to accustom toddlers to a good source of fiber in their diets—a practice that may prevent disease in later life. A deficiency of dietary fiber in adult diets has been implicated in constipation, diverticulosis, gallstones, obesity, ischemic heart disease, intestinal polyps, hiatus hernia, and colonic cancer [42]. Burkitt and coworkers encourage an increase in dietary fiber, particularly cereal fiber in childhood [12]. They recommend brown or whole-meal bread together with fiber-rich cereals, especially in children who tend to be constipated (see Chap. 8). The presence of fiber in a food will vary with the age of the food, the plant source, and the amount of processing. For example, white flour contains about 3.5 gm of dietary fiber per 100 gm while 13.5 gm are found in 100 gm of whole-grain flour. Thus, simply altering the type of bread can increase the fiber content by 25 percent.

For the most part, protein is found to be adequate in the diets of preschoolers. Between the ages of 1 and 3 years, children require 23 gm per day or about 1.76 gm/kg [32]. In the Preschool Nutrition Survey, Owen questioned whether protein was "oversold" because many children were getting more protein than they needed [51]. Crawford and associates found protein intakes consistently high at all ages between 6 months and 6 years despite lower caloric levels [16]. They found that 50 percent of the children between the ages 2 and 6 drink low-fat milk, nonfat milk, or a mixture of these milks. They speculated that this practice would decrease caloric intake but increase protein intake. With an increase in protein intake, there is an increased requirement for vitamin B_6.

In a study of vitamin B_6 nutriture of 24 preschoolers, 16 to 17 percent had estimated intakes of less than two-thirds of the RDA [35]. Nine percent of the children seemed to have inadequate vitamin B_6 status as indicated by plasma pyridoxal phosphate levels below 8.5 mg per milliliter. The vitamin B_6 intakes and plasma pyridoxal phosphate levels of children on vitamin supplements were significantly higher. Although the number of children in this study were limited, below-standard vitamin B_6 intakes for preschoolers were also found in the Nationwide Consumption Survey [64]. Thus, for those children not taking supplements, inclusion of good dietary sources of vitamin B_6 is important. Vitamin B_6 is found in wheat germ, organ and muscle meats, pork, whole grain cereals, and bananas.

Energy needs between the ages of 1 and 3 years range from 900 to 1,800 kcal per day (tenth to ninetieth percentile of energy intake—a midpoint of 1,300 kcal per day [32] (see Appendix 1). For children who need increased calories (e.g., children with failure to thrive (see Chap. 9), small amounts of energy-dense foods can be added to their diets (Table 6-7). These children should not be drinking low fat or skim milk.

Beal found the erratic food intakes of toddlers to be associated with changes in growth rate [5]. In fact, poor growth (determined by height measurement) is much more common than obesity in this age group [68]. Although unpredictable appetites make supplying nutrient needs

Table 6-7. Energy Content of Selected Energy-Dense Foods

Type	Calories per tbsp
Powdered, skim milk	25
Powdered, whole milk	31
Evaporated milk, undiluted	41
Condensed milk	64
Cream, heavy, fluid	52
Sour cream	26
Butter, margarine	36
Mayonnaise	101
Oil (corn)	126
Cream cheese	33
Cheese spread*	41
Peanut butter	86
Wheat germ	36
Orange juice crystals, dehydrated	54
Grape juice, frozen, concentrated, sweet, undiluted	52

Note: These foods can be added to foods in small amounts but care must be taken not to overwhelm appetites or digestive systems.
*High in sodium—190 mg per tbsp
Data from J. A. Pennington and H. H. Church, *Food Values of Portions Commonly Used* (13th ed.). Philadelphia: Lippincott, 1980.

a challenge, toddlers, for the most part, are well nourished except for possible deficiencies in calcium, zinc, and vitamins A, C, B_6. The toddler is particularly at high risk for iron deficiency anemia. When calcium needs are being met by dairy products, riboflavin and vitamin A levels are more assured. When heme sources of iron, whole grains, and wheat germ are used, iron, zinc, and B_6 are also provided. When citrus fruits or juices or juices fortified with vitamin C are encouraged, vitamin C stores are repleted and iron absorption is enhanced. Thus, with the proper food sources, nutrient needs can be met (see Table 6-14). With respect to supplementation, the Committee on Nutrition of the American Academy of Pediatrics advises that there is little basis for routine vitamin and mineral supplementation in normal children, especially as the growth rate decreases after infancy. One exception, of course, is fluoride for children without a fluoridated water supply (see Table 5-9). There are some situations, however, in which vitamin supplementation is recommended [3]:

1. Children and adolescents from deprived families, especially those suffering from parental neglect or abuse
2. Children and adolescents with anorexia, poor and capricious appetites, or poor eating habits; also, children on dietary regimens to manage obesity

3. Pregnant teenagers
4. Children and adolescents consuming vegetarian diets without adequate dairy products (vitamin B_{12} is particularly needed)

In order for nutrient needs to be met through diet, special care must be given to food selection, preparation, and the environment. For diet alone to be sufficient, there must be adequate parental education and responsibility. When these prerequisites are missing, vitamin-mineral supplementation should be used. Also, when toddlers are being difficult about the food they will eat, a period of vitamin-mineral supplementation can prevent food battles and relieve mealtime stress. The results of a study of the nutrient intakes of children in the second and sixth grades point to the advisability of supplementing children with vitamins and minerals (including iron) provided the daily supplements do not exceed the recommended allowances [17]. One cannot assume without an evaluation that children are getting enough nutrients from their diets. One also should not assume that vitamins are the panacea for good nutrition. Supplementation is often misused; indeed, one study showed no relationship between the use and need for vitamin supplements [17]. Therefore, the need for supplementation must be decided for each child individually.

DIETARY RISK FACTORS AND THE TODDLER DIET

Because of the growing consensus that the pathological process that results in atherosclerosis begins in childhood, there is a concern about the cholesterol content of the toddler diet and for the safety of cholesterol restriction. Moderate cholesterol consumption is necessary developmentally for the production of bile salt and cell membranes [29, 56]. The cholesterol content of breast milk is high. To date, however, no significant difference in serum cholesterol level has been found when bottle- and breast-fed infants are compared after one year [33] (see Chap. 5).

Friedman and Goldberg evaluated children ranging from birth to age 3 fed a low–saturated fat and low-cholesterol diet [34]. The diet averaged 200 mg of cholesterol per day and provided polyunsaturated–saturated fat ratio of approximately 1 : 1. A matched control group of 3-year-olds not fed the restricted diet was compared with respect to differences in percentile of height and weight, head circumference, skinfold thickness, total serum protein, and hemoglobin. The number of sick visits and failures on the Developmental Screening Test were also quantitated. The only significant difference was a lower serum cholesterol in the experimental group. Diet failed to alter other measured variables.

Eggs and, to some extent, red meat were the dietary components mostly responsible for the association between dietary cholesterol and

Table 6-8. Cholesterol and Fat Content of Selected Foods

Type	Amount	Fat (gm)	Cholesterol (mg)
Beef cuts	1½ oz	7.5	35
Liver (calf, fried)	1½	6.6	204
Bacon (cured, cooked)	2 slices	9.0	13
Bologna	1 oz	8.2	15
Chicken (light meat)	1½ oz	1.45	25.6
Fish	1½ oz	2.7	25–35
Peanut butter	1 tbsp	7.2	—
Egg (boiled)	1 (medium)	5.5	262
Milk, whole (3.25% fat)	8 oz	8.1	34
Milk, lowfat			
(1% fat with nonfat milk solids)	8 oz	2.4	10
Cheese, cheddar	1 oz	9.1	30

Data from J. A. Pennington and H. H. Church, *Food Values of Portions Commonly Used* (13th ed.). Philadelphia: Lippincott, 1980, and R. M. Feeley, et al. Cholesterol content of foods. *J. Am. Diet. Assoc.* 61:134, 1972.

serum cholesterol in 6-year-olds [17]. Whole milk, butter, and cheese intakes were not significantly related. Of practical interest, the activity level during childhood and serum cholesterol level at age 6 were inversely related.

Although a diet devoid of cholesterol is not recommended, there is no evidence of harm from a moderate restriction of cholesterol and fat. Control of these substances appears warranted especially in view of the evidence that atherosclerosis begins in childhood. Cholesterol can be controlled by the use of 1 or 2 percent fat milk, cereal with milk versus eggs for breakfast, and more chicken, fish, or vegetarian-type dinners with beans, lentils, or tofu. Table 6-8 lists the cholesterol and fat content of selected foods.

Like cholesterol, sodium is another nutrient causing concern in the pediatric population. There is increasing evidence that decreased intakes of sodium in childhood may help to prevent hypertension in later life. From birth, the prevention of obesity and the avoidance of a high-sodium diet should be considered for children, especially those born into hypertensive families [26].

In societies where there is little or no sodium in the diet, hypertension is virtually absent [45, 52]. Hypertension most likely would be absent from a population with extremely low levels of sodium intake (less than 400 mg per day) [52]. Data suggest that the time of life when an individual is exposed to high sodium intake also may be important. From experimental work on rats, Dahl and coworkers have postulated a critical time period in early life during which a high salt intake may be particularly harmful [19].

Table 6-9. Sodium Intakes with Age
Compared to Safe and Adequate Intakes

Group	Sodium (mg)	Estimated Safe and Adequate* Daily Dietary Intakes of Sodium (mg)
6 MONTHS		
White	622	
Black	831	
Oriental	611	
		250–750
1 YEAR		
White	1,168	
Black	1,426	
Oriental	1,074	
2 YEARS		
White	1,453	
Black	1,885	
Oriental	1,471	
		325–975
3 YEARS		
White	1,537	
Black	1,998	
Oriental	1,466	

*Because there is less information on which to base allowances, these figures are not given in the main table of RDA and are provided here in the form of ranges of recommended intakes.
Data from Food and Nutrition Board, *Recommended Daily Dietary Allowances,* Revised 1980, National Academy of Sciences, National Research Council, and D. B. Crawford, J. H. Hankin, and R. L. Hunneman, Environmental factors associated with preschool obesity III. Dietary intakes, eating patterns and anthropometric measurements. *J. Am. Diet. Assoc.* 72:589, 1978.

Although there is no evidence yet for a critical stage concerning sodium intake in humans, a prudent approach to sodium is warranted. Sodium intake is relatively low when infants are fed human milk, prepared formula, and infants' foods, but it increases greatly with the progression to cow's milk and table food (see Chap. 5). The impact of table foods on sodium intake is not due to the amount of food consumed but rather to the amount of salt in selected foods [73]. Crawford and associates found that, black children had consistently higher intakes of sodium at all ages. Their high intakes were possibly related to the frequent use of undiluted canned soups [17]. Sodium intake tends to increase with age and often exceeds the National Research Council recommendations for sodium (Table 6-9; Appendix 3). Thus the impact of salt-free commercial infant foods is small and of short duration.

With respect to salt preference, experiments with adults showed that discrimination, sensitivity, perceived intensity, preference, and responses to salt were independent behavioral measures [53]. How-

Table 6-10. Sodium Content of Commonly Used Toddler Foods

Food	Amount	Sodium (mg)
American cheese	1 oz	318
Bologna	1 slice	374
Bugles (General Mills)	1 oz	272
Cheese Goldfish (Pepperidge Farm)	10 pieces	117
Chicken rice soup (canned)	1 serving (218 gm)	730
Oyster Crackers	10	145
Potato Sticks	1 oz	280
Pretzel (3 ring)	1	54
Ritz (Nabisco)	3 crackers	97
Spaghetti with tomato sauce and cheese	1 serving (250 gm)	955
Tomato soup (canned) made with water	1 serving (198 gm)	805
Tortilla Chips (Frito-Lay)	1 oz	99

Data from J. A. Pennington and H. H. Church, *Food Values of Portions Commonly Used* (13th ed.). Philadelphia: Lippincott, 1980.

ever, there are few data on the development of salt preference in children. Foman found no differences in intake of salted infant food over unsalted food [31]. However, by age 2 it appears that heavier use of salt in some foods, such as soup, increases the amount consumed [8]. By 4 years, salty pretzels are preferred to plain pretzels. It would appear that salt preference is a learned behavior that is influenced by the type of food to which the child is exposed [7]. Therefore, children can and should be accustomed to foods without added salt (e.g.) unsalted crackers and popcorn). Canned soups and other canned foods such as spaghetti and high-sodium foods such as luncheon meats should be used prudently (Table 6-10).

Careful consideration should also be given to the use of table salt. Although iodized salt is a major contributor of iodine, other incidental sources such as dough conditioners, alginates, and dyes along with natural sources in seafood and milk contribute an abundance of iodine to the diet. Therefore replacing salt with herbs, spices, and lemon juice should not compromise iodine status. When there is a concern for adequate iodine, as there is for people living in endemic goiter regions around the Great Lakes in the United States, a reduction in salt intake could possibly pose a problem. Families living in these regions should be made aware of this and encourage foods that are high in iodine.

As a nation, we use too much salt. Adults consume an estimated 20 to 50 times the amount of salt needed and, as seen in Table 6-10, infants and toddlers far exceed their requirements as well. Because Americans consume more sodium than they need, the USDA's Food Safety and Inspection Service, in conjunction with the FDA and the Heart, Lung, and Blood Institute, has launched a program to educate

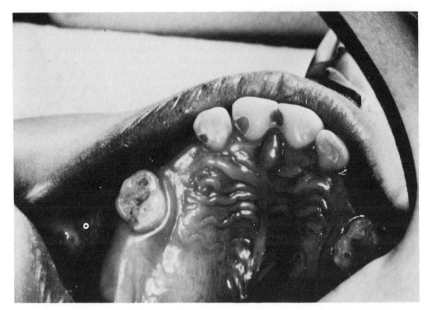

Figure 6-2. Nursing bottle caries in an 18-month-old breast-fed toddler. This condition usually occurs in prolonged bottle feeding. (Courtesy of Norman Budde, D.M.D.)

consumers about sodium in the diet, to encourage sodium labeling of food products, and to research ways of decreasing the sodium content of processed foods.

The sugar content of the American diet must also be decreased. Although the pathological potential of sugar in dental disease has been demonstrated with certainty, there is much speculation (but no definitive evidence) about its role in obesity, alteration in blood lipids and glucose metabolism, chronic nonspecific diarrhea, recurrent abdominal pain in childhood, and disturbances in childhood behavior.

Carbohydrates provide an essential substrate for bacterial initiation of dental caries [47]. The decreasing order of cariogenicity of carbohydrates is sucrose, glucose, maltose, lactose, fructose, and sorbitol. Certain acidogenic bacteria in dental plaque, such as streptococci and lactobacilli, act upon monosaccharides and disaccharides producing lactic acid, which decalcifies the enamel. Parents who add sugar to milk or formula create a greater risk for dental caries. The greatest carious activity in the primary teeth occurs between the ages of 4 and 8 years, but young children who fall asleep while sucking a bottle or those breast-feeding or bottle-feeding for prolonged periods are candidates for caries (Fig. 6-2). During sleep, the rate of sucking, swallowing, and salivary secretion decreases so that carbohydrates present

Table 6-11. Nutritious Snacks

Food	Examples
Thirst quenchers	Fruit juices; milk; protein shake (½ cup milk, ½ cup orange juice, ¼ cup powdered milk); milkshakes made with milk and fruit (i.e., bananas and milk, or yogurt and fruit); Popsicles made from fruit juice
Finger fruits	Orange sections; banana disks; apple, pear, or peach slices; pineapple chunks; dried apricots, dates, raisins, figs;* cherries; berries
Finger vegetables	Cherry tomatoes; carrot and celery sticks; cucumber and zucchini wedges; green pepper strips
Spread-ons	Peanut butter; nut butters; yogurt or tofu dips
Other	Yogurt with fruit and wheat germ sprinkled on top; cottage cheese with cinnamon spread on raisin toast and broiled; whole grain crackers or toast; popcorn without salt (sprinkle lightly with Parmesan cheese)
Occasional sweets	Pumpkin, squash or custard pie; oatmeal, peanut butter, molasses, or gingerbread cookies

*Dried fruits are retentive on tooth surfaces and are therefore cariogenic. These are best given with meals so that children can brush afterward.
Adapted from Cronk, C., and Howard, R. B. Growth and Nutrition. In R. B. Howard and N. H. Herbold, *Nutrition in Clinical Care* (2nd ed.). New York: McGraw-Hill, 1982.

in the juice or milk remain in contact with the teeth for a prolonged period of time and promote the formation of lactic acid. Thus, children should not be put to bed with bottles containing milk or juice. Also, because it appears that postnatal experiences can influence response to sweets [6], attention should be given to the sugar content of toddlers' diets.

Among preschoolers Crawford and associates found that 87 percent of mothers reported their children like sweets the best, but only 15 percent wished that their children would eat fewer sweets [16]. So although parents may like their children to eat fewer sweets, they seem to continue to provide them. Also, the use of presweetened cereals is pervasive. Some of these cereals are more than 50 percent sugar. Obviously, parents need some concrete guidelines concerning the use of sugar in their children's diets. They should be encouraged to read labels and to select foods with lower sugar content, such as homemade juice pops instead of Popsicles or fruits packed in natural juices. In addition, parents need some direction in selecting nutritious snacks (Table 6-11). They also need help in developing a functional rather than a rigid approach to sugar intake. Parents should be aware that if they become obsessive about sugar restriction, this can make sugar-containing foods all the more attractive to children. Sugar can then become a tool that children use to manipulate their anxious parents.

When foods with sugar are allowed, they should be presented with meals because it is usually easier to get children to brush and floss their teeth after a meal. Sticky and chewy varieties of sugary foods should be avoided along with other foods or candies (lollipops, gum with sugar, breath mints) that maximize the exposure of teeth to sugar. Fluoride is the active agent in caries prevention. Therefore, fluoridated water should become part of meals, and juice concentrate versus canned, bottled, or reconstituted juices should be used to take advantage of fluoridated water supplies. Children without access to a fluoridated water supply should be given a fluoride supplement (See Table 5-9).

Whether or not sugar in the toddler diet contributes to obesity is speculative, but the presence of obesity among preschoolers is real. The prevalence varies from 7 percent [66] to 12.2 percent depending on the criteria used [37]. Although a single cause of preschool obesity cannot be isolated, families that provide good role models are important in prevention (See Chap. 10). Family therapy is increasingly recognized as a major component in combatting weight problems in children. It appears that eating disorders are more likely to surface when parents exhibit some form of status discrepancy, limit the communication within the family and with friends, direct children without an awareness of developmental needs, and inconsistently use foods to exhibit affection and discipline [39]. The probability of successful treatment for obesity is increased by improving family-living and parenting skills, but attention to diet and exercise must be incorporated into the therapy program. Attention to diet and exercises should be an ongoing part of well-child care and become important to family members. Energy (calorie) control should be encouraged as part of prudent food selection (Table 6-12); families should be encouraged to be active together. In certain conditions such as Prader-Willi syndrome or Down syndrome where excessive weight becomes manifest in early childhood, weight reduction may be necessary. However, weight loss should not exceed 1 pound of body weight per week.

During the early years, games and toys that promote movement should be selected for toddlers, and their burgeoning interests should be directed toward athletics. Parents should be encouraged to walk, run, swim, and dance with their children. In order to promote prudent diets, they should be encouraged to screen all food brought into their household according to the Dietary Guidelines for Americans (Table 6-13). It is possible to meet the toddlers' nutrient needs and control dietary risk factors by using these guidelines.

Table 6-12. Food Selection for Energy Control

Food	Amount	Energy (kcal)	Food	Amount	Energy (kcal)
Milk, whole (3.7% fat)	8 oz	161	Milk, low fat (1% fat)	8 oz	102
Cottage cheese (2% fat)	½ cup	101	Cottage cheese (1% fat)	½ cup	81
Cube steak	1 oz	74	Chicken, light meat, no skin	1 oz	47.4
Hamburger, medium fat, cooked	1 patty (85 gm)	224	Hamburger, lean fat, cooked	1 patty (86 gm)	140
Sugar Frosted Flakes (Kellogg)	1 cup	141	Puffed Rice (Quaker)	1 cup	54
Vienna Finger Sandwich (Sunshine)	1 cookie	72	Graham cracker	1 cracker	27
Blueberry Muffin	1 average	112	White, enriched bread, toast	1 slice	62
French toast	1 slice	119	Cinnamon raisin bread	1 slice	68
Margarine	1 tsp	36	Diet margarine	1 tsp	16
Mayonnaise	1 tbsp	101	Diet mayonnaise	1 tbsp	50
Orange juice drink	4 oz	65.5	Orange juice (2 oz juice + 2 oz water)	4 oz	28

Data from J. A. Pennington and H. H. Church, *Food Values of Portions Commonly Used* (13th ed.). Philadelphia:Lippincott, 1980.

Table 6-13. Dietary Guidelines for Americans

Eat a variety of food
Maintain ideal weight
Avoid too much fat, saturated fat, and cholesterol
Eat foods with adequate starch and fiber
Avoid too much sugar
Avoid too much sodium
If you drink alcohol, do so in moderation

Source: U. S. Department of Agriculture and Health, Education and Welfare. *Nutrition and Your Health: Dietary Guidelines for Americans.* Washington, D.C.: U. S. Government Printing Office, 1981.

THE DIETARY GUIDELINES AND TODDLERS

The Dietary Guidelines for Americans [65] evolved from the Dietary Goals for the United States first issued by the Senate Select Committee on Nutrition in 1977 [69]. The Dietary Goals recommend specific dietary levels for the type and amount of fat, protein, and carbohydrate and the amount of cholesterol and sodium to be consumed with the recommendation to achieve energy balance. They produced a vigorous debate on the benefits and possible nutritional risks that might come about from such specificity. In the summer of 1979, the first Surgeon General's Report on Health Promotion and Disease Prevention was published [67]. It stated that given what is already known or strongly suspected about the relationship between diet and disease, Americans would probably be healthier if they followed certain dietary guidelines. At this time, the Dietary Guidelines were jointly released by the USDA and the Department of Health, Education, and Welfare. While the Dietary Guidelines for Americans are more general than the Dietary Goals, arguments against them center on the role of the government in issuing dietary advice and the lack of conclusive evidence on the role of saturated fat and cholesterol in heart disease and sodium intake in hypertension. However, with mounting evidence concerning diet and heart disease and recent information on the relationship of sugar, salt, fat, and alcohol to cancer [48], there is more support for the Dietary Guidelines. With respect to applicability of the guidelines for children, the Select Panel for the Promotion of Child Health stated, "the Panel finds the guidelines to be prudent advice to Americans about nutritionally sound diets and applicable to the needs of children and pregnant women" [68]. However, because of the multiplicity of influences on the food intake of children, parents need more advice than the Dietary Guidelines. They need a strategy to control the amount of fat, salt, and sugar in their families' diet. It is not enough to say "eat less fat, salt, and sugar" without providing more specific advice.

Table 6-14 summarizes toddler food needs and provides suggestions for avoiding dietary risk factors.

Table 6-14. Toddler Foods and Dietary Risk Factors

Food Group	Servings Per Day	Toddler Serving Size	Dietary Risk Control
MILK OR EQUIVALENTS ½ cup milk equals: 2 tbsp powdered milk ¼ cup evaporated milk	3 or more	4–6 oz	Use lower fat milk products
1 oz of cheese[a]		½–¾ oz	
1 serving custard (4 servings from 1 pint milk) ½ cup milk pudding ½ cup yogurt		¼–½ cup	
MEAT, FISH, POULTRY OR EQUIVALENTS 1 oz of meat equals:	2	1–2 oz	Use more chicken, fish. Bake, broil, and trim visible fat. Avoid processed meats (luncheon meat) and canned meats due to high fat and sodium contents. Avoid cured meats due to nitrates
1 egg		1	Limit to 3 eggs per week
1 oz cheese		½–¾ oz	Use low-fat cheese (i.e., Swiss or skim mozarella)
4 tbsp cottage cheese		1–2 tbsp	Use low-fat cottage cheese
4 tbsp peanut butter		1–2 tbsp	Use unsalted and without added corn syrup. Sandwiches can be made with a variety of nut butters and fruit (i.e., peanut butter and minced apple on whole grain bread)
1 cup legumes (beans, garbanzos, lentils, peas)		¼–⅓ cup	
4 oz soy cheese or curd		1 oz	Vegetarian casseroles can be made with tofu or complementary proteins such as beans and rice
1½ tbsp nuts and seeds[b]		½–1 tbsp	

Table 6-14 (Continued)

Food Group	Servings Per Day	Toddler Serving Size	Dietary Risk Control
VEGETABLES AND FRUITS	4 or more		
Vegetables include:			
1 green or yellow daily		4 tbsp (cooked)	Avoid canned vegetables or let them stand in water before cooking to remove some of the salt
Fruit juice include:			
citrus daily		4 oz	Avoid fruit drinks
Fruit:			
canned		4–8 tbsp	Use canned fruits packed in natural juices
raw		½–1 (small)	Use for snacks and desserts to promote fiber in the diet
GRAINS, WHOLE GRAINS, ENRICHED	3–4		
Whole grain or enriched white bread		½–1 slice	Whole grain higher in fiber
Cooked cereal		¼–½ cup	
Ready-to-serve dry cereals		½–1 cup	Select cereals with low sugar contents
Spaghetti, macaroni, noodles, rice		¼–½ cup	Use whole grain pasta, brown rice
Crackers		2–3	Select crackers without salted tops

[a]When cheese is used as a milk equivalent, it cannot be counted as a meat equivalent also.
[b]Since children do not develop good rotary chewing until about age 2½ years, nuts and seeds should be presented as butters until good chewing skills are developed.

VEGETARIAN DIETS FOR TODDLERS

Vegetarianism has been gaining a new acceptance over this past decade. Many of these so-called new vegetarians [20] were once omnivores and belonged to philosophical and quasi-religious groups during the 1960s [54]. There is much individuality in their food proscriptions as well as in the reasons they espouse vegetarianism. Although health appears to be the overriding incentive, they are drawn to vegetarianism for ethical, metaphysical, ecological, and political reasons, as well as by their own food preferences [20]. They practice varying degrees of vegetarianism usually with emphasis on natural or organically grown foods, and embrace a spectrum of diets and lifestyles that defy classification.

Traditionally, the term *vegetarianism* was used to describe an individual whose diet consisted mainly of plant foods (one who abstained from the consumption of meat, fowl, and fish with or without the additional proscription on eggs or dairy foods). Vegetarians could be classified according to their consumption of animal foods (Table 6-15). But in today's culture the term *vegetarian* is used loosely and may be used to describe one who only avoids red meat. Thus, there is a need to clarify the extent of food proscriptions and other idiosyncratic convictions that might influence food intake.

In general, as vegetarian diets become less restrictive, the probability of meeting nutrient requirements increases. Vegetarianism, per se, is not a concern, but the extremism with which it is practiced and the age at which it begins may present problems. The attendant nutritional risks increase as animal products are excluded. Therefore, children in vegetarian families where dairy products (lactovegetarians) and eggs (lacto-ovovegetarians) are consumed can meet all of their nutrient needs, but iron levels may be insufficient.

Although iron is contained in legumes, green leafy vegetables, whole and enriched grains, cereals and breads, and some nuts and dried fruits consumed by vegetarian children, the small amount con-

Table 6-15. Classification of Vegetarians

Type	Food Allowed
Lacto-ovovegetarians	Milk, eggs, cheese, vegetables, fruits, grains, nuts, legumes
Lactovegetarian	Milk, cheese, vegetables, fruits, grains, nuts, legumes
Total vegetarian or vegan	Vegetables, fruits, grains, nuts, legumes
Fruitarian	Raw or dried fruit, nuts, honey, olive oil

sumed and the availability of the nonheme iron in foods are the cause for concern. Ascorbic acid and reducing sugars enhance iron absorption, but milk, eggs, and cheese may depress the intake of nonheme iron, further compromising iron. Because of the lack of heme iron in the diet, vegetarian children should be monitored for iron deficiency and maintenance doses of iron may be needed. Monson and coworkers determined how to calculate absorbable iron from different types of meals [46].

Unlike lacto-vegetarian or lacto-ovovegetarian children, the vegan (total vegetarian) child or vegan macrobiotic child is presented with more serious health risks (see p. 137). Dwyer and coworkers found that preschool children consuming a macrobiotic diet ingested marginal amounts of vitamin D, calcium, and phosphorus. These children were more likely to have possible signs of rickets [22]. In addition, macrobiotic children differed in size from other vegetarian children, with deficits in length, weight, and hemoglobin [21]. Another study analyzing 24-hour recalls of vegetarian children found deficiencies of riboflavin, vitamin D, vitamin B_{12}, and calcium in macrobiotic children, especially vegan macrobiotics [23]. Again, vegan macrobiotic children were found to have the lowest intake of vitamins B_{12} and D in an analysis of preschoolers consuming different kinds of vegetarian diets.

Reports on children with vegan diets vary from physical measurements within normal limits [24] to below standard growth [36]. However there are dietary risks to consider with all vegan children. Before explaining these risks to parents, the motivating force drawing them to vegetarianism shoud be understood so that foods supporting the nutritional needs of the child as well as the social and psychological needs of the parents can be selected. A major problem in meeting the nutrient needs is the small stomach volume of the child. The bulk of the unprocessed food and the amount that a toddler must consume to obtain adequate nutrition makes it difficult for the child to eat enough to meet energy needs, which then compromises protein status. To provide the needed energy and spare the protein reserved for growth, a small amount of vegetable oils (which also provide essential fatty acids that are minimally present in some vegan diets), mashed avocado, or margarine fortified with vitamin A can be added to toddler foods. To further protect the protein, special attention must be given to the use of complementary proteins at meals, such as rice with legumes. By combining the essential amino acids that are limited in one food but present in another, the biological value of the protein can be improved (Table 6-16).

Complementing proteins works in theory, but the developmental characteristics of the toddler, known for finicky appetite and unrefined

Table 6-16. Complementary Proteins

Food group	Complementary proteins
Legumes	Legumes and rice Soybeans, rice, and wheat Beans and wheat Soybeans, corn, and milk Beans and corn Soybeans, wheat, and sesame seeds Soybeans, peanuts, and sesame seeds Soybeans, sesame seeds, and wheat
Grains	Rice and legumes Corn and legumes Wheat and legumes Rice and milk Wheat and cheese Wheat and milk Wheat, peanuts, and milk Wheat, sesame seeds, and soybeans Brewer's yeast and rice
Vegetables	Lima beans, Peas, Brussels sprouts, Cauliflower, Broccoli } and sesame seeds, brazil nuts, mushrooms
Nuts and seeds	Peanuts, sesame seeds, and soybeans Sesame seeds and beans Sesame seeds, soybeans, and wheat Peanuts and milk Peanuts and sunflower seeds Peanuts, wheat, and milk Sesame seeds, wheat, and soybeans

Source: Howard, R. B., and Herbold, N. H. *Nutrition In Clinical Care* (2nd ed.). New York: McGraw-Hill, 1982. Adapted from F. M. Lappe, *Diet for a Small Planet*, Friends of the Earth/Ballantine Books, Inc., New York, 1971.

chewing skills, can make getting the proper mix of amino acids a more complicated task. However, when a wide variety of plant proteins such as seeds and legumes are included, the amino acid pattern of the children's diets is likely to be satisfactory [36].

All legumes should be cooked and mashed. Nuts should be presented as butters (i.e., peanut butter) to spread on bread, and cereals and grains should be milled to maximize nitrogen absorption.

Obtaining adequate vitamin B_{12} from an all-plant diet is as challenging as obtaining adequate protein. Because there are no vegetable sources of vitamin B_{12}, vegan children are very much at risk for deficiencies. An all plant diet needs vitamin B_{12} supplementation. Even if a child continues to be breast-fed, if the mother is a vegan and has been so for some time, there is a risk of vitamin B_{12} deficiency [70]. Vegan mothers should receive vitamin B_{12} supplements. Other sources of vitamin B_{12} for vegan children are soy milk supplements with B_{12} and nutritional yeast. Although some parents are opposed to commercial formulas because of the processing, these soy formulas provide a readily available source of vitamin B_{12} and protein as well as other vitamins and minerals. Soy formulas must be well processed to inactivate the enzyme inhibitors present in raw soybeans. Also, they must be supplemented with L-methionine to maximize the protein quality [30]. For this reason, home-prepared formulas made from grinding soybeans are of dubious nutritional value. They do not provide a source of vitamin B_{12} unless they are fortified. If yeast is used as a source of vitamin B_{12}, it must be grown on a proper media or fortified with vitamin B_{12}. The yeast can be added to soy formulas or foods consumed by the toddler. Yeast also contains some protein, B vitamins, choline, and trace elements. However, it does not help offset the notable deficit of vitamin D in vegan toddlers who do not drink a supplemented soy formula. (The endogenous production of vitamin D cannot be counted on to replace the dietary inadequacy.)

When parents are opposed to using a soy formula, a vitamin D supplement (400 IU daily) or fish oil must be used to prevent deficiencies, and other dietary sources of calcium and riboflavin must be found. Unfortunately, large volumes of plant food must be consumed to achieve the amount of riboflavin and calcium found in one cup of milk (which increases the phytate and oxylate content of the diet) (Table 6-17). The phytates in whole grains and nuts tend to form zinc-phytate complexes that inhibit zinc absorption. Recently, an equation for assessing dietary zinc bioavailability was developed that can be used to estimate the relative risk of zinc inadequacy [49]. Phytates also inhibit calcium absorption. In addition, some vegetables, notably spinach, chard, and beet greens, contain oxalic acid that combines with calcium oxalate and is excreted in the feces. Phytates and oxalates are not likely to interfere with calcium utilization if their concentrations in the diet are low relative to the calcium content of the diet. However, with vegan diets the ratio is high, so this is another added nutritional concern. The high fiber content increases the transit time through the gut, and phytate content can additionally interfere with the absorption of phosphorus and iron. Thus, phosphorus and iron are further compromised because the nature of the vegan diet lends itself to a diet already low in rich sources of phosphorus (milk, meat, fish, poultry, eggs) and contains no heme food sources of iron. As with other deficiencies in vegan diets, an awareness of the potential prob-

Table 6-17. Calcium and Riboflavin in Plant Food
Equivalent to One Cup of Milk

Calcium Equivalents to 291 mg Ca	Riboflavin Equivalents to 0.395 mg B$_2$
1 cup calcium-fortified soy milk	1 oz fortified cereal
1 cup broccoli, collards	1 avocado
1 cup almonds	1¼ cups broccoli
1¼ cup turnip greens	1¼ cups mushrooms, fresh
1½ cup kale, mustard greens	1¼ cups turnip greens, cooked
1⅔ cup sunflower seeds	1½ cups winter squash
2 cups beet greens	1¾ cups asparagus
2 cups quick cooking, enriched farina	1¾ cups spinach, cooked
3 cups dried beans	2 cups brussels sprouts
3 pieces enriched cornbread	2¼ cups okra

Adapted from *Vegetarian Nutrition.* National Dairy Council, Rosemont, Ill. 60018, 1979.

lem can prevent deficiencies and preserve the beneficial qualities that vegetarian diets can offer, including the opportunity to control weight and the dietary risk factors of saturated fat, cholesterol, and sodium. Table 6-18 summarizes the foods and amounts that can be used in diets of vegetarian children to achieve optimal nutritional status.

Dwyer and colleagues studied the diets of 39 preschoolers consuming different types of vegetarian diets. They found that the type and amount of carbohydrate, fat, and protein and the amount of sodium and cholesterol provided by their diets were closer to levels suggested by the Dietary Goals than amounts found in the diets of nonvegetarian children [24]. Serum cholesterol levels were low for the group. Similar beneficial effects have been found with adults. In fact, compared to a normal mixed diet, the vegan diet contained a high polyunsaturated-saturated ratio, a low concentration of saturated fat and cholesterol, and a high concentration of dietary fiber and plant sterols. It was felt that these factors probably contributed to such findings as low blood pressure and normal to low body weights for age among vegans [1]. It appears that lacto-ovovegetarian diets may be beneficial in the control of bone mineral losses in later years [44]. Bergan and Brown found "new vegetarians" to be lean and well nourished, except for potential problems with riboflavin and iron [9].

Vegetarian diets may be the diet of the future on a planet with limited resources and an expanding population. Vegetarian diets are no longer considered fad diets but are becoming part of our culture and are here to stay. Children can grow and thrive on well-planned vegetarian diets.

Table 6-18. Food Sources for Vegetarian Toddlers

Food Group	Food Sources	Standard Servings	Toddler Servings
Milk (3 toddler servings, 2–3 standard servings)	Milk	1 cup	½–¾ cup
	Soy milk	1 cup	½–¾ cup
	Cottage cheese	4 tbsp	1–2 tbsp
	Cheese	1 oz	½–¾ oz
	Yogurt	1 cup	½–¾ cup
Vegetable protein* (2 toddler servings)	Cooked legumes (beans, soybeans, lentils, chick peas)	1 cup	¼ serving
	Textured vegetable protein,	20–30 gm, dry	
	meat analogues,	2–3 oz	
	soy cheese or curd (tofu)	4 oz	
	Peanut butter, nuts, seeds	4 tbsp 1½ tbsp	¼ serving
Animal protein (3 week)	Eggs	1	1
Fruits and vegetables (4 or more toddler servings) Fruits (include citrus daily)	Cooked fruit	½ cup	4 tbsp
	Raw fruit	1 cup	½ cup
	Dried apricots	5 halves	2–3 halves
Vegetables (include dark green, deep yellow daily)	Cooked vegetables	½ cup	4 tbsp
	Raw vegetables	1 cup	Few pieces
Grains, (Whole grain or enriched, 3–4 toddler servings)	Whole grain or enriched bread	1 slice	½–1 slice
	Cooked cereal	½–¾ cup	¼–½ cup
	Ready-to-serve dry cereal	¾–1 cup	½–1 cup
	Spaghetti, macaroni, rice, noodles	½–¾ cup	¼–½ cup
	Crackers	4	2–3
Energy sources (added to foods to provide sufficient energy and protect protein reserved for growth)	Fat: margarine, butter, vegetable oils, avocado		
	Sweeteners: molasses, maple syrup, honey, sugar, apple butter, fruit preserves		

Table 6-18 (Continued)

Food Group	Food Sources	Standard Servings	Toddler Servings
Other nutrient sources	Brewer's yeast: vitamin B_{12}, other B vitamins, protein, choline		
	Fish oil: vitamin D		
	Bone meal: Calcium, phosphorus, protein		

Note: Standard servings are provided to indicate the amount considered appropriate to provide the needed nutrients from each food group.
*Vegetarian recipes that utilize complementary protein can be found in a variety of cookbooks; for example: Ewald, E. B. *Recipes for a Small Planet.* New York: Ballantine Books, 1973, and Robertson, L., et al. *Laurel's Kitchen.* Petaluma, California: Nilgiri Press, 1981.
Data from Vhymeister, I. B., et al. Safe vegetarian diets for children. *Pediatr. Clin. North Am.* 24(1):207, 1977, and Smith, E.V. A guide to good eating the vegetarian way. *J. Nutr. Ed.* 7:109, 1978.

CONCLUSION

Toddler autonomy, nutrient needs, and dietary risk factors can combine forces at mealtime to confront parents. In this milieu, parents may be tempted to simply open a can "to get dinner over," or their "nagging nutritional conscience" may prompt them to prepare a nourishing meal. For their conscience to win out, they need to know that nutrition is important to their family's health.

When mothers were asked, "Who has been advising you on how to feed your child at his or her present age?" most mothers, responded, "no one" or "the doctor" [4]. Parents need guidance in choosing foods for their toddlers so that nutrient needs can be met without creating dietary risk factors. Parents must be made aware of the importance of restricting excess fat, salt, sugar, and additives. Pediatricians are in a position to guide this process and set the course for nutritional health.

REFERENCES

1. Abdulla, M., et al. Nutrient intake and health status of vegans. *Am. J. Clin. Nutr.* 34:2464, 1981.
2. Action for Children's Television. Personal communication, Nov. 1982.
3. American Academy of Pediatrics Committe on Nutrition. Vitamin and mineral supplement needs in normal children in the United States. *Pediatrics* 66:1015, 1980.
4. Andrew, E., et al. Infant feeding practices of families belonging to a pre-paid practice health care plan. *Pediatrics* 65:978, 1980.
5. Beal, V. Dietary intake of individuals followed through infancy and childhood. *Am. J. Public Health* 51:1107, 1961.

6. Beauchamp, G. K. Ontogenesis of taste preference. Presented at the Fifth International Organization for the Study of Human Development. Campione, Italy, May, 1980.
7. Beauchamp, G. K. The development of taste in infancy. In J. T. Ond, L. J. Filer, G. A. Leveille, A. Thompson, and W. B. Weil (Eds.), *Infant and Early Childhood Feeding.* New York: Academic Press, 1981. Pp. 413-426.
8. Beauchamp, G. K., and Maller, O. The Development of Flavor Preference in Humans: A Review. In M. R. Kare, and O. Maller (Eds.), *The Chemical Senses and Nutrition.* New York: Academic Press, 1977. Pp. 292-315.
9. Bergan, J. G., and Brown, P. T. Nutritional status of new vegetarians. *J. Am. Diet. Assoc.* 76:151, 1980.
10. Berkelhamer, M., et al. Kwashiorkor in Chicago. *Am. J. Dis. Child.* 129:1240, 1975.
11. Brown, P. T., and Bergan, J. G. The dietary status of the new vegetarians. *J. Am. Diet. Assoc.* 67:455, 1975.
12. Burkitt, D., et al. Dietary fibre in under- and overnutrition in childhood. *Arch. Dis. Child.* 55:803, 1980.
13. Centers, R., and Centers, J. Social character, types and beliefs about child rearing. *Child Dev.* 34:69, 1963.
14. Clarke, F. C. Consumer buying habits: A study revisited. *Snack Food,* p. 28, April 1978.
15. Cook, C. C., and Payne, I. R. Effects of supplements on the nutrient intake of children. *J. Am. Diet. Assoc.* 74:130, 1979.
16. Crawford, P. B., et al. Environmental factors associated with pre-school obesity. III. Dietary intake, eating patterns and anthropometric measurements. *J. Am. Diet. Assoc.* 72:589, 1978.
17. Crawford, P. B., et al. Serum cholesterol of 6-year-olds in relation to environmental factors. *J. Am. Diet Assoc.* 78:41, 1981.
18. Crest shows restaurant type influences dollar sales. *N.R.A. News* 17:A (No. 6), 1977.
19. Dahl, L. K., et al. Effects of chronic excess salt ingestion: Modifications of experimental hypertension in the rat fed by variations of salt. *Circ. Res.* 22:11, 1968.
20. Dwyer, J. T., et al. The new vegetarians. *J. Am. Diet. Assoc.* 62:503, 1973.
21. Dwyer, J. T., et al. Pre-schoolers on alternative life style diets. *J. Am. Diet. Assoc.* 72:264, 1978.
22. Dwyer, J. T., et al. Risk of nutritional rickets among vegetarian children. *Am. J. Dis. Child.* 133:134, 1979.
23. Dwyer, J. T., et al. Mental age and I.Q. of predominantly vegetarian children. *J. Am. Diet. Assoc.* 76:142, 1980.
24. Dwyer, J. T., et al. Nutritional status of vegetarian children. *Am. J. Clin. Nutr.* 35:204, 1982.
25. Edidin, D. V., et al. Resurgence of nutritional rickets associated with breast feeding and special dietary practices. *Pediatrics* 65:232, 1980.
26. Ellison, R. C., et al. Pediatrics aspects of essential hypertension. *J. Am. Diet. Assoc.* 80:1, 1982.
27. Eppright, E. S., et al. Eating behavior of the preschool child. *J. Nutr. Ed.* 1:16, 1969.
28. Federal Trade Commission. *Staff Report on T.V. Advertising to Children.* Washington, D.C., Feb. 1978.
29. Fomon, S. J. A pediatrician looks at early nutrition. *Bull. N.Y. Acad. Med.* 47:569, 1971.
30. Fomon, S. J. *Infant Nutrition* (2nd ed.). Philadelphia: Saunders, 1974. Pp. 378-390.

31. Fomon, S. J., et al. Acceptance of unsalted strained foods by normal infants. *J. Pediatr.* 76:242, 1970.
32. Food and Nutrition Board. *Recommended Dietary Allowances* (rev. 9th ed.). Washington, D.C.: National Academy of Sciences, 1980.
33. Friedman, G., and Goldberg, S. J. Concurrent and subsequent serum cholesterol of breast and formula fed infants. *Am. J. Clin. Nutr.* 28:42, 1975.
34. Friedman, G., and Goldberg, S. J. How safe is a modified fat diet in infancy. *Pediatrics* 58:655, 1978.
35. Fries, M. E., et al. Vitamin B_6 status of a group of pre-school children. *Am. J. Clin. Nutr.* 34:2706, 1981.
36. Fulton, J. R., et al. Pre-school vegetarian children. *J. Am. Diet. Assoc.* 76:360, 1980.
37. Ginsberg-Fellner, F., et al. Overweight and obesity in pre-school children in New York City. *Am. J. Clin. Nutr.* 34:2236, 1981.
38. Hambridge, K. M., et al. Zinc nutrition of pre-school children in the Denver Head Start Program. *Am. J. Clin. Nutr.* 29:734, 1976.
39. Hertzler, A. Obesity-impact of the family. *J. Am. Diet. Assoc.* 79:525, 1981.
40. Hertzler, A., et al. Classifying cultural food habits and meanings. *J. Am. Diet. Assoc.* 80:421, 1982.
41. Kawla, J. Marketing snack food. *Marketing Communications*, May 1978. P. 48.
42. Lebenthal, E., et al. Carbohydrates in pediatric nutrition, consumption, digestibility and disease. *Adv. Pediatr.* 28:99, 1981.
43. Lozoff, B., and Farnloff, A. A. Kwashiorkor: In Cleveland. *Am. J. Dis. Child.* 129:710, 1975.
44. Marsh, A. G. Cortical bone density of adult lacto-ovo-vegetarian and omnivorous women. *J. Am. Diet. Assoc.* 76:148, 1980.
45. Meneely, G. R. and Attarbee, H. D. High sodium-low potassium environment and hypertension. *Am. J. Cardiol.* 38:768, 1978.
46. Monson, E. R., et al. Estimation of available dietary iron. *Am. J. Clin. Nutr.* 31:134, 1978.
47. Newbrun, E. Sucrose, the archcriminal of dental caries. *J. Dent. Child* 35:239, 1969.
48. Nutrition and Cancer National Research Council, Committee on Diet. *Nutrition and Cancer.* Washington, D.C.: National Academy Press, 1982.
49. Oberleas, D., and Harland, B. F. Phytate content of foods: Effect on dietary zinc bioavailability. *J. Am. Diet. Assoc.* 79:433, 1981.
50. One member in 94% of all U.S. families eats out every 2.8 days says Crest report. *N.R.A. News* 16:D (no. 10), 1977.
51. Owen, G. M. A study of nutritional status of pre-school children in the United States. 1968–1970. *Pediatrics* 53 (Suppl.): 1, 1974.
52. Page, L. B. Appraisal and reappraisal of the cardiac therapy. Epidemiologic evidence on the etiology of human hypertension and its possible prevention. *Am. Heart J.* 91:421, 1976.
53. Pangborn, R. M., and Pecone, S. D. Taste perception of sodium chloride in relation to dietary intake of salt. *Am. J. Clin. Nutr.* 35:510, 1982.
54. Position paper on the vegetarian approach to eating. *J. Am. Diet. Assoc.* 77:61, 1980.
55. Public Health Service, National Center for Health Statistics. *Preliminary Findings of the First Health and Nutrition Examination Survey. U.S. 1971-1972.* DHEW Publication No. (HRA) 75-1229. Hyattsville, Maryland, 1979.
56. Reiser, R., and Sidelman, Z. Control of serum cholesterol hemostasis by cholesterol in the milk of the suckling rat. *J. Nutr.* 102:1009, 1972.

57. Shannon, B. M., and Parks, S. C. Fast Foods: A perspective on their nutritional impact. *J. Am. Diet. Assoc.* 76:242, 1980.
58. Sherlock, P., and Rothchild, E. D. Scurvy produced by Zen macrobiotic diet. *J.A.M.A.* 199:794, 1967.
59. Ted Tse, C. S. Food products containing tartrazine. *N. Engl. J. Med.* 306:681, 1982.
60. Twelfth annual state of the snack food industries report. *Snack Food Magazine.* June, 1980.
61. U.S. Department of Agriculture. *Farm Index,* Oct. 1979.
62. U.S. Department of Agriculture. U.S. Food Expenditures 1954–1978. *Agricultural Economics Report 431,* 1979.
63. U.S. Department of Agriculture. Warning: Organic foods may contain chemicals. *Food News for Consumers,* June, 1982.
64. U.S. Department of Agriculture, Service and Education Administration. *Food and Nutrition Intake of Individuals in One Day in the United States. 1977-78. Nationwide Food Consumption Survey.* USDA Preliminary Report No. 2, Spring, 1977–September, 1980.
65. U.S. Department of Agriculture and U.S. Department of Health, Education and Welfare. *Nutrition and Your Health. Dietary Guidelines for Americans.* Washington, D.C.: U.S. Government Printing Office, 1979.
66. U.S. Department of Health, Education and Welfare, Health Services and Mental Health Administration. *Ten State Nutrition Survey 1968-1970.* DHEW Publication No. (HMS) 372-8310 through 72-8133. Atlanta: Centers for Disease Control. U.S. Food Expenditures 1954-1978. U.S.D.A. Agricultural Economics Report 431, 1979.
67. U.S. Department of Health, Education, and Welfare. Public Health Service, Office of the Assistant Secretary for Health and Surgeon General. *Surgeon General's Report on Health Promotion and Disease Prevention: Healthy People.* DHEW (PHW) Publication No. 79-55071. Washington, D.C.: U.S. Government Printing Office, 1979. Pp. 33-52 and 131.
68. U.S. Department of Health and Human Services (Public Health Service). *Better Health for Our Children. A National Strategy: The Report of the Select Panel for the Promotion of Child Health.* Vol. I. Publication No. 79-55071. Washington, D.C.: U.S. Government Printing Office, 1979.
69. U.S. Senate, Select Committee on Nutrition and Human Needs. *Dietary Goals for the United States* (2nd ed.). Washington, D.C.: U.S. Government Printing Office, 1977.
70. Vitamin B_{12} deficiency in the breast fed infant of a strict vegetarian. (Nutrition Reviews). *N. Engl. J. Med.* 37:142, 1979.
71. Wakefield, L. M., and Merrow, S. B. Interrelationships between selected clinical and sociological measurements of preadolescent children from independent low income families. *Am. J. Clin. Nutr.* 20:29, 1967.
72. Yankelovitch, D., Skelly, F., and White, A. Supermarket Shoppers in a Period of Economic Uncertainty. A nationwide poll presented at the Food Marketing Institute convention. Chicago, Illinois, 1982.
73. Yeung, D. L., et al. Sodium intakes of infants in the United States. *Pediatrics* 68:444, 1981.

7. The Evaluation of Nutritional Status

Patricia M. Queen

To evaluate the nutritional status of the population of the United States, three major surveys were sponsored by the Department of Health, Education, and Welfare [21, 24, 30]. Despite food surpluses, these surveys indicate that some Americans continue to suffer from poor nutrition or are at nutritional risk. This is of special concern in the pediatric population, where problems of retarded growth, iron deficiency anemia, and dental caries exist.

Unfortunately, in pediatric populations across the nation, these nutritional problems continue and may go undetected until obvious symptoms become manifest. Because nutritional assessment often is not a routine part of well-child care and is sometimes overlooked in hospitals, children may exist in suboptimal states of nutrition chronically. Even when assessments are undertaken, errors in technique or failure to properly integrate the data gathered from the medical history, clinical examination, growth measurements, and laboratory and diet evaluations may cause conditions to be overlooked.

This chapter reviews for the practitioner the practical techniques of nutritional assessment. A complete assessment requires the collection of four types of data: anthropometric, clinical, biochemical, and dietary. Because there is no single complete measurement of nutritional status, a standardized approach to nutritional assessment is necessary to identify deficiencies. Public concern about the quality of food and the adequacy of nutrition will force the health provider to include nutritional assessment as an integral part of routine pediatric care.

LEVELS OF NUTRITIONAL ASSESSMENT

The evaluation techniques used for nutritional assessment depend on the goals of the program and, to some degree, the environment. The needs of a child coming to an office for a routine physical examination differ considerably from the needs of a child in an acute care facility. Table 7-1 summarizes three levels of nutritional assessment (minimal, mid-level, and in-depth), which may be used singly or in combination to assess nutritional status. Children who are at nutritional risk require a mid-level or in-depth assessment. Table 7-2 is a summary of factors found in children at nutritional risk.

Factors in the family and child's medical history can help determine the degree of nutritional risk and alert the practitioner to the need for nutritional assessment. For example, a child in a family with a positive history of inherited disease, birth defects, growth problems, recurrent infections, hyperlipidemia, or hypertension is at high nutritional risk. The child's social environment may also be significant: children in

Table 7-1. Levels of Nutritional Assessment for Infants and Children

| Level of Approach | History | | Clinical Evaluation | Laboratory Evaluation |
	Dietary	Medical and Socioeconomic		
BIRTH TO 24 MONTHS				
Minimal	Source of iron Vitamin supplement Milk intake (type and amount)	Birth weight Length of gestation Serious or chronic illness Use of medicines	Body weight and length Gross defects	Hematocrit Hemoglobin
Mid-level	Semi-quantitative Iron-cereal, meat, egg yolks, supplement Energy nutrients Micronutrients: calcium, niacin, riboflavin, vitamin C Protein Food intolerances Baby foods (processed commercially); home cooked	Family history: diabetes, tuberculosis Maternal height, prenatal care Infant immunizations, tuberculin test	Head circumference Skin color, pallor, turgor Subcutaneous tissue paucity, excess	RBC morphology Serum iron Total iron binding capacity Sickle cell testing

In-depth Level	Quantitative 24-hour recall Dietary history	Prenatal details Complications of delivery Regular health supervision	Cranial bossing Epiphyseal enlargement Costochondral beading Ecchymoses	Same as above, plus vitamin and appropriate enzyme assays; protein and amino acids; hydroxyproline, etc., should be available
FOR AGES 2 TO 5 YEARS				
	Determine amount of intake	Probe about pica; medications	Add height at all levels Add arm circumference at all levels Add triceps skinfolds at in-depth level	Add serum lead at mid-level Add serum micronutrients (e.g., vitamins A, C, folate) at in-depth level

Source: Christakis, G. (Ed.). *Nutritional Assessment in Health Programs.* Washington, D.C.: The Public Health Association, Inc., 1978.

Table 7-2. Children at Nutritional Risk

Area of Assessment	Evaluation
Growth	Significant change in weight or height Height for age, 5th percentile Weight for height below 5th percentile, less than 90% standard above 95th percentile, more than 120% standard
Condition/disease	Disease or condition of major organ system Inborn errors of metabolism Food allergies Failure-to-thrive Dental caries Oral-facial anomalies Prematurity Neuromuscular disorders Surgery Burns
Laboratory	Hemoglobin, less than 11 gm/dl Albumin, serum, less than 2.5 gm/dl
Environment	Inadequate income, food supply No facilities for food storage, preparation Poor sanitation

families with alcohol or drug abuse are at high risk [13]. In addition, the emotional climate of the home is important. Studies have shown that neglected or emotionally deprived children may not grow as well as happy or secure children [22].

The child's history should include growth data from birth on height, weight, and head circumference. The parent's height and weight are also included to estimate growth potential. Pertinent information gathered from the medical history including presenting complaints, parental concerns, and medical problems can be incorporated with the nutritional history (Table 7-3).

When gathering information for the nutritional history, dietary data are collected by one of three methods: the 24-hour recall (Table 7-4), the 3- to 7-day food record (Table 7-5), or food frequency lists (Table 7-6). These methods vary in reliability, validity, and depth [11, 14]. The method of choice depends on the level of assessment needed. The accuracy of these methods depends on the interviewing skills of the clinician and the reliability of the informant. The advantages and problems associated with each method are presented in Table 7-7. It should be noted that the process of nutritional assessment usually involves several health team members (i.e., pediatrician, nurse, and nutritionist), and therefore, the responsibility for both data collection and follow-up should be clearly outlined.

Table 7-3. Nutritional Assessment of Children

Patient _____   Date _____

Birth date _____   Age _____

Informant _____

Presenting nutritional problem(s) _____

_____

Current concern (parental) _____

_____

Growth

Height _____ (_____ %)   Head circumference _____ (_____ %)

Weight _____ (_____ %)   Fat-fold measure _____

Birth weight _____ lb _____ oz   Birth length _____ inches

Has weight gain since birth been: Satisfactory? _____ Slow? _____ Fluctuating? _____

Has there been recent weight: Gain? _____ Loss? _____ Neither _____

Mother's height _____ ft _____ in   Weight _____ lb

Father's height _____ ft _____ in   Weight _____ lb

As compared with siblings at the same age, patient is: Larger _____ Same size _____ Smaller _____

Pertinent laboratory findings _____

Nutrition history

Has the patient taken vitamin-mineral supplements?

Yes _____ No _____ Kind _____ At what age? _____

Has the patient been prescribed medication(s)? Yes _____ No _____

Kind _____ Reason _____ At what age? _____

Indicate if there have been problems with the following:

	Patient	Family	Comment
Colic	_____	_____	_____
Spitting up	_____	_____	_____
Appetite	_____	_____	_____
Food allergies	_____	_____	_____
Diarrhea	_____	_____	_____

Table 7-3 (Continued)

Constipation   _____   _____   _____

Vomiting   _____   _____   _____

Anemia   _____   _____   _____

Dehydration   _____   _____   _____

Failure to thrive   _____   _____   _____

Unusual cravings   _____   _____   _____

Overweight   _____   _____   _____

Need for special diet   _____   _____   _____

Feeding history

Who fed the child? _____

Was the child difficult to feed? Yes _____ No _____

How long did feedings take? _____

Was there any early feeding intervention? Yes _____ No _____

Was the child: Breast-fed _____ Formula-fed? _____ Formula: _____

Was the child fed: On demand? _____On hourly schedule? _____

At what age was the child weaned: From breast? _____ From bottle? _____

Did the child suck his/her thumb? Yes _____ No _____

   Did the child use a pacifier? Yes _____ No _____

Indicate if there were early difficulties with the following:

		Comment
Sucking	_____	_____
Swallowing	_____	_____
Chewing	_____	_____
Tongue control	_____	_____
Lip control	_____	_____

Table 7-3. (Continued)

Developing feeding milestones

	Age	Comment
Baby food introduction	_____	_____
Junior foods	_____	_____
Finger feeding	_____	_____
Cup drinking	_____	_____
Weaning	_____	_____
Whole table foods	_____	_____
Use of spoon	_____	_____
Independent feeding	_____	_____
Self-preparation of food	_____	_____

Feeding environment

Is the child fed: Alone? _____ With family? _____

Who feeds the child? _____Other that may feed or care for the child at mealtime: _____

The child eats: Alone _____ With family _____

Does the child care for himself/herself at the table? Yes _____ No _____

Does the child serve himself/herself food? Yes _____ No _____

Does the child generally finish all food served? Yes _____ No _____

Does the child ask for second helpings? Yes _____ No _____

How long is the usual eating period? _____

Where does the child eat: Breakfast? _____ Lunch? _____ Dinner? _____

Number of persons eating together at: Breakfast _____ Lunch _____ Dinner _____

Who prepares: Breakfast? _____ Lunch? _____ Dinner? _____

Is the child's behavior during mealtimes: Acceptable? _____ Disruptive? _____

  Dawdling? _____ Distractible? _____

Is the rule for eating: Clean plate? _____ Taste everything? _____

  Other: _____

How many times does the family dine out during the month? _____

Table 7-3 (Continued)

How often is shopping done for food? _____

How much money is spent on food each week? _____

Are food stamps used? Yes _____ No _____

Present eating habits

Child's appetite is: Excellent _____ Fair _____ Poor _____ Fluctuating _____

Has there been recent appetite: Increase? _____ Decrease? _____

When is the child most hungry? _____

Does the child know when he/she is full? Yes _____ No _____

What is the usual snacking pattern? _____

Are the child's food habits similar to those of other family members? Yes _____ No _____

Does the child get up during the night or early morning to eat or drink? Yes _____ No _____

Is the child's acceptance of foods: Good? _____ Fair? _____ Poor? _____

   Rigidly selective? _____

What are the child's food dislikes? _____

What is the child's favorite food? _____

Dental factors

Does the child have regular dental check-ups? Yes _____ No _____

Does the child brush and floss teeth regularly? Yes _____ No _____

Is the local water supply fluoridated? Yes _____ No _____

Is a fluoride supplement taken? Yes _____ No _____ Age _____

   Kind _____

Does the child receive topical fluoride applications? Yes _____ No _____

Are sweets included as: Part of meals? _____ Snacks? _____

Present food intake

24-h recall
1- to 3-day food record
General recall of usual food pattern

Table 7-3 (Continued)

Time   *Amount*   *Type of food*

Does the weekend food pattern vary from the usual food intake during the week?

Yes _____ No _____ Comment _____

Comments regarding food intake: _____

_____

_____

_____

Analysis of food intake:

Total fluid _____

kcal _____ kcal/kg _____ kcal/cm _____

Protein, gm _____ Protein, gm/kg _____

Vitamins/minerals _____

Impressions:

Recommendations:

Summary:

Source: Developmental Evaluation Clinic, The Children's Hospital, Boston, Ma.

Table 7-4. 24-Hour Recall

Name _____

Date and time of interview _____

Length of interview _____

Date of recall _____

Day of the week of recall _____

       1-M   2-T   3-W   4-Th   5-F   6-Sat   7-Sun

"I would like you to tell me everything you (your child) ate and drank from the time you (he) got up in the morning until you (he) went to bed at night and what you (he) ate during the night. Be sure to mention everything you (he) ate or drank at home, at work (school), and away from home. Include snacks and drinks of all kinds and everything else you (he) put in your (his) mouth and swallowed. I also need to know where you (he) ate the food, and now let us begin."

What time did you (he) get up yesterday? _____

Was it the usual time? _____

What was the first time you (he) ate or had anything to drink yesterday

morning? _____

Where did you (he) eat? (list on form which follows)

Now tell me what you (he) had to eat and how much?

(Occasionally the interviewer will need to ask:)

   When did you (he) eat again? Or, is there anything else?

   Did you (he) have anything to eat or drink during the night?

Was intake unusual in any way? Yes _____ No _____

(If answer is yes) Why? _____

   In what way? _____

What time did you (he) go to bed last night?

Do(es) you (he) take vitamin or mineral supplements?

   Yes _____ No _____

(If answer is yes) How many per day? _____

Table 7-4 (Continued)

Per week? _____

What kind? (Insert brand name if known)

Multivitamins _____

Ascorbic acid _____

Vitamins A and D_____

Iron _____

Other _____

Also note:
Fluid intake in infants and children, especially in handicapped children with increased losses or children drinking excessive amounts
Serving size (i.e., teaspoon, infant teaspoon, etc.)
Method of food preparation
Use of condiments, flavorings added to milk, margarine, jelly, jam
Source: *Screening Children for Nutritional Status.* PHS Publication No. 2158, U.S. Department of Health, Education, and Welfare, 1971.

Table 7-5. Directions for Recording 3- to 7-Day Diet Diary

1. Use standard measuring cups and spoons for all servings. All measurements are level.
2. Utensils needed:
     1 set standard measuring spoons
     1 set standard measuring cups
     1 standard glass measuring cup
3. Equivalent measures:
     3 teaspoons = 1 tablespoon
     16 tablespoons = 1 cup
     1 fluid ounce = 2 tablespoons
     1 jar *strained* fruits, vegetables, vegetables and meat, and desserts (4½ oz) = 9 tablespoons
     1 jar *junior* fruits, vegetables, vegetables and meat, and desserts (7½ oz) = 15 tablespoons
     1 jar *strained* or *junior* meat (3½ oz) = 7 tablespoons
     1 jar *strained* or *junior* high meat dinner (4½ oz) = 9 tablespoons
4. The exact amount of all food the child has eaten during the specified three days prior to the clinic visit should be recorded at the time it is eaten.

Table 7-5. (Continued)

5. Amount of formula or milk consumed should be recorded in ounces. Included amount used with cereal.
6. Cereals should be measured as served (baby cereals in tablespoon portions, level measurements, dry; cooked cereals in tablespoon or cup portions, level measurements, after cooking; dry cereals in level cup portions or tablespoons).
7. Amount of fruit juice taken should be recorded in ounces. Whole fruits should be recorded as number and size (small, medium, or large); strained and junior fruits should be recorded in level tablespoon or teaspoon portions.
8. Vegetables should be measured as served (strained and junior vegetables in level tablespoon or teaspoon portions; cooked vegetables in cup portions).
9. Meats should be measured as served (strained and junior meats in level tablespoon portions; chopped table meats in level tablespoon portions [1 oz = 2 tbsp]; whole meats should be recorded with approximate measurements of size, such as 1 pork chop 2" x 3" x ½").
10. Bread: state number of slices; cookies and crackers: give brand name and number eaten.
11. Fats: record in level teaspoons or tablespoons—include those used in cooking.
12. Desserts: describe size of portion.
13. Miscellaneous: remember to include gravies, sodas, candy, chips, and snack foods.
14. Describe method of food preparation (e.g., fried, baked, broiled).
15. List amount of ingredients in mixed dishes.

Note: Seven days provides more representative information because weekends are included.
Source: Developmental Evaluation Clinic, The Children's Hospital, Boston, Ma.

Table 7-6. Food Frequency Record

How many times per week do you eat the following foods (at any meal or between meals)? Circle the appropriate number:

Bacon	0 1 2 3 4 5 6 7 >7, specify _____
Tongue	0 1 2 3 4 5 6 7 >7, specify _____
Sausage	0 1 2 3 4 5 6 7 >7, specify _____
Luncheon meat	0 1 2 3 4 5 6 7 >7, specify _____
Hot dogs	0 1 2 3 4 5 6 7 >7, specify _____
Liver—chicken	0 1 2 3 4 5 6 7 >7, specify _____
Liver—other	0 1 2 3 4 5 6 7 >7, specify _____
Poultry	0 1 2 3 4 5 6 7 >7, specify _____
Salt pork	0 1 2 3 4 5 6 7 >7, specify _____

Table 7-6. (Continued)

Pork or ham ⸺ 0 1 2 3 4 5 6 7 >7, specify ⸺

Bones (neck or other) ⸺ 0 1 2 3 4 5 6 7 >7, specify ⸺

Meat in mixtures (stew,
tamales, casseroles, etc.) ⸺ 0 1 2 3 4 5 6 7 >7, specify ⸺

Beef or veal ⸺ 0 1 2 3 4 5 6 7 >7, specify ⸺

Other meat ⸺ 0 1 2 3 4 5 6 7 >7, specify ⸺

Fish ⸺ 0 1 2 3 4 5 6 7 >7, specify ⸺

Cheese and cheese dishes ⸺ 0 1 2 3 4 5 6 7 >7, specify ⸺

Eggs ⸺ 0 1 2 3 4 5 6 7 >7, specify ⸺

Dried bean or pea dishes ⸺ 0 1 2 3 4 5 6 7 >7, specify ⸺

Peanut butter or nuts ⸺ 0 1 2 3 4 5 6 7 >7, specify ⸺

How many servings per day do you eat of the following foods? Circle the appropriate number:

Bread (including sandwich),
toast, rolls, muffins (1 slice
or 1 piece is 1 serving) ⸺ 0 1 2 3 4 5 6 7 >7, specify ⸺

Milk (including on cereal or
other foods) (8 ounces is 1
serving) ⸺ 0 1 2 3 4 5 6 7 >7, specify ⸺

Sugar, jam, jelly, syrup (1 tsp
is 1 serving) ⸺ 0 1 2 3 4 5 6 7 >7, specify ⸺

Butter or margarine (1 tsp is 1
serving) ⸺ 0 1 2 3 4 5 6 7 >7, specify ⸺

How many times per week do you eat the following foods (at any meal or between meals)?
Circle the appropriate number:

Fruit juice ⸺ 0 1 2 3 4 5 6 7 >7, specify ⸺

Fruit ⸺ 0 1 2 3 4 5 6 7 >7, specify ⸺

Cereal—dry ⸺ 0 1 2 3 4 5 6 7 >7, specify ⸺

Cereal—cooked or instant ⸺ 0 1 2 3 4 5 6 7 >7, specify ⸺

Pancakes or waffles ⸺ 0 1 2 3 4 5 6 7 >7, specify ⸺

Potato ⸺ 0 1 2 3 4 5 6 7 >7, specify ⸺

Other cooked vegetables ⸺ 0 1 2 3 4 5 6 7 >7, specify ⸺

Raw vegetables ⸺ 0 1 2 3 4 5 6 7 >7, specify ⸺

Macaroni, spaghetti, rice, or
noodles ⸺ 0 1 2 3 4 5 6 7 >7, specify ⸺

Ice cream, milk pudding,
custard, or cream soup ⸺ 0 1 2 3 4 5 6 7 >7, specify ⸺

Sweet rolls or doughnuts ⸺ 0 1 2 3 4 5 6 7 >7, specify ⸺

Crackers or pretzels ⸺ 0 1 2 3 4 5 6 7 >7, specify ⸺

Cookies ⸺ 0 1 2 3 4 5 6 7 >7, specify ⸺

Pie, cake, or brownies ⸺ 0 1 2 3 4 5 6 7 >7, specify ⸺

Potato chips or corn chips ⸺ 0 1 2 3 4 5 6 7 >7, specify ⸺

Candy ⸺ 0 1 2 3 4 5 6 7 >7, specify ⸺

Soft drinks, Popsicles, or
Kool Aid; sherbets ⸺ 0 1 2 3 4 5 6 7 >7, specify ⸺

Table 7-6. (Continued)

Instant Breakfast _____ 0 1 2 3 4 5 6 7 >7, specify _____

Artificially sweetened
  beverage _____ 0 1 2 3 4 5 6 7 >7, specify _____

Coffee or tea _____ 0 1 2 3 4 5 6 7 >7, specify _____

Beer _____ 0 1 2 3 4 5 6 7 >7, specify _____

Wine _____ 0 1 2 3 4 5 6 7 >7, specify _____

Whiskey, vodka, rum,
  scotch, gin _____ 0 1 2 3 4 5 6 7 >7, specify _____

What specific kinds of the following foods do you eat most often?

Fruit juice _____

Fruit _____

Vegetables _____

Cheese _____

Cooked or instant cereal _____

Dry cereal _____

Milk _____

Cream or cream substitute _____

Butter or margarine _____

Salad dressings _____

Source: *Screening Children for Nutritional Status*. PHS Publication No. 2158, U.S. Department of Health, Education, and Welfare, 1971.

Table 7-7. Methods for Evaluating Dietary Data

Type	Level of Assessment	Advantages	Disadvantages
24-hour recall	Minimal; qualitative and quantitative	Rapid; overview of diet with data on specific amounts of nutrients	One 24-hour period not necessarily a typical pattern
Food frequency	Minimal; qualitative	Rapid; overview of diet, highlights problem nutrients	No data on the specific amount of food consumed per day by an individual
3–7 day food record	In-depth; qualitative and quantitative	More reliable; provides information on specific nutrients over time	Relies heavily on parental accuracy and cooperation; time consuming

Table 7-8. Basic Food Groups for Children

Food Group	Serving Size	Recommended No. of Servings/Day
Milk	1 cup milk, yogurt, or calcium equivalent: 1½ slices (1½ oz) cheddar cheese* 1 cup pudding 1¾ cups ice cream 2 cups cottage cheese*	3
Meat	2 oz cooked, lean meat, poultry, fish, or protein equivalent: 2 eggs 2 slices (2 oz) cheddar cheese ½ cup cottage cheese 1 cup dried beans, peas 4 tbsp peanut butter	2
Fruit, vegetable	½ cup cooked or juice 1 cup raw 1 medium sized whole (e.g., apple, banana)	4
Grain (whole grain, fortified, enriched)	1 slice bread 1 cup ready-to-eat cereal ½ cup cooked cereal, pasta, grits	

*Count cheese as serving of either milk or meat, not both simultaneously. Equivalents complement but do not replace foods from the four food groups. Amounts should be determined by individual caloric needs.
Source: *A Guide to Good Eating*. Rosemont, Ill.: National Dairy Council, 1977.

DIETARY ASSESSMENT

Once the dietary information is collected, it is assessed for adequacy. Again, the level of assessment is determined by the level of need. A cursory method is to group the foods consumed into the Basic Four Food Groups: milk or equivalent, meat or equivalent, fruit-vegetable, and grains (Table 7-8). A more meaningful method of assessment includes an analysis of specific nutrients. Information on food composition is gathered from tables such as:

"Composition of Foods; Raw, Processed and Prepared," *USDA Handbook* (Series for Several Food Categories). Washington, D.C.: USDA, 1975-1976
"Nutrition Values of American Foods in Common Units," *USDA Handbook 454*. Washington, D.C.: USDA, 1975

Food Values of Portions Commonly Used," J.A. Pennington and H.H. Church, Philadelphia: Lippincott, 1980

The total nutrient intake is calculated and then compared to the Recommended Dietary Allowances (RDA) [7]. The diet is considered below standard when less than two-thirds of the RDA for a specific nutrient is present. Hand calculation of dietary data is time consuming, and a detailed dietary analysis is usually used when the services of a registered dietitian are available or in a research setting. Computers with nutrient data banks are now available in universities but are usually unavailable to practitioners. However, in some communities nutritional consultation firms provide this service on a fee basis.

The common sources of error leading to miscalculations of dietary data are summarized in Table 7-9. Often, food composition tables do not contain the specific brands used by a client; this information must be requested from the manufacturer. Another problem in determining food composition is encountered when families use ethnic foods or homemade recipes.

The nutrients to be analyzed should be determined according to the child's growth, clinical findings, and laboratory findings. In routine screening for infants and toddlers, iron is the nutrient most at risk (see Appendix 4). The diets of toddlers also are often found to be low in calcium, zinc, and vitamins A and C, so a review for foods containing these nutrients is in order. The diet of the child with poor growth but showing no other clinical or biochemical abnormalities should be evaluated for energy and protein. When deficient or excess nutrients are discovered, nutrition counseling is recommended.

Table 7-9. Common Sources of Error
Leading to Miscalculation of Dietary Data

---

1. Mistakes in converting a household portion to a weighed amount (e.g., 1 cup to 100 gm)
2. Arithmetic mistakes converting food intake into nutrient values
3. Use of food table values that are estimated rather than actual laboratory analysis amounts for nutrient content
4. Use of food table average values that may not reflect nutrient variations due to seasonal differences and methods of processing, cooking, and storage
5. Frequent ingredient changes in processed food products
6. Wide variability in combined-ingredient recipes (e.g., baked goods, casseroles)

Data from: Wellman, N. S. The Evaluation of Nutritional Status. In R. B. Howard and N. H. Herbold (Eds.), *Nutrition in Critical Care* (2nd ed.). New York: McGraw-Hill, 1982.

GROWTH ASSESSMENT

Growth increments in weight, height, and head circumference are extremely rapid before birth and during the first few years of postnatal life (Fig. 7-1). The rates of normal weight gain and increase in length per day are presented in Table 7-10. A normal 1-month-old infant grows approximately 1 mm per day in length and gains 30 gm per day, while at 3 years of age, a child grows 0.2 mm per day and gains 5 gm per day [6]. Thus, children grow at a slower rate with increasing age.

Normal development is associated with a predictable rate of increase in height. However, there are certain factors that will influence the rate. Among those factors associated with height are the sex of the child, birth order, length of gestation, age of the parents, mother's smoking habits during pregnancy, and parental education, occupation, and income. Parental stature is the major influence and should be considered routinely [29]. With respect to parental influence on growth, birth length relates predominately to maternal size. However, by 2 years of age the length correlates best to mean parental height, reflecting the genetic growth factors of both parents. This phenomenon, described by Smith and associates [28] as "lagging down," occurs in mid-infancy.

The anthropometric measurements commonly used in nutritional assessment are summarized in Table 7-11. Also presented are the advantages, disadvantages, reproducibility, and interpretation of these measurements.

HEIGHT, LENGTH, AND WEIGHT

Tables 7-12 and 7-13 present the guidelines for measuring weight, length, and height. In calculating gains in stature after 2 years of age, it is important that measurements represent length (subject recumbent) or that serial measurements represent height (subject standing). For infants, satisfactory measurement of length requires adequate equipment and two examiners (Fig. 7-2). An examining table inexpensively modified as described by Falkner [4] will provide a suitable apparatus. Otherwise, a portable measuring board can be purchased or constructed [5].

The standing position is used for measuring older children (Fig. 7-3). If the child is knock-kneed, the medial borders of the knees should touch each other with the heels slightly separated. If the buttocks are markedly protuberant, the child should be vertically positioned with only the buttocks in contact with the wall [26]. Children with scoliosis, cerebral palsy, or other disorders may require recumbent length measurement (stretching the child as straight as possible). Sitting height or crown-rump length may be determined in infants and children whose legs are severely deformed [25, 26] (see Chap. 11).

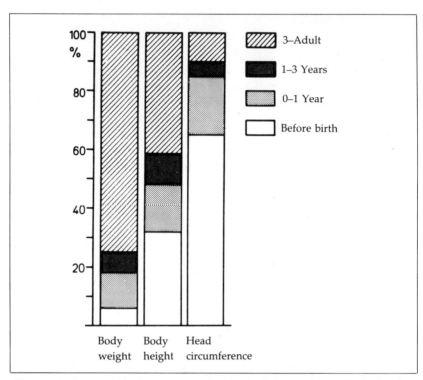

Figure 7-1. Growth in body parameters during development. (From Vahlquist, B. The Young Child: Normal. In D. B. Jelliffe and E. F. Jelliffe (Eds.), Human Nutrition—A Comprehensive Treatise. *Vol. 2. Nutrition and Growth. New York: Plenum Press, 1979.)*

Table 7-10. Gains in Length and Weight of Reference Children

	Males			Females	
Age	Length (mm/day)	Weight (gm/day)	Age	Length (mm/day)	Weight (gm/day)
0–1 mo	1.03	29.3	0–1 mo	0.94	26.0
1–2 mo	1.13	35.2	1–2 mo	1.10	28.6
2–3 mo	1.06	29.9	2–3 mo	0.94	24.3
3–4 mo	0.80	20.8	3–4 mo	0.77	18.6
4–5 mo	0.65	16.6	4–5 mo	0.65	16.1
5–6 mo	0.57	15.2	5–6 mo	0.63	15.0
6–9 mo	0.52	12.6	6–9 mo	0.51	11.2
9–12 mo	0.42	10.7	9–12 mo	0.43	10.0
12–18 mo	0.34	7.2	12–18 mo	0.32	8.7
18–24 mo	0.26	6.1	18–24 mo	0.29	6.2
2–3 yr	0.22	5.7	2–3 yr	0.24	6.0
3–4 yr	0.21	5.5	3–4 yr	0.20	5.1

Source: Fomon, S. J., Haschke, F., Ziegler, E. E., and Nelson, S. E. Body composition of reference children from birth to age 10 years. *Am. J. Clin. Nutr.* 35:1171, 1982.

Table 7-11. Anthropometric Measurements Applied in Nutritional Assessment

Measurements	Age Groups	Nutritional Indication	Reproducibility	Advantages	Disadvantages	Observer Error	Interpretation (Percentage of Standard)
Weight	All	Present nutritional status; under and over	Good	Common in use	Difficult in field, cannot tell body composition, need accurate age, height related (insensitive)	<100 gm in children <250 gm in adults	<60 severe malnutrition 60–80 moderate malnutrition 80–90 mild malnutrition 90–110 normal 110–120 overweight >120 obese
Height	All	Chronic under-nutrition	Good	Common in use, Simple to do in field	Other factors play a role	≤ 0.5 cm <3.0 cm in adults	<80 dwarf 80–90 short 93–105 normal >105 giant
Head circumference	0–4 yr	Intrauterine and childhood nutrition (chronic under-nutrition)	Good	Simple	Other factors play a role (e.g., brain development)	<0.5 cm	

Table 7-11. (Continued)

Measurements	Age Groups	Nutritional Indication	Reproducibility	Advantages	Disadvantages	Observer Error	Interpretation (Percentage of Standard)
Mid-arm circumference	All	Present under and over-nutrition	Fair	Simple, age independent, child need not be stripped, suitable for rapid survey	No limits for over-nutrition, No standard for adult	<0.5 cm	<75 severe malnutrition 75–80 moderate malnutrition 80–85 mild malnutrition >85 normal
Skinfold thickness, subscapula or triceps	All	Present under and over-nutrition	Fair	Measures body composition, detects obesity in adults	Needs expensive caliper, difficult with child and in the field. ? ethnic differences	1.0–1.5 mm	Similar to weight
Weight/height/age ratio	All	Present under and over-nutrition	Good	Index of body build, age independent 1–4 years and adults	Need proper scales, need trained personnel		<75 severe malnutrition 75–85 moderate malnutrition 85–90 mild malnutrition 90–110 normal 110–120 overweight >120 obese

Adapted from McLaren, D. S. Nutritional Assessment. In D. S. McLaren, and D. Burman (Eds.), *Textbook of Paediatric Nutrition* (2nd ed.). New York: Churchill Livingstone, 1982.

Table 7-12. Guidelines for Measuring the Weight of Infants and Children

Infant's Weight	Child's Weight
1. Remove outer clothing including shoes, caps, or bonnets. Infants may remain in dry diapers.	1. After balancing the scale, and with the weights placed in the zero position, have the child stand in the center of the scale, feet slightly apart.
2. After the scale has been balanced and the weights are in the zero position, place the undressed infant in the center of the scale.	2. Move the lower weight away from zero until the marker drops below the center point. Then slide the weight back toward zero until the marker is above the center point.
3. Move the lower weight away from zero until the marker drops below the center point. Then move the weight back toward zero until the marker is just above the center point.	3. Move the weight on the upper beam away from zero until the marker is centered. You may need to move the upper weight back and forth a few times until the scale is balanced.
4. Move the upper weight away from zero until the marker is centered. You may need to move the upper weight back and forth a few times until the scale is balanced.	4. Read the weight measurement to the nearest ¼ pound (100 gm) and jot it down.
5. Read the weight measurement to the nearest ½ ounce (10 gm). Repeat the measurement until you get two weights that agree within ½ ounce (10 gm).	5. Have the child step off the scale and return the weights to zero. Repeat the measurement until you get two readings that agree within ¼ pound (100 gm).
6. Record the second reading that agrees within ½ ounce (10 gm) on the child's chart right away.	6. Record the second measurement that agrees within ¼ pound (100 gm) on the child's chart.
7. When you are finished, return both the upper and lower beam weights to zero.	7. When you are finished, return both the upper and lower beam weights to zero.

Modified after *Nutritional Screening of Children.* PHS (DHHS) Publication No. (HSA) 81-5114, 1981.

Table 7-13. Guidelines for Measuring
the Infant's Length and Child's Height

Infant's Length	Child's Height
1. Lay the child down face up on the measuring board. The body must be straight, lined up with the measuring board.	1. Remove all outer clothing, including hats and shoes. Measure the child in his or her underclothing.
2. Have an assistant or the parent hold the infant's head firmly against the headboard until the measuring is completed.	2. Have the child stand on a bare flat surface with heels slightly apart, and back as straight as possible. Heels, buttocks, and shoulder blades should touch the wall or measuring surface. Eyes should be straight ahead, arms at sides, and shoulders relaxed. Be sure that the child's knees are not bent and that the heels are not lifted from the floor.
3. With one hand, hold the infant's knees, completely straightening the infant's hips and knees.	3. Slowly, lower the movable headboard until it touches the crown (or top) of the head firmly. Make sure the headboard is not just resting on the hair but is actually touching the top of the head and is level.
4. With the other hand, move the footboard until it is resting firmly against the infant's heels. The toes should point directly up.	4. Check the child's position, read the height measurement to the nearest ⅛ inch (1 mm) out loud, and jot it down.
5. Read the measurement to the nearest ⅛ inch (1 mm) and jot it down.	5. Take the headboard away, check the child's position, and repeat the measurement as many times as necessary, jotting down the height until you get two readings that agree within ¼ inch (½ cm).
6. Slide the footboard away from the infant's heels and start again. To be sure you were correct, measure the child's length and jot it down as many times as necessary until you get two readings that agree within ¼ inch (½ cm).	6. Record the second measurement that agrees within ¼ inch (½ cm) on the child's chart at once.
7. Record the final measurement on the child's chart right away.	

Modified after *Nutritional Screening of Children*. PHS.DHHS Publication No. (HSA) 81-5114, 1981.

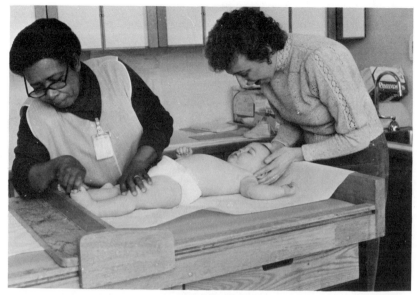

Figure 7-2. Technique for determining recumbent length. Note use of measuring board and correct placement of the child by two attendants.

HEAD CIRCUMFERENCE

Head circumference is a good index of brain growth, although it is usually taken on infants and young children as a screening test for microcephaly and macrocephaly [18]. Head circumference is measured in children up to 36 months of age with a nonstretchable tape measure graduated in millimeters. Either a flexible narrow steel tape or commercially available tape (Ross Laboratories, Columbus, Ohio) should be used for accuracy. The tape is applied firmly around the head above the supraorbital ridges (or the most prominent part of the frontal bulge) and over the occipital circumference. Large amounts of hair should be excluded and care should be taken to ensure that the plane of the tape is the same on both sides of the head [19].

SKINFOLD MEASUREMENT

In the United States between 1963 and 1974, skinfold thicknesses and upper arm girths were measured systematically on children age zero to 17 years. These children were included in the United States Ten-State Nutrition Survey and the National Health and Nutrition Examination Survey (NHANES) conducted by the National Center for Health Statistics (NCHS). Published percentiles were compiled for triceps skinfold (TSF) as shown in Table 7-14.

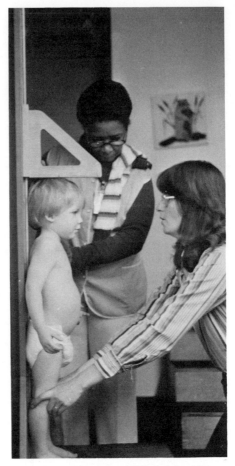

Figure 7-3. Technique for determining the child's height. Note use of the measuring apparatus and correct positioning of the child looking straight ahead with heels flat against the wall.

In relation to data interpretation, it must be stressed that these percentiles describe the skinfold thickness of American children and should not be considered "norms" or "standards." Owen [20] questions the use of skinfold measurements in general pediatric practice (see Chap. 10, Anthropometric Measurements). However, the TSF is a noninvasive method of assessing the amount of body fat and can help clarify the relationship between weight and height [3, 20]. While weight-for-height is the most widely used index of adiposity, it fails to differentiate muscle and soft tissue from fat and may be unreliable in young children [16, 27]. A direct relationship between weight-for-height and fatness cannot be assumed.

Table 7-14. Percentiles for Triceps Skinfold for Whites of the United States

Age Group (yr/mo)	Triceps Skinfold (mm)					
	Males			Females		
	5th	50th	95th	5th	50th	95th
0/0–0/4	4	8	15	4	8	13
0/5–0/9	5	9	15	6	9	15
1/0–1/9	6	10	16	6	10	16
2/0–2/9	6	10	15	6	10	16
3/0–3/9	6	10	15	7	11	15
4/0–4/9	6	9	14	7	10	16

Data from Frisancho, A. R. Triceps skinfold and upper arm muscle size norms for assessment of nutritional status. *Am. J. Clin. Nutr.* 27:1052, 1974, and Frisancho, A. R. New norms of upper limb fat and muscle areas for assessment of nutritional status. *Am. J. Clin. Nutr.* 34:2540, 1981.

Triceps skinfold is measured to the nearest tenth of a millimeter with Lange skinfold calipers having the pressure of 10 gm/mm^2 of contact surface area. Inexpensive plastic calipers that operate on the principle of pressure applied by the examiner may be used although they are less accurate than the Lange skinfold calipers. The measurement is taken on the back of the right arm midway between the point of the acromion and olecranon process while the arm hangs relaxed. The calipers are applied to a double fold of skin and subcutaneous fat is picked up 1 cm above the site of measurement between the left thumb and index finger of the examiner. The skinfold is lifted from the underlying muscle surface and is shaken gently to be certain that muscle has not been included. The caliper is then applied at the level of the horizontal mark below the thumb and index fingers of the left hand (Fig. 7-4). The caliper jaws are held in place while the measurer counts for 3 seconds. The reading is taken and recorded to the nearest millimeter. Independent TSF measurements are taken and the mean figure derived from the multiple measurements is used for the final skinfold value [9, 10]. Decreased TSF (below the fifth percentile) suggest malnutrition or depleted fat stores and excessive thicknesses (greater than the ninety-fifth percentile) indicate obesity.

Mid-Arm Muscle Circumference (MAMC)

Indications for obtaining mid-upper-arm muscle circumference include: (1) abnormal weight of a child due to nonnutritional causes (e.g., ascites) and (2) muscle estimation (e.g., protein status of infants and children on special diets or medications, or because of possible protein energy malnutrition) [32].

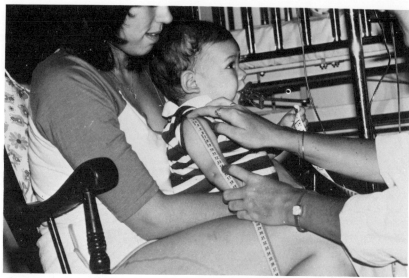

A

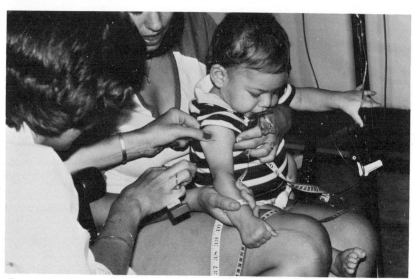

B

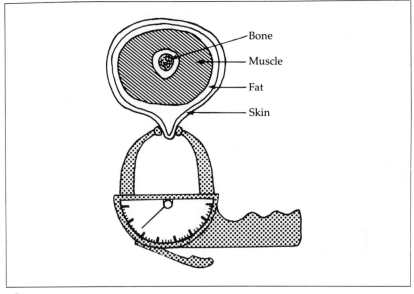

C

Figure 7-4. Measurement of triceps skinfold thickness. A. Location of the midpoint of the upper arm. B. Application of the Lange calipers for measurement of triceps skinfold. C. Representation of the tissues of the arm (bone, fat, muscle, and skin) and measurement of skinfold thickness.

The MAMC is measured to obtain an index of fat mass and muscle mass. Several studies suggest that this measurement may be more sensitive than weight in detecting nutritional changes. The technique for obtaining the MAMC is described by Frisancho [9]. The measurement is made at the level of the TSF site using a measuring tape with the right arm hanging relaxed. The tape is fitted snugly around the arm and the circumference is recorded to the nearest mm (Fig. 7-5). The arm circumference corrected for TSF measures the cross-sectional muscle and bone area at this level.

The MAMC derived from the arm circumference and TSF measurement is an indirect gross indicator of lean body or muscle mass [12]. MAMC is calculated by subtracting the TSF measurement (multiplied by 3.14) from the arm circumference. Published percentiles for American infants and children are shown in Table 7-15. For example, a 2-year-old male who has a TSF of 10 mm and an upper arm circumference of 170 mm will have a MAMC of 139 mm (170 − [10 × 3.14]), which is above the fiftieth percentile. On the other hand, a decreased MAMC (below the fifth percentile) would indicate muscle wasting due to malnutrition.

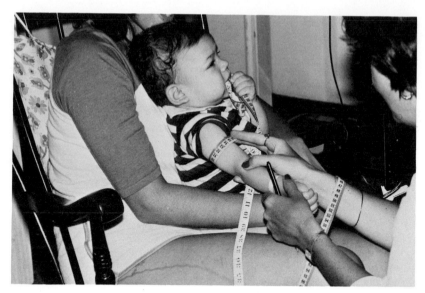

Figure 7-5. Measurement of mid-arm circumference.

Table 7-15. Percentiles of Upper Arm Circumference and Estimated Upper Arm Muscle Circumference for Whites of the United States

Age Group (yr/mo)	Arm Circumference (mm)			Arm Muscle Circumference (mm)		
	5th	50th	95th	5th	50th	95th
MALES						
0/0–0/4	113	134	153	81	106	133
0/5–0/9	128	152	175	100	123	146
1/0–1/9	142	159	183	110	127	147
2/0–2/9	141	162	185	111	130	150
3/0–3/9	150	167	190	117	137	153
4/0–4/9	149	171	192	123	141	159
FEMALES						
0/0–0/4	107	127	150	86	104	126
0/5–0/9	125	146	170	97	117	135
1/0–1/9	138	156	177	105	124	143
2/0–2/9	142	160	184	111	126	147
3/0–3/9	143	167	189	113	132	152
4/0–4/9	149	169	191	115	136	157

Data from: Frisancho, A. R. Triceps skinfold and upper arm muscle size norms for assessment of nutritional status. *Am. J. Clin. Nutr.* 27:1052, 1974, and Frisancho, A. R. New norms of upper limb fat and muscle areas for assessment of nutritional status. *Am. J. Clin. Nutr.* 34:2540, 1981.

GROWTH INTERPRETATION

Measurements of height, weight, and head circumference should be obtained at birth, every 2 months up to the age of 1, and every 6 months up to the age of 3. Thereafter, height and weight measurements should be obtained at yearly intervals unless further evaluation is indicated. The most representative growth charts are those of the National Center for Health Statistics (NCHS) published in 1976 [17], which were developed from a cross section of the United States population. These charts comprise length for age (birth to 36 months), stature for age (2 to 18 years), head circumference (birth to 36 months), weight for age (birth to 18 years), and weight for length/stature (birth to prepubertal). The percentiles range from the fifth to ninety-fifth percentile with the fiftieth percentile being used as the standard (see Appendix 2).

Measurements of growth parameters are plotted on the NCHS growth charts. To use the charts, one plots points that represent the child's age on the horizontal axis and weight, length, or head circumference on the vertical axis.

The best interpretation of a child's growth is made from serial observations rather than measurements at a single point in time. Two measurements permit calculation of growth during a defined period of time while a one-time measurement gives only size. The larger the number of serial observations, the more reliable is the judgment on normalcy of growth [19]. Although growth charts are not constructed for separately identified cohorts of children, it is assumed that children maintain their relative size during growth (i.e., small children tend to continue to be small [in the lower percentiles] and larger children continue to be near the upper percentiles). However, there are many exceptions to this rule. For example, children with Down syndrome are often characterized by deficient growth levels. For this reason, special growth charts may be more applicable for specific groups of children [2] (see Appendix 2). It must be realized that percentile lines on growth charts are smoothed averages and that individual patterns are less smooth due to variation and measurement error [19].

Including weight for length/stature on a separate chart overcomes the problem of interpretation between the percentiles of weight for age and length/stature for age. Weight for length/stature gives an index of current nutritional status, while length/stature for age provides an index of past nutritional history. Thus, a child may be classified as having acute or chronic undernutrition by these criteria [31].

In general, children may be at nutritional risk if their length/stature or weight is below the fifth percentile (<90 percent of standard) or if their weight is greater than the ninety-fifth percentile (>120 percent of standard).

GROWTH ASSESSMENT IN THE PREMATURE INFANT

The postnatal growth pattern of premature infants warrants attention. When plotting the infant's growth on the NCHS growth chart, the length, weight, and head circumference must be corrected for post-menstrual age. To correct for gestational age, the number of weeks of prematurity (based on 40 weeks gestation) are subtracted from the child's chronological age. In general, premature infants will catch up to normal weight by 24 months, head circumference by 18 months, and length by 3½ to 5 years, at which time correction is no longer needed [1]. For example, a child who is 12 months old but was born at 32 weeks gestation will have a corrected age of 10 months.

ABNORMAL GROWTH

Any deviation from normal growth is defined as abnormal growth or a failure to grow at a rate consistent with age. Children displaying abnormal growth patterns show major changes in their individual growth pattern but do not necessarily fall below the fifth percentile or above the ninety-fifth percentile on the growth charts. Children with abnormal growth must be differentiated from those with an endocrine disorder (Fig. 7-6) or other conditions causing growth retardation (Table 7-16).

In many cases, the basis for poor physical growth will not be defined; these children will grow within their constitutional limitations. For example, children with chromosomal aberrations or fetal alcohol syndrome are usually height stunted and nutritional intervention will not change the rate of growth. Nutrition is just one part of the growth complex interwoven with genetic and environmental factors; however, it should not be overlooked in efforts to maximize growth or promote catch-up growth.

CATCH-UP GROWTH

Catch-up growth is a process seen in young children following a period of growth retardation when the cause of the growth deficit is no longer present. It consists of a rapid increase in weight gain followed by an increase in height until the original or normal growth pattern is achieved [8]. Examples of this phenomenon include recovery from malnutrition (Fig. 7-7) and celiac disease (Fig. 7-8). In chronic disease or malnutrition, growth is slowed and the growth curve crosses into lower percentiles. If the cause of the disease of nutritional deficit is corrected, the growth trend is reversed.

The capacity for catch-up growth depends on the duration, timing, and severity of restriction [15, 23]. Furthermore, the developmental stage of the tissue involved (e.g., head circumference) appears to be a critical determinant of the effects of feeding the child on catch-up growth. Catch-up growth in head circumference seems to exist only

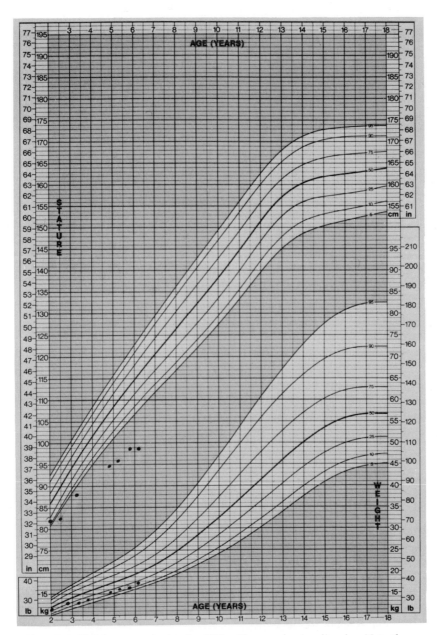

Figure 7-6. Serial measurements of a child with an endocrine disorder. Note the decrease in height increment without a decrease in weight.

Table 7-16. Causes of Growth Retardation

I. Malnutrition
  A. Secondary to chronic infection or systemic disease
  B. Nutritional deprivation
II. Genetic short stature
  A. Familial
  B. Chromosomal abnormalities
    1. Trisomies 13, 18, 21
    2. Gonadal dysgenesis
III. Constitutional delay in growth and sexual maturation
IV. Systemic diseases
  A. Cardiovascular
    1. Congenital heart disease (cyanotic or acyanotic)
    2. Acquired heart disease (rheumatic)
  B. Respiratory
    1. Asthma
    2. Cystic fibrosis
  C. Urinary
    1. Chronic renal insufficiency
      a. Congenital (obstructive anomaly of the urinary tract)
      b. Acquired (chronic glomerulonephritis or pyelonephritis)
    2. Renal tubular acidosis
      a. Isolated
      b. With other abnormalities or tubular function (e.g., Fanconi syndrome)
  D. Gastrointestinal
    1. Malabsorption syndromes (celiac syndrome, cystic fibrosis, parasites)
    2. Regional enteritis
    3. Hepatic insufficiency
  E. Hematologic
    1. Chronic anemia (congenital or acquired)
  F. Skeletal and reticuloendothelial
    1. Chondrodystrophies
    2. Mucopolysaccharidoses
    3. Gangliosidoses
    4. Rickets
      a. Nutritional vitamin D deficiency
      b. Insensitivity to vitamin D
      c. Hypophosphatasia
    5. Diseases of the spine (congenital or acquired)
    6. Brachymetacarpal dwarfism
      a. Albright's hereditary osteodystrophy (pseudo- and pseudopseudohypoparathyroidism)
        1. With and without abnormalites of serum calcium and phosphorus
  G. Endocrinologic
    1. Hypopituitarism
    2. Hypothyroidism
    3. Hypoadrenocorticism
    4. Hyperadrenocorticism (spontaneous or iatrogenic)
    5. Ganglioneuroma
  H. Central nervous
    1. Mental retardation of varied etiology
V. Inborn errors of metabolism
  A. Aminoaciduria and aminoacidemias
  B. Ketoacidurias
VI. Primordial dwarfism
  A. Intrauterine growth retardation
    1. Associated with placental insufficiency (toxemia, idiopathic)
    2. Assocated with intrauterine infections (e.g., rubella, cytomegalic inclusion disease, toxoplasmosis)
  B. Progeria
  C. Dwarfism with or without associated anomalies (e.g., Seckel, Cockayne, Silver)

Source: Root, A. W., Bongiovanni, A. M., and Eberstein, W. R. Diagnosis and management of growth retardation with special reference to the problem of hypopituitarism. *J. Pediatr.* 78:737, 1971.

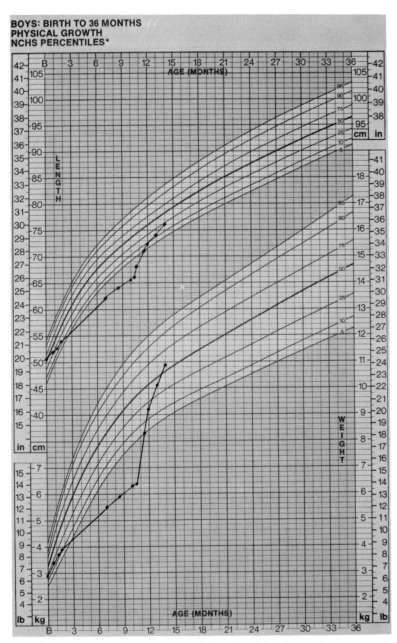

Figure 7-7. Serial measurements of length and weight of a child with failure to thrive and subsequent catch-up growth.

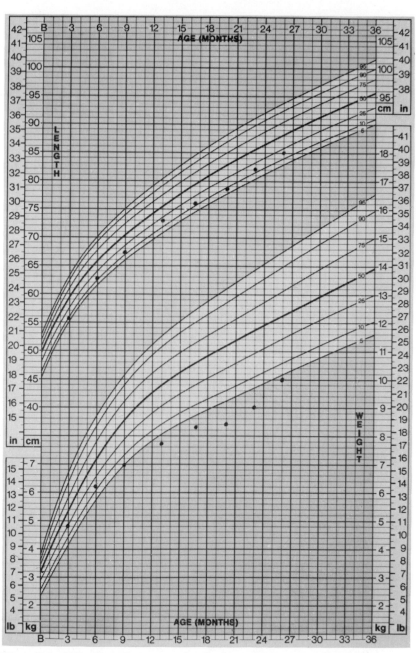

Figure 7-8. Girl with celiac disease. Note the decrease in weight gain that occurred at 6 months of age when cereals were added to her diet and the increase in weight gain following initiation of a gluten-free diet at 20 months.

in the first 6 to 8 months of postnatal life. An initial retardation of weight may take up to 24 months to compensate for, while catch-up in length may take up to 3½ years. However, catch-up in weight and length may occur at later ages independent of whether there is catch-up in head circumference in the first months of life [1].

CONCLUSION

The evaluation of nutritional status is not completed with a single test but with a compilation of anthropometric, biochemical, clinical, and dietary data. Children with overt malnutrition are easy to detect and can often fit neatly into Waterlow's classification of malnutrition (Table 7-17). However, children in the pediatric population are more often affected by subclinical malnutrition—a more difficult entity to diagnose. The diagnosis of malnutrition is confounded by the progressive nature of insidious deficiency disease, the range of individual nutrient requirements, inadequate measurement tools, and lack of comparative standards. Despite the poor state of the art, monitoring the nutrients known to be at risk in certain children can prevent further depletion and promote well-being. Table 7-18 summarizes the signs of nutrient deficiency in children known to be at risk.

Children identified as nutrient deficient are in need of nutritional counseling by a qualified practitioner who can provide diet therapy while considering the child's feeding ability, food preferences, behavior, and family resources and who also has a knowledge of government programs and community agencies (see Appendix 9). Programs such as the Food Stamp Program and the Special Supplemental Feeding Program for Women, Infants, and Children (WIC) are available for those who meet the criteria. The evaluation of nutritional status is the first step toward nutritional counseling. It will play an increasing role in the health care of the developing child and should, in this era, be an integral part of routine pediatrics.

Table 7-17. Waterlow Classification of Malnutrition

Grade of Malnutrition	Weight for Height[a] (percent of standard)	Height for Age[b] (percent of standard)
0	>90	>95
1	81–90	90–95
2	70–80	85–89
3	<70	<85

Note: Weight for height versus height for age differentiates acute from chronic malnutrition or the duration of nutritional deprivation.
Adapted from [a]Waterlow, J. C. Classification and definition of protein-calorie-malnutrition. *Br. Med. J. [Clin. Res.]* 2:566, 1972, and [b]Waterlow, J. C. Some aspects of childhood malnutrition as a public health problem. *Br. Med. J. [Clin. Res.]* 4:88, 1974.

202

Table 7-18. Nutritional Evaluation

Nutrient	Diet Sources	Signs of Deficiency		Conditions that Place Children At Risk
		Clinical	Laboratory	
Protein	Meat, fish, poultry, eggs, milk, milk products (including yogurt, cheese), vegetable protein: dried peas, beans, lentils, oil seeds (i.e., sunflower), nut butters, meat analogues, tofu	Hair: dull, dry, sparse, dyspigmented, pluckable, loss of curl, flag sign; moon facies; emaciation; edema; decreased muscle strength and wasting; enlarged fatty liver; flaky skin rash; poor growth	Decreased serum protein, serum albumin, prealbumin, transferrin, hemoglobin, creatinine-height index; delayed hypersensitivity on skin tests	Protein-restricted diet; amino acid disorders; vegan diet; malabsorption; increased needs with surgery, burns, stress; low income
Fat	Oils, mayonnaise, margarine, butter, shortening, salad dressing, bacon, animal protein (i.e., whole milk, eggs, cheese)	Sparse hair growth; skin: dry, flaky (like sandpaper); poor wound healing; loss of subcutaneous fat; poor growth	Decreased serum carotene, platelet count (linoleic acid), plasma lipids. Increased 72-hour fecal fat excretion	Malabsorption; malignancies involving gastrointestinal lymphatic drainage; gluten-sensitive enteropathy; cystic fibrosis, biliary atresia, biliary obstruction; short bowel syndrome; long-term hyperalimentation; intestinal lymphangiectasia; vegan diets
Vitamin A	Liver, fish oil, whole milk, egg yolk, fortified margarine and cereals, butter	Eyes: Bitot spots, soft cornea, dry eye membranes; skin: follicular hyperkeratosis	Decreased plasma, vitamin A, carotene, retinol	Gluten-sensitive enteropathy; chronic liver disease: biliary atresia, cirrhosis; cystic fibrosis

Vitamin	Sources	Deficiency symptoms	Laboratory findings	Predisposing conditions
Provitamin A (carotene)	Dark green and deep yellow fruits and vegetables			
Vitamin D	Fortified milk and milk products (including yogurt, cheese), sunlight exposure	Head: frontal and parietal bossing, thin skull bones, craniotabes, open anterior fontanel; beading of ribs (rachitic rosary); legs: bow-legs, knock-knees; flared wrists	Decreased serum clacium (early and late), phosphorus, vitamin D, bone age Increased alkaline phosphatase, urinary amino acids	Gluten-sensitive enteropathy; chronic liver disease; biliary atresia; cirrhosis; chronic renal disease; cystic fibrosis; antiseizure medications
Vitamin E	Vegetable oils, wheat germ, cereals, legumes, green leafy vegetables	Deficiency symptoms rare; in premature infants: irritability, edema, hemolytic anemia; ataxia; peripheral neuropathy	Decreased plasma tocopherol Increased peroxide hemolysis	Prematurity; cystic fibrosis; steatorrhea; abetalipoproteinemia
Vitamin C (ascorbic acid)	Citrus fruits, juice, other fruits (strawberries, melon, cantaloupe, acerola, papaya, guava, black currants), rose hips, vegetables (tomatoes, cabbage, potatoes)	Infantile scurvy: frog's leg position, dry rough skin, irritability, lip tenderness, extreme sensitivity in arms and legs; bleeding, spongy gums; loose teeth; skin: petechia, dry; delayed wound healing; swollen joints; aching bones; normochromic anemia	Decreased serum ascorbic acid, alkaline phosphatase, urine ascorbic acid	Unsupplemented cow's milk formula; Feingold diet

Table 7-18 (Continued)

Nutrient	Diet Sources	Signs of Deficiency		Conditions that Place Children At Risk
		Clinical	Laboratory	
Thiamine (B₁)	Whole grain products, enriched grain products, wheat germ, pork, legumes, nuts, brewer's yeast	Beriberi; infants: congestive heart failure; cyanosis; tachycardia; vomiting; sensory loss; motor weakness; calf tenderness, cardiac enlargement; anorexia	Decreased urine thiamine, erythrocyte transketolase Increased blood pyruvate and lactate	Beriberi (rare) found in developing countries where children subsist on polished rice
Riboflavin (B₂)	Milk, milk products (including yogurt and cheese), green leafy vegetables, organ meats, enriched grain products	Scaling around nostrils; glossitis; photophobia; cheilosis; scrotal and vulval dermatosis; redness and fissuring of eyelid corners	Decreased urine riboflavin, plasma riboflavin, RBC count, glutathione reductase	Deficiency (rare) found in conjunction with other B vitamin deficiencies; vegan diets; unsupplemented milk free diets
Niacin	Meat, fish, poultry, whole grain and enriched grain products, peanut butter	Pellagra; glossitis; redness and fissuring of eyelid corners; dermatitis (Casal's necklace, rash around neck); diarrhea; dementia; change in nerve cell function	Decreased urine N-methyl, nicotinamide, plasma nicotinamide Increased RBC count	Pellagra (rare)
Pyridoxine (B₆)	Meat (especially liver, beef, pork), bananas, whole grain products, wheat germ	Glossitis; stomatitis; cheilosis; microcytic anemia; muscle weakness; mental depression	Decreased RBC count, SGPT, SGOT, plasma PALP Decreased urine B₆ and/ or pyridoxic acid Increased urine excretion of xanthurenic acid in response to tryptophan load test	Toddler diets can be deficient in B₆, unsupplemented formulas

B$_{12}$	Meat, fish, poultry, eggs, milk, cheese, fortified cereal, fortified soy milk, brewer's yeast	Neurological symptoms; hyperpigmentation; glossitis; filiform papillary atrophy; pernicious anemia; macrocytic anemia	Decreased hemoglobin, reticulocyte count, serum B$_{12}$ Increased MCH, MCV	Vegan diets; breast-fed children of vegan mothers; regional enteritis; short bowel syndrome
Folic acid	Green leafy vegetables, whole grain products, wheat germ, organ meats, legumes, milk (except goat's milk), brewer's yeast	Glossitis; filiform papillary atrophy; hyperpigmentation; gastrointestinal disturbances; macrocytic anemia	Decreased hemoglobin, serum folate	Idiopathic steatorrhea; gluten-sensitive enteropathy; chronic infectious enteritis; hemolytic anemia; liver disease; malignancy; myeloproliferative disease; drugs: methotrexate, pentamidine, phenytoin, aminopterin
Calcium	Milk, milk products, green leafy vegetables (collard greens, mustard, turnip greens, kale, spinach), shellfish, salmon, sardines, tofu (processed with calcium), bone meal, black strap molasses	Reproduce symptoms of rickets	Decreased calcium (may be normal), serum phosphorus (may be normal), urine calcium, urine phosphorus, bone age; increased serum alkaline phosphatase	Gluten-sensitive enteropathy; acute pancreatitis; malabsorption; cystic fibrosis; milk-free diets; vegan diets; toddler diets; diets lacking calcium sources

Table 7-18 (Continued)

Nutrient	Diet Sources	Signs of Deficiency		Conditions that Place Children At Risk
		Clinical	Laboratory	
Iron	Heme soures: beef, chicken, fish, lamb, liver, pork; nonheme sources: whole grain or enriched grains, dairy products, eggs, soluble iron supplements	Pale skin and eye membranes; smooth tongue; spoon nails (brittle, ridged); behavioral changes: short attention span, lassitude, fatigue, weakness, irritability; microcytic hypochromic anemia	Decreased hemoglobin, MCH, MCHC, MCV, serum transferrin saturation, serum iron; increased total iron-binding capacity	Chronic blood loss (i.e., parasites in intestine); decreased food intake (poverty, esophagitis); malabsorption; toddler diets; unsupplemented infant diets
Zinc	Meat, liver, eggs, seafood, oysters, cereals, legumes	Anorexia; growth retardation; short stature; delayed wound healing; dermatitis; hypogeusia; hypogonadism; lethargy, depression	Decreased serum zinc, red blood cell zinc, hair zinc, urine zinc, serum alkaline phosphatase, glucose tolerance	Sickle cell anemia; malabsorption; chronic renal disease; upper respiratory infections; malignant neoplasms; toddler diets; parenteral nutrition

Data from: Dietz, W. H., Jr., Personal Communication. Jan. 1983, Howard, R. B., and Herbold, N. H. (Eds.). *Nutrition in Clinical Care.* New York: McGraw-Hill, 1982, and Wallach, J. *Interpretation of Diagostic Tests* (3rd ed.). Boston: Little, Brown, 1978.

REFERENCES

1. Brandt, I. Growth Dynamics of Low-Birth-Weight Infants with Emphasis on the Perinatal Period. In F. Falkner and J. M. Tanner (Eds.), *Human Growth 2. Postnatal Growth*. New York: Plenum, 1978.
2. Cronk, C. E. Growth of children with Down's syndrome: Birth to age 3 years. *Pediatrics* 61:654, 1977.
3. Cronk, C. E., and Roche, A. F. Race- and sex-specific reference data for triceps and subscapular skinfolds and weight/stature. *Am. J. Dis. Child.* 35:347, 1982.
4. Falkner, F. Office measurement of physical growth. *Pediatr. Clin. North Am.* 8:13, 1961.
5. Fomon, S. J. *Infant Nutrition*. Philadelphia: Saunders, 1974.
6. Fomon, S. J., Haschke, F., Ziegler, E. F., and Helson, S. E. Body composition of reference children from birth to age 10 years. *Am. J. Clin. Nutr.* 35:1169, 1982.
7. Food and Nutrition Board, National Research Council. *Recommended Dietary Allowances* (9th ed.). Washington, D.C.: National Academy of Sciences, 1980.
8. Forbes, G. B. A note on the mathematics of "catch-up" growth. *Pediatr. Res.* 8:929, 1974.
9. Frisancho, A. R. Triceps skinfold and upper arm muscle size norms for assessment of nutritional status. *Am. J. Clin. Nutr.* 27:15, 1974.
10. Frisancho, A. R. New norms of upper limb fat and muscle areas for assessment of nutritional status. *Am. J. Clin. Nutr.* 34:2540, 1981.
11. Gersonitz, M., Madden, J. P., and Snucklas-Wright, H. Validity of the 24-hour dietary recall and seven-day record for group comparisons. *J. Am. Diet. Assoc.* 73:48, 1977.
12. Hooley, R. A. Clinical nutritional assessment: A perspective. *J. Am. Diet. Assoc.* 77:682, 1980.
13. Kanawati, A. A., and McLaren, D. S. Failure to thrive, in Lebanon. *Acta. Paediatr. Scand.* 62 [Suppl.]:571, 1973.
14. Karvetti, R. L., and Knuts, L. R. Agreement between dietary interviews. *J. Am. Diet. Assoc.* 79:654, 1981.
15. Martorell, R., Yarbrough, C., Klein, R. E., and Lechtig, A. Malnutrition, body size, and skeletal maturation: Interrelationships and implications for catch-up growth. *Hum. Biol.* 51:371, 1979.
16. McLaren, D. S. Nutrition Assessment. In D. S. McLaren and D. Burman (Eds.), *Textbook of Paediatric Nutrition* (2nd ed.). New York: Churchill Livingstone, 1982.
17. National Center for Health Statistics (NCHS), U.S. Department of Health, Education, and Welfare. *NCHS Growth Curves for Children: Birth to 18 Years.* Series 11, No. 165, DHEW Publication No. (PHS) 78-1650, 1977.
18. Nellhaus, G. Head circumference from birth to 18 years. *Pediatrics* 41:106, 1968.
19. Owen, G. M. The assessment and recording of measurements of growth of children. *Pediatrics* 57:461, 1973.
20. Owen, G. M. Measurement, recording, and assessment of skinfold thickness in childhood and adolescence: Report of a small meeting. *Am. J. Clin. Nutr.* 35:629, 1982.
21. Owen, G. M., Kram, K. M., Garry, P. J., Lowe, J. E., and Lubin, A. H. A study of nutritional status of preschool children in the United States, 1968–1970. *Ped. Suppl.* 53:594, 1974.
22. Patton, R. G., and Gardner, L. I. Influences of family environment on growth: The syndrome of maternal deprivation. *Pediatrics* 30:957, 1962.

23. Prader, A., Tanner, J. M., and von Harnack, G. A. Catch-up growth following illness or starvation. An example of developmental canalization in man. *J. Pediatr.* 62:646, 1973.
24. *Preliminary Findings of the First Health and Nutrition Education Survey. U.S., 1971–1972.* DHEW Publication No. (HSA) 74-1219-1, 1974.
25. Roche, A. F. Growth assessment in abnormal children. *Kidney Int.* 14:369, 1978.
26. Roche, A. F. Growth assessment of handicapped children. *Ross Dietetic Currents* 6:25, 1979.
27. Sanchez, C. L., and Jacobson, H. N. Anthropometry measurements, a new type. *Am. J. Clin. Nutr.* 31:1116, 1978.
28. Smith, D. W., Troug, W., Rogers, J. E., Greitzer, L. J., Skinner, A. L., McCann, J. J., and Harvey, M. A. Shifting linear growth during infancy: Illustration of genetic factors in growth from fetal life through infancy. *J. Pediatr.* 89:225, 1976.
29. Tanner, J. M., Goldstein, H., and Whitehouse, R. H. Standards for children's height at ages 2-9 years allowing for height of parents. *Arch. Dis. Child.* 45:755, 1970.
30. *Ten-State Nutrition Survey in the United States. 1968–1970.* DHEW Publication No. (HSM) 72-8129 through 72-8134, 1972.
31. Waterlow, J. C. Classification and definition of protein-calorie malnutrition. *Br. Med. J.* 2:566, 1972.
32. Zerfas, A. J. Office assessment of nutritional status. *Pediatr. Clin. North Am.* 24:253, 1977.

8. The Infant at Nutritional Risk

Janis Maksimak, Martin Maksimak, Jeffrey A. Biller,
Julie R. Ingelfinger, David H. Perlmutter, Frances J. Rohr,
Harry Shwachman, and Harland S. Winter

Infancy is a time of rapid growth. By the age of 2 years most healthy children almost quadruple their birth weight. Because of this growth, good nutrition is important and becomes more so if medical problems develop, since the stress of an illness markedly increases nutrient needs. In addition, diet may itself be the only treatment, as with inborn errors of metabolism or gluten-sensitive enteropathy, or may be part of the treatment, as in renal disease or congenital heart disease.

In this chapter, some of the medical conditions that place the child at nutritional risk and their nutritional management are examined by clinical practitioners who agree that nutritional therapy must be coupled with nutritional counseling to make it effective.

Congenital Heart Disease
Janis Maksimak

Congenital malformations of the heart take a variety of forms and are caused by many prenatal factors, including genetic, infectious, metabolic, and teratogenic. Alterations in the flow of blood and the transport of oxygen are common to all lesions. Congestive heart failure, cyanosis, acidosis, pulmonary hypertension, repeated infections, and growth retardation may result. Any of these sequelae may contribute to growth failure, but many infants who seem to be well do not grow adequately.

ETIOLOGY OF GROWTH FAILURE
In data collected by the New England Regional Infant Cardiac Program, 19 percent of children with congenital heart disease weighed less than 2500 gm at birth. By 5 years of age, 21 percent were still in less than the fifth percentile for weight [1]. Percentages varied with the type of congenital heart disease. Specifically, infants with transposition of the great vessels at birth tended to be normal in size, whereas over 14 percent of infants with a ventricular septal defect are small for gestational age. Although the severity of the cardiac defect contributes to the hypoxia, hypermetabolism, malabsorption, and other factors of growth, correction of one single factor rarely reverses growth failure entirely. As the severity of the cardiac failure increases, the amount of oxygen consumed per kilogram of body weight also increases. In these children, the amount of total body fat is decreased,

which results in an increase in the relative proportion of the lean body mass. Thus, adequate caloric needs may be as high as 150 to 180 kcal/kg per day.

Malabsorption may also be a factor in the poor growth of these children. Infants who have hypothermia at the time of surgery frequently have diarrhea postoperatively. Diarrhea may be related to disaccharidase intolerance presumably due to damage of the intestinal brush border. Although the underlying congenital heart disease may result in intestinal epithelial cell injury, the brush border enzymes seem to return to normal in the postoperative period. Because of this, it is suggested that in the first week or two following surgery, infants receive a sucrose- or glucose-containing formula [4]. There is also evidence that children with cyanotic congenital heart disease have mild degrees of fat malabsorption [2]. Nevertheless, fat restriction is rarely recommended because fat is a high energy food and dietary restriction may result in inadequate caloric intake. Attention should be given to more easily absorbable forms of fats such as medium chain triglycerides and polyunsaturated oils.

Hypoxia may also be a factor in growth failure, but the severity of growth retardation does not correlate with the degree of hypoxia. This is a complicated issue because if the child's heart disease is surgically corrected at an early age, the possibility for catch-up growth appears to be greater.

One of the most significant factors in the growth failure of children with congenital heart disease is the maintenance of adequate calories. The amount of energy required to nurse from the breast or the bottle may result in dyspnea, fatigue, and cyanosis. These children have periods of excellent intake followed by periods of low caloric intake. For the health provider to be encouraged by a few days of good appetite or to begin intervention after a day or two of poor intake does not allow for variability in daily eating habits. Some have suggested that the rate of gastric emptying may be delayed in children with congenital heart disease. This problem may cause early satiety and intermittent emesis. Changes should be made only after a prolonged period of observation in which the ranges of intake have been established.

Parents are often justifiably concerned about the weight gain of their children. Feeding times are fraught with anxiety. At feedings when the infant would normally be nurtured, parents must watch for signs and symptoms of congestive heart failure. The potential cyanotic episodes, dyspnea, and cough all contribute to parental anxiety at mealtimes. These concerns can become important issues and must be discussed in an open, supportive forum.

Anticipatory guidance should be offered to the parents of infants and children with congenital heart disease. Parents should learn to positively reinforce good food behaviors with attention and praise while quietly and calmly ignoring negative behaviors. Pediatricians working in conjunction with the family's cardiologist can provide support in dealing with the cyanosis, gagging, and vomiting that are frequently encountered when feeding an infant with congenital heart disease.

TREATMENT

The objective in managing the infant with congenital heart disease is to provide adequate calories, protein, and other nutrients without exceeding fluid limits or solute load. As previously mentioned, when compared to healthy babies of similar ages, infants with congenital heart disease have a greater caloric need per kilogram. The average infant formula of 20 kcal per ounce is often inadequate. Commercially prepared formulas with a caloric density of 24 kcal per ounce are available or standard formulas such as SMA or Similac PM 60/40, both low in sodium and with easily absorbable oils, may be supplemented with Polycose or medium chain triglycerides to provide 25 to 30 calories per ounce. Standard formulas should not be concentrated by adding less water than recommended. This limits free water and may result in serious problems for the child with limited intake or increased losses due to diarrhea or vomiting (see Appendix 3). Close dietary supervision is needed because additives may dilute the protein content of the formula needed for optimal growth, exceed the renal solute load, or lead to steatorrhea or carbohydrate-induced diarrhea.

If the infant fatigues during bottle-feedings or has difficulty controlling swallowing and respiration, small amounts of strained infant foods from a spoon or thickened liquids from a cup (formula may be thickened with fruit or cereal) may impose less stress on the infant and promote better intake.

Continuous nasogastric enteral feedings have also been reported to be of benefit in the child with congenital heart disease who is failing to thrive. A small nasogastric feeding tube is placed into the stomach and an appropriate formula is infused over a 24-hour period. Nasogastric tubes are replaced every 3 days and formula-containing tubes and bottles are replaced daily. In one study [3], initial infusion rates ranged between 100 to 150 ml/kg per day that provided 70 to 120 kcal/kg per day. Eventually, children tolerated as high as 150 kcal/kg per day. Complications from gastroesophageal reflux and tube-induced esophagitis were not noted.

Although commercial manufacturers no longer add salt to baby foods, when the infant begins taking semisolid foods, the sodium content must be considered. Foods should be selected with calories and the overall nutrient contribution in mind. If baby food is home-prepared, foods used in the preparation should be selected with the sodium content in mind, and no salt should be added in cooking. To increase the calories, small amounts of Polycose, MCT (medium chain triglycerides), or polyunsaturated oil can be mixed into the food.

With congestive heart failure, fluid intake is a concern. Most cardiologists prefer to encourage oral intake and control fluids with diuretics. This avoids caloric deprivation in the guise of fluid restriction. A potassium-sparing diuretic such as spironolactone or triamterene may be used in combination with chlorothiazide or furosemide. Potassium supplements are often needed because the child cannot eat enough high potassium foods (i.e., bananas and orange juice) to replace potassium losses.

Children with congenital heart disease deserve special and individualized considerations. By selecting appropriate types of foods and means of delivery, growth potential may be maximized.

Renal Disease
Julie R. Ingelfinger

NUTRIENT ALTERATIONS
Much of the kidneys' work load is determined by the composition of the food and the amount of nutrients an individual ingests. For that reason nutritional factors must be considered to understand renal function in health and disease [31]. Under normal circumstances, the kidneys are the major organs responsible for homeostatic functions such as conservation and excretion of water and solutes, maintenance of normal acid base and electrolyte balance, and excretion of the waste products of metabolism. When renal disease is present, these functions still belong to the kidneys, though a number of adjustments take place to maintain homeostasis. In addition, endocrine functions of the kidneys such as hydroxylation of vitamin D and production of renin, erythropoietin, and prostaglandins may indirectly affect nutrition.

Renal disease often leads to changes in human nutritional status. In uremia, a number of alterations in the metabolic state occur, including decrease in cell mass, increases in extracellular fluid, total body water, and often sodium, and decrease in body fat. Lean body mass also decreases. Vitamin D metabolism is disordered, and cortisol, growth hormone, and insulin levels are often increased, while somatomedin is decreased [31]. Serum zinc, copper, protein, amino acids, and the ratio of essential to nonessential amino acids (as well as valine to glycine) may decrease [31]. Along with these metabolic abnormalities, patients tend to exhibit behavioral changes—anorexia and decreased intake of nutrients. Thus, energy intake is often deficient. In renal disease, additional factors that affect nutrition may be involved, such as altered taste sensation [51] and abnormal gastrointestinal function. Apparently unrelated problems such as the necessity for multiple medications for hypertension and metabolic bone disease may affect nutrition [15, 18, 37–39]. Food may come to have a psychological meaning for children as they use the ingestion or non-ingestion of meals and snacks for attention [53].

ENERGY

Children with renal insufficiency frequently have a low energy intake for age and/or height [11, 14, 31, 36]. This is especially true in very young children where usual energy requirements (percentage of RDA) are 115 kcal/kg per day between 0 and 6 months of age, 105 kcal/kg per day from 6 to 12 months, and 100 kcal/kg per day for the 1- to 3-year-old [53]. Indeed, many groups have tried to relate the decreased energy intake in chronic renal failure patients to the frequently seen growth retardation. This is not always possible, because other factors contribute to the growth failure—metabolic bone disease (secondary hypoparathyroidism) [42], acidemia [54], abnormal vitamin D metabolism [13, 16], and other, less clear parameters. Nevertheless, spontaneous food intake of children with chronic renal disease is often inadequate for catch-up growth [53]. Growth rates have correlated with energy intake in some groups [7, 49], but there is also evidence that calorie utilization may be impaired in some patients [12].

With protein-calorie malnutrition, energy requirements for repair and restoration of homeostasis increase. There are certain similarities between uremia and protein-calorie malnutrition. Children recovering from malnutrition require 140 to 160 kcal/kg per day, and their catch-up growth is related to their caloric intake [31]. Increased energy requirement may also be present because of inefficient utilization; even with supplementation, calorie requirements are high.

PROTEIN

In renal insufficiency, plasma levels of urea and other nitrogen-containing compounds rise. Some of these compounds are toxic and are associated with metabolic abnormalities. Malaise and anorexia are also associated with severe renal insufficiency [40]. For that reason, protein intake in patients with renal insufficiency has frequently been restricted. This can lead to symptomatic improvement as well as decreased intake of phosphorus and nitrogen. Such observations led to the use of the Giordano-Giovanetti diet, which was a very high-calorie diet for adults, containing 20 gm of high biological value protein or essential amino acids [29, 30]. However, others suggested that this amount of protein in a high-calorie diet could lead to negative nitrogen balance and that twice the amount of high biological value protein was needed for positive balance [53].

In the United States, normal children ingest a large amount of protein. In order for protein intake to be diminished below 100 percent of RDA, energy intake would need to be decreased by approximately one-half. In children with severe renal insufficiency, energy intake may be so decreased that this is the case. An excess protein intake might increase urea generation, promote inefficient nitrogen utilization, and cause problems; however, if high protein might improve nitrogen retention in children, the results could be beneficial. For the child on chronic hemodialysis, it has been unclear until recently whether liberalized protein intake would enhance nutrition or whether it was still preferable to limit protein intake, compensating with very high energy levels. Recently, Grupe and colleagues showed that raising protein intake was correlated with improved protein balance when protein represents 12 percent of the available total energy [34]. Thus, with adequate energy intake, the use of high-quality protein (i.e., in eggs or meat) is beneficial, and further restriction may not be necessary.

Because nonessential amino acids are manufactured in the human, low-protein diets supplemented with keto acids or essential amino acids, together with adequate calorie intake, have been studied as a means for lessening the degree of urea production and promoting positive nitrogen balance [23, 52]. Individuals on such diets maintain positive nitrogen balance without increasing urea levels. Reports of such diets in children are still very limited at this time, and in view of some early data [8, 41], nitrogen balance may be positive, but growth in height and intracellular water do not seem to increase.

In the dialyzed child, some protein loss occurs [43]. In hemodialysis this is not significant, but with peritoneal dialysis, major protein loss may occur (primarily albumin but also some immunoglobulins and amino acids) [43]. Smaller amounts of large protein molecules are lost in the dialysate because they do not pass as freely through the peritoneal membrane. However, the amount of protein lost does not require supplementation in the average dialyzed child.

It is important to note that the optimal daily allowances of protein in the daily diet and the ratio of essential to nonessential amino acids has not been established for infants or young children with renal disease [22, 31, 53]. There are no definitive recommendations for the use of essential amino acids or ketoanalogs of amino acids in children [5, 6, 31, 53]. Because urea is the major toxic by-product of protein metabolism, the consideration of nitrogenous substances in the diet of the child with renal disease becomes important. An optimal balance must be found between excess nitrogen and toxic by-products and inadequate nitrogen and malnutrition. For normal children, the recommended daily allowance for protein ranges between 0.8 and 2 gm/kg, as shown in Table 8-1. When a child has a glomerular filtration rate greater than 25 percent of normal for age, protein intake should correspond to the RDA. With an extremely decreased glomerular fil-

Table 8-1. Dietary Intake for Pediatric Dialysis Patients

Parameter	Suggested Daily Intake
Calories	Approximately 100 cal/kg, depending on deficit, activity
Fluid	Approximately 20 ml/kg plus urine output from previous day (insensible water loss and prior day urine output)
Protein	Approximately 0.8–2 gm protein per kg
Na^+	1–2 gm/day depending on presence or absence of hypertension, edema, body size (70–100 mEq/m²/day or 2–3 mEq/kg/day)
K^+	1–2 gm/day depending on size (< 1 mEq/kg/day)
$PO_4^=$	400–600 mg/day in infants and younger children; 600–800 mg/day in older children and adolescents

tration rate (GFR), a lower protein diet has generally been recommended. High biological value protein is preferred and is found in such sources as eggs, meat, and fish. The studies of Grupe and colleagues would suggest that restriction may not be necessary [33, 34].

For the child on dialysis, Grupe and colleagues [34] found a linear correlation between net protein balance and protein intake with neutral balance predicted at a daily intake of protein of 0.3 gm per centimeter of height. Though there was no correlation between protein intake and protein catabolic rate (PCR) in the patients studied as a whole, there was a positive correlation between protein intake and PCR when those in positive and negative balance were grouped. Even more important, children in positive nitrogen balance had a lower PCR at each level of protein intake and thus a lower urea generation rate, indicating a lesser dialysis requirement. Thus, increased protein intake may be necessary in the young child with dialysis to produce positive protein balance and thus increase the potential for height and growth. Further studies in this area are needed at this time.

Protein Utilization in Nephrotic Syndrome

In contrast to end-stage renal disease, excess protein losses by the kidney may occur if there is a normal glomerular filtration rate, yet heavy proteinuria [32]. Childhood nephrotic syndrome is one such entity affecting very young children. With active nephrosis, up to 70 percent of total protein intake may be lost in the urine as albumin and other plasma proteins. Immunoglobulins and complement may also be lost in the urine depending upon the selectivity of the protein. In addition, decreased production and utilization of these proteins may occur within the body. This constellation of problems may effectively drain the protein stores of the body, and lead to tissue wasting, malnutrition, impaired immunity, and the severe edema so often seen. Hyperlipidemia is associated and may be related. In a child with steroid-responsive nephrotic syndrome, the average time to respond is 14 to 17 days; long-term nutritional problems related to protein loss are uncommon. However, some youngsters may not respond for 4 to 12 weeks, or the child may be steroid resistant and be faced with ongoing long-term protein losses. With active nephrosis, some patients also have malabsorption.

When treating a child with nephrosis, large amounts of high quality protein are advisable. Generally, supplementation with amino acids or keto acids is not necessary. Very occasionally, enteral or parenteral alimentation can be considered in severe malnutrition.

ABNORMALITIES IN CARBOHYDRATE METABOLISM

Renal failure defects in cellular glucose metabolism lead to an increase in gluconeogenesis, a decrease in glycolysis, and a decrease in glycogen synthesis [47]. There is an elevated ratio of insulin to glucose during glucose tolerance testing and it has generally been felt that there is a peripheral insensitivity to insulin [24, 26]. With these defects, there is an inefficiency of glucose utilization and relative glucose intolerance. Nonetheless, it has been felt that glucose and other carbohydrates are protein sparing and decrease endogenous protein catabolism and the production of urea. Thus, in chronic renal failure, high-carbohydrate diets have been recommended. It has been estimated that, to minimize endogenous protein catabolism, the basal carbohydrate intake should be 75 gm of glucose per square meter daily. Adding products such as Polycose to the diet of a child in renal failure may be helpful in supplementing caloric intake.

Reversal of some of the carbohydrate metabolic abnormalities may be achieved through dialysis. Improvement in glucose tolerance following dialysis may suggest that uremic toxins are factors for insulin resistance; as yet, none has been isolated.

Carbohydrate supplements may be ingested as hard candy, gumdrops, jelly, honey, jam, sugar, or Popsicles. Polycose, a powder polymer of glucose, is a protein-free carbohydrate that can be mixed with formula or drinks. Controlyte is a protein-free carbohydrate supplement supplying 1,000 kcal in 7 ounces of powder, which can also be added to drinks or used in cooking. A high-calorie, low-electrolyte beverage called Cal-Power is a drink that supplies 775 kcal/8 ounces. Hycal is a similar beverage that provides 425 kcal/175 ml.

LIPID ABNORMALITIES

Hyperlipidemia and hypertriglyceridemia are common findings in renal failure and appear to be more pronounced in patients on dialysis [10, 24, 25]. A high frequency of vascular disease in patients with chronic renal insufficiency has been reported (including a relatively young population) [46]. However, in young children with chronic renal failure, no direct complications have been reported.

In adults on maintenance dialysis, triglyceride levels increase. This abnormality places a limit on the use of fat for protein sparing. The exact cause for the hyperlipidemia is unclear, though some have suggested that nitrogen retention may be involved. For instance, cysteine levels are increased in the plasma of uremic patients [44]. It is a nonessential amino acid originating from demethylation of methionine through homocystine and cystathionine [19]. This pathway is stimulated in uremia [20]. Serum homocystine is increased as a result of the excessive demethylation of methionine in uremics. In an unrelated syndrome, homocystinuria, there is a deficiency of the enzyme cystathionine synthetase (which leads to the accumulation of homocystine) [19]. This syndrome is associated with an increase of vascular accidents due to rapidly advancing atherosclerosis. Thus, in uremic patients this metabolic pathway may result in abnormalities in lipid metabolism.

Abnormalities in lipid metabolism are commonplace in active nephrotic syndrome with normal renal function [17]. Hypercholesterolemia and hypertriglyceridemia are hallmarks of the disease. The etiology of the hyperlipidemia is unknown at this time and may be related to the hypoproteinemia [9] or to altered lipoprotein lipase activity [45]. Although the hyperlipidemia is worrisome, patients in remission have normal cholesterol and triglyceride levels. Thus, most childhood nephrotics do not have constant lipid abnormalities. For the child with unresponsive and active nephrosis, the question of how to treat this problem is absolutely unresolved.

SODIUM

In renal failure, the abilities to retain and excrete sodium may be impaired. Children with renal tubular abnormalities may waste sodium [21, 35]. Such patients include those with relatively normal renal function who have renal dysplasia or medullary cystic disease. Some patients with pyelonephritis or interstitial nephritis also waste sodium. In the recovery phase of acute renal failure during diuresis, much sodium, as well as water, may be excreted. Occasional patients with severe renal insufficiency due to interstitial and tubular problems continue to waste sodium. Rather than providing a set figure for sodium replacement, it is important to remember that even in infants with renal disease, it is worthwhile to determine urine sodium losses so that daily sodium intake may be adjusted. When reduction of salt intake is sudden in such children, extracellular fluid is not maintained, further decreasing glomerular filtration rate and rapidly leading to accumulation of waste products and possibly uremic symptoms. Thus, those caring for children with renal disease who are salt wasters should be alerted to the possibility that even short periods of decreased sodium intake may lead to acute changes in renal function and potential morbidity.

In some children with renal disease, however, the ability to excrete a sodium load is impaired [48]. A result of this is positive sodium balance, and for each 3 gm (130 to 140 mEq) of sodium retained, the patient must retain a liter of water in the body in order to maintain isotonicity. If a child with decreased ability to excrete a sodium load takes in a high salt burden, it is possible to become volume expanded very rapidly. For most children with chronic renal insufficiency, salt should be restricted to approximately 2 mEq/kg per day. This sort of restriction is also helpful for a child with edema-forming nephropathy, such as various forms of nephrotic syndrome. If the physician is unsure as to whether a child with renal disease is a sodium waster or a sodium retainer, it is helpful to collect a 24-hour urine specimen under stable conditions in order to assess sodium requirement.

POTASSIUM

The safe and adequate daily dietary intake of potassium is about 650 mg per day for the first 6 months of life, 850 mg per day for the second 6 months of life, and 1,100 mg per day for a child between ages 1 and 3 [53]. Hyperkalemia is generally only a problem with acute and severe renal failure or with the development of end-stage renal disease because the renal tubules increase potassium secretion with advancing renal insufficiency. In addition, there is evidence that the intestinal tract secretes more potassium with renal disease.

The mechanisms for potassium secretion operate near or at maximum levels in chronic renal insufficiency, and sudden addition of potassium by an acute catabolic event (such as a GI bleed) or by dietary indiscretion can cause hyperkalemia. Patients with chronic renal failure may require dietary restriction and possibly potassium binding agents. One binding agent, a sodium and potassium exchange resin (Kayexalate) [28], is given in sorbitol with vehicles such as Kool-Aid or cranberry juice to make it more palatable. One gram of Kayexalate will bind approximately 1 mEq (39 mg) of potassium and release an equivalent amount of sodium. In someone receiving a great deal of Kayexalate, hypernatremia or volume expansion may occur. Dialysis may control chronic hyperkalemia.

Potassium wasting may occur in some forms of renal disease [48]. In patients with renal tubular disease or chronic pyelonephritis, hypokalemia may occur. In patients on lactose or corticosteroids, potassium wasting also may occur. Patients with chronic glomerulonephritis receiving diuretic medication may also become potassium depleted. Potassium levels and urinary excretion of potassium should be monitored in order to prevent chronic hypokalemia, which may cause weakness, systemic effects, and a secondary hypokalemic nephropathy.

VITAMINS

Vitamin deficiency states may occur in renal disease [39]. This group of nutritional disorders may stem from a number of conditions including anorexia, dietary restriction, altered metabolism, altered excretion, and altered synthesis. The need for replacement must be constantly kept in mind with a child with renal disease.

Vitamin D is converted to its active form in the kidney. Initially, cholecalciferol is converted to 25-hydroxycholecalciferol in the liver and then is converted to the active metabolite 1,25-dihydroxycholecalciferol in the kidney. The inability of the chronically diseased kidney to hydroxylate vitamin D may lead to calcium/phosphorus imbalance and play a role in metabolic bone disease. The use of dihydrotachysterol, cholecalciferol, vitamin D, or the active metabolite may circumvent this problem [13].

Folic acid deficiency has also been reported in patients with renal disease [53]. Low levels of folate may result from inadequate intake, destruction of the vitamin during food preparation and from the removal of folic acid by dialysis. Even prior to dialysis, 1 mg per day of folic acid should be supplied to patients with chronic insufficiency [27].

Low levels of ascorbic acid have been reported in patients on dialysis [27]. Children on dialysis are limited in vitamin C intake by the restriction of citrus fruits, leafy vegetables, and other fruits high in potassium. Thus, inadequate intake is to be expected, and losses through dialysis occur as well. B vitamins are water soluble and are removed during dialytic therapy [27]; intake is usually inadequate. In addition, pyridoxine metabolism is altered in the uremic state, with low levels being reported in the plasma and red blood cells. B complex vitamins are generally supplemented in a multivitamin form. A child on dialysis should receive 50 to 100 mg of ascorbic acid and 25 to 50 mg of pyridoxine [48]. In practice, the administration of a vitamin complex such as 1 ml of Polyvisol, a chewable Polyvisol tablet, or, in a child who can swallow, Famprin forte or Nephrocaps.

MINERALS

Calcium balance is generally negative in children with chronic renal failure. Specific restrictions of dairy products is usually prescribed and anorexia further decreases calcium intake. In addition, calcium absorption from the intestinal tract is depressed. Because 1,25-dihydroxycholecalciferol is decreased as mentioned above, active transport of calcium is decreased in the gastrointestinal tract. Once the calcium/ phosphorus product is below a dangerous level in children with hyperphosphatemia, calcium supplementation in the form of calcium lactate or Neo-Calglucon may be helpful [48].

In addition to hypocalcemia or a decreased calcium balance, hyperphosphatemia is a chronic problem in the child with end-stage renal disease. The hypocalcemia may be further aggravated by a reciprocal decrease in plasma-ionized calcium due to hyperphosphatemia. For each small decrement in renal function, there is an undetectable rise in plasma phosphate at first and a proportional decrease in phosphate excretion [50]. This combination of events stimulates the parathyroid gland to secrete an increased amount of parathyroid hormone, which, in turn, increases the amount of calcium and phosphate reabsorbed from bone [50]. The renal excretion of phosphate may rise in order to decrease renal phosphorus reabsorption. Development of metabolic bone disease may be an end result [50]. It has been shown that phosphate intake, which is related to protein intake, may be limited by the addition of phosphate binders to the diet.

Dosages for vitamin D supplements, calcium supplements, and phosphate binders are given in Table 8-2. An aggressive program should be begun by the time the GFR has fallen to 50 percent of its normal level.

Additional deficiencies of zinc, copper, and iron have been reported in children with renal disease [31, 51]. In the child with renal insufficiency, zinc and copper intake should be encouraged insofar as possible. However, zinc, commonly found in shellfish and meats, and copper, commonly found in nuts, raisins, shellfish, organs such as liver, and legumes, may be difficult to give a patient who is restricted in intake of those foods because of other problems such as hyperkalemia. Hence, supplementation of these minerals has been tried. In patients who are going to be hemodialyzed, iron supplementation is of dubious benefit. Most patients will receive blood transfusions and, in the long run, could become iron-overloaded rather than iron-depleted. Altered taste acuity which is common in renal insufficiency, may be related to zinc deficiency. However, the role of zinc supplementation in possibly improving appetite is, as yet, unknown.

ADDITIONAL FEEDING TECHNIQUES

Because of severe anorexia, the young infant or very young child may, in spite of all possible encouragement, have inadequate intake for positive nitrogen balance. In such instances, gavage-feeding the infant may be necessary. If it is carried out enthusiastically with home training, it can result in good increase in weight and height even in the

Table 8-2. Vitamins, Phosphate Binders, and Calcium Supplements

Vitamin D Supplements	Dose — Physiological (μg/day)	Dose — Pharmacological (μg/day)	Strength		Maximum Effect
Vitamin D_2 Calciferol, Drisdol	10	200–600	Liquid / Capsules / Tablets	200 μg/ml / 1,250 μg	qd for 30 days
Dihydrotachysterol Hytakerol	20	125–400	Liquid / Capsules / Tablets	250 μg/ml / 1,000 μg/ml / 125 μg / 200 μg / 400 μg	qd for 15 days
25-OHD_3 Calderol	5	1–2 (μg/kg/day)	Tablets	20 μg / 50 μg	qd for 15 days
1,25-dihydroxyvitamin D_3 Rocaltrol	0.5	0.015–0.050 (μg/kg/day)	Tablets	0.25 μg	bid for 3 days

222

Table 8-2 (Continued)

Multivitamin Supplements	Vitamin A (IU)	Vitamin D (IU)	Vitamin E (IU)	Vitamin C (mg)	Folic Acid (mg)	Thiamine (mg)	Ribo-flavin (mg)	Niacin (mg)	Vitamin B_6 (mg)	Vitamin B_{12} (mcg)	Iron (ferrous fumarate) (mg)	Calcium (mg)	Iodine (mg)
POLY-VI-SOL													
Drops (1.0 ml) without iron	1,500	400	5	35	—	0.5	0.6	8.0	0.4	2.0	—	—	—
Drops (1.0 ml) with iron	1,500	400	5	35	—	0.5	0.6	8.0	0.4	2.0	10	—	—
Chewable tablet without iron	2,500	400	15	60	0.3	1.05	1.2	13.5	1.05	4.5	—	—	—
Chewable tablet with iron	2,500	400	15	60	0.3	1.05	1.2	13.5	1.05	4.5	12	—	—
FAMPRIN FORTE	4,000	400	—	100	1.0	2.0	2.0	10.0	0.8	8.0	60	240	0.15
FLINTSTONES													
Chewable tablet	2,500	400	15	60	0.3	1.05	1.20	13.5	1.05	4.5	—	—	—
NEPHROCAPS	—	—	—	100	0.95	1.5	1.7	20.0	10.0	6.0	—	—	—

Trade name	Form	Description	Composition				
			$Al(OH)_3$ (mg)	Na^+ (mg)	K^+ (mg) (mEq)	P (mg) (mEq)	Ca (mg) (mEq)
PHOSPHATE BINDERS							
ALTERNAGEL	Suspension (5 ml)	Slightly lemon flavored, white liquid; pleasant tasting, high potency	600	<2	0	0	0

Amphojel	Suspension (5 ml)	Chalky, mint flavored, white liquid	320	6.9	0	
	Tablets 0.3 gm	Aspirin-sized white tablets	300	1.4	0	
	0.6 gm	Nickel-sized white tablets	600	1.8	0	
Alu-Cap	Capsule	Easy to open and mix with food or fluid	475		0	
Basaljel	Capsule	Easy to open and mix with food or fluid	500	2.8	0	
	Suspension	White liquid	400	1.8	0	
Dialume	Tablet	Large, capsule-sized	500		0	
Nephrox	Suspension (5 ml)	Watermelon flavored, pink liquid with chalky aftertaste; mineral oil 10% by volume	320		0	
CALCIUM SUPPLEMENTS						
Calcium Lactate	Tablets	325 mg Ca lactate/tablet				60 (1.5)
Neo-Calglucon	Suspension (5 ml)	1,800 mg calcium glubionate				115 (2.9)
Cal-Sup	Tablets	750 mg calcium carbonate/ tablet				300 mg
Titralac	Suspension (5 ml) Tablets	1,000 mg calcium carbonate 420 mg calcium carbonate/ tablet				

Source: Compiled by N. Spinozzi, R.D., Renal Dietician, The Children's Hospital, Boston, Ma.

uremic infant. In some instances where gavage-feeding is not possible, gastrostomy and hypercaloric formula have been shown to promote good health.

CONCLUSION

Most dietary parameters are altered in childhood renal disease. Current dietary management is made difficult by insufficient knowledge of how renal disease alters many of these parameters and how they interact with one another. Dietary recommendations need to be carefully monitored, considered, and reviewed over time in order to maintain proper nutrition in the face of chronic renal disease.

Liver Disease

Martin Maksimak

The liver plays a crucial role in many aspects of the maintenance of nutritional well-being. In order to fully understand the interrelationship of nutrition and liver disease, one must first have a basic understanding of the physiological functions performed by the liver and how those functions develop in the fetus and neonate [55].

Hepatic parenchymal cells perform a remarkably broad spectrum of vital functions. Among these are participation in the maintenance of glucose homeostasis and removal of excess nitrogen from amino acids via the synthesis of urea. Enzyme systems in the liver also are responsible for the conversion of certain vitamins and hormones to their active forms and for the detoxification of various drugs and harmful substances. Many serum proteins with important functions are of hepatic origin. These include albumin and certain coagulation and complement proteins.

The secretion of bile by the liver subserves several essential functions. Bilirubin and other breakdown products of hemoglobin, as well as many detoxified compounds, are excreted in the bile. Furthermore, bile acids, synthesized by hepatocytes from cholesterol, are secreted in the bile, and are crucial in the digestion and absorption of fats. Most of the bile acids secreted are recovered by reabsorption in the terminal ileum, enter the portal circulation, and are extracted by the liver for reutilization. Some or all of the hepatic functions discussed above may be altered in the child with liver disease.

Before discussing specific pathophysiological processes and their nutritional ramifications, it will be useful to review the impact of development in liver function. Although the placenta and maternal liver provide most of the excretory and detoxification functions needed in utero, the infant's liver is required for intrauterine survival. Furthermore, even with complete in utero development of the necessary enzymatic systems, adaptation must still occur after birth for the child to thrive. In infants born prematurely, the rate at which this postnatal adaptation occurs is inversely related to gestational age.

Bile acid–dependent fat digestion and absorption are not fully developed in the neonate. While in adults the intrahepatic circulation of bile salts is extremely efficient and minimal amounts of bile acid are lost in the stool, in the neonate, the intrahepatic circulation is less efficient, bile flow is diminished, and bile acid synthesis is decreased. As a result, intraluminal bile salt concentrations are below critical levels and fat absorption is inefficient. In the premature infant, these defects are more marked. The absorption of cholesterol, saturated fatty acids, and vitamins A, D, E, and K are very dependent on bile salts and, therefore, these substances are particularly apt to be malabsorbed in the term and, especially, in the premature neonate. On the other hand, medium chain triglycerides (and unsaturated fatty acids) are not dependent on bile salts for their assimilation and are a reliable caloric source. By 3 to 5 months of age, the healthy full-term child will achieve efficient fat absorption. In the premature infant, the time necessary for maturation is longer [59].

The discussion of the interaction of nutrition and childhood liver disease can be simplified by focusing on general categories of liver disease rather than specific disease entities. The following discussion will center on cholestasis, acute liver failure, and chronic liver failure.

CHOLESTASIS

Cholestasis can be simply defined as diminished bile flow and is characterized by an elevation of the level of conjugated bilirubin in the serum. As Table 8-3 indicates, cholestasis may accompany a number of acute and chronic insults to the liver in the neonate and infant. These include lesions that obstruct the biliary tree such as extrahepatic biliary atresia, lesions associated with hypoplasia of the intrahepatic biliary tree such as Alagille's syndrome, and lesions that affect the ability of the hepatocyte to secrete bile such as viral hepatitis and metabolic diseases. For completely obstructive lesions, surgery is indicated, but in prolonged, nonsurgical cases of cholestasis, careful nutritional management is vital.

The major nutritional efforts relevant to cholestasis are directed at correcting the abnormal fat digestion and absorption resulting from altered bile acid metabolism. The pathophysiological principles are the same as those that pertain to fat metabolism in the neonate and premature infant, although the nutritional costs are much higher. The ratio of medium chain to long chain dietary triglycerides should be increased. Fat-soluble vitamins, as noted above, are dependent on bile acids for their absorption. Therefore, two to four times the recommended daily allowance of these vitamins should be given to children with cholestasis.

Table 8-3. Causes of Neonatal Cholestasis

Infections
  Hepatitis B, hepatitis A (?), non-A, non-B hepatitis (?), rubella, toxoplasmosis, cytomegalovirus, varicella, herpes, echo 14, listeriosis, treponema
Toxic conditions
  Total parenteral nutrition, sepsis (*E. coli*, urinary tract infection)
Hemolysis
  Hemoglobinopathy, red cell membrane defects, Coombs-positive hemolytic anemia, hematoma
Secretory defects
  Dubin-Johnson syndrome, Rotor syndrome
Intrahepatic obstruction
  Arteriohepatic dysplasia (Alagille's syndrome), Byler disease, familial benign recurrent cholestasis, congenital hepatic fibrosis, Caroli's disease, non-syndrome intrahepatic biliary hypoplasia/atresia
Extrahepatic obstruction
  Biliary atresia, bile plug or stone, perforation at bile duct
Intestinal obstruction
  Pyloric stenosis
Metabolic disease
  Tyrosinemia, Wolman's disease, Niemann-Pick disease, Gaucher's disease, galactosemia, fructosemia, glycogenosis IV, trihydroxy-coprostanic acidemia, cystic fibrosis, alpha-1-antitrypsin deficiency, trisomy 21, Turner's syndrome, Zellweger's syndrome

Not only is vitamin D poorly absorbed in children with cholestasis, but the liver is necessary for its conversion to the active metabolite [58]. Thus, vitamin D supplementation in children with cholestasis is very important to prevent the development of rickets [56]. If there is a significant degree of loss of hepatic parenchymal function, it may be necessary to administer vitamin D in a form that does not require hydroxylation by the liver, either as 25-hydroxycholecalciferol or 1,25-dihydroxycholecalciferol.

Because of poor absorption and activation of vitamin D and loss of dietary calcium related to fat malabsorption, dietary calcium intake should be between 50 and 200 mg of elemental calcium per kilogram per day. Dietary phosphorus may also need to be supplemented (up to 25 to 50 mg of elemental phosphorus per kilogram per day) [57].

The symptoms of vitamin E deficiency are becoming increasingly recognized in children with cholestatic liver disease. Prominent among these is neuromuscular impairment. Serum vitamin E levels, the peroxide hemolysis test, and thorough neurological examination help monitor children for possible vitamin E deficiency. In children with hyperlipidemia, the ratio of vitamin E to total serum lipid most accurately reflects vitamin E sufficiency. Supplementation of vitamin E may be successful orally through use of alpha-tocopherol acetate or succinate, but parenteral therapy may be necessary.

Medical approaches to the problem of cholestasis involve the administration of agents designed to increase bile flow. Phenobarbital in a dose of 5 to 10 mg/kg per day has been shown to increase bile flow. Cholestyramine, an orally administered resin, binds intraluminal bile acids and makes them unavailable for reutilization. As a result, the availability of bile acids decreases, and the stimulus for the liver to synthesize more bile acids is increased. With further bile acid synthesis, the flow of bile is increased. Cholestyramine is most effective when given before the first meal of the day so that bile acids stored in gallbladder bile can be effectively bound.

ACUTE LIVER FAILURE

Certain insults to the liver result in the immediate paralysis of hepatic function, leading to a state of acute liver failure. This is most commonly seen in children as a result of Reye's syndrome, fulminant viral hepatitis, toxin-induced hepatitis, or during an acute exacerbation or final phase of chronic liver disease. Regardless of the exact cause of liver failure, nutritional management is crucial so that metabolic derangements are minimized. Serum glucose levels may fall if hepatic generation of glucose via gluconeogenesis or glycogenolysis in damaged hepatocytes is insufficient. This may necessitate administration of glucose intravenously in amounts necessary to maintain normal serum glucose levels. Failure to detoxify excess nitrogen may result in an elevation of serum ammonia levels and is associated with encephalopathy. Although the exact cause of hepatic coma in the setting of liver failure is unknown, measures to decrease serum ammonia levels by restriction of exogenous sources of protein may result in clinical improvement. Patients with acute liver failure should receive no protein until recovery begins. Other measures that may result in normalization of serum ammonia levels include the use of neomycin, which reduces ammonia production by urea-splitting bacteria, and lactulose, which decreases ammonia absorption from the colon. The selective use of branched-chain amino acids has been reported to improve the central nervous system manifestations of hepatic coma while contributing to a positive nitrogen balance. Inability of the liver to produce normal amounts of essential serum proteins may result in hypoalbuminemia and attendant fluid and electrolyte problems as well as coagulopathy and bleeding. Careful monitoring of sodium, potassium, and water balance is critical in caring for patients with acute liver failure as is monitoring for possible accompanying renal failure. From the above discussion, it is evident that nutrition is one of the few tools available to the physician to help manage patients with acute hepatic failure.

CHRONIC LIVER FAILURE

Even in infancy and childhood, chronic liver disease may develop. Among the causes are metabolic diseases such as alpha-1-antitrypsin deficiency, viral infections, prolonged extrahepatic biliary obstruction, or unknown factors as in some cases of chronic active hepatitis. Children with chronic liver disease, particularly cirrhosis, may face many of the problems discussed in the section on acute liver failure, but usually on a partial and more prolonged basis. In addition, chronic liver failure may present unique problems.

Metabolic abnormalities may require continual correction over extended periods of time. Type I glycogen storage disease is an example in which frequent or continuous enteral glucose supplements or starch can make a dramatic difference in morbidity by compensating for the liver's inability to mobilize glycogen and maintain serum glucose levels. A variety of lesions may lead to failure to convert excess nitrogen to urea, either as a result of loss of parenchymal tissue (cirrhosis) or from portosystemic shunts created surgically or occurring spontaneously. To control symptoms of chronic encephalopathy, protein restriction may be necessary. In the infant, protein intake should be approximately 1.0 to 1.5 gm/kg of body weight per day and in the older child, 0.5 to 1.0 gm/kg of body weight per day. In addition to protein restriction, lactulose can be administered on a chronic basis to decrease ammonia.

Chronic hypoalbuminemia, because of decreased production of albumin by the liver, may contribute to fluid retention as ascites, peripheral edema, and serum electrolyte abnormalities, especially hyponatremia. Control of these problems in the patient with chronic liver disease often requires both pharmacological and nutritional intervention. Dietary sodium should be moderately restricted without compromising caloric intake. Initial diuretic therapy generally consists of an agent such as spironolactone or triamterene to antagonize the hormone aldosterone. A second agent with another renal site of action, such as furosemide, can be added to this. Water restriction is usually unnecessary and potentially dangerous and should therefore be avoided except in rare cases. The efficacy of the therapy can be monitored by measuring body weight and urine and serum electrolyte levels.

Thus, proper nutrition is crucial in the management of the metabolic derangements and fluid and electrolyte abnormalities that accompany chronic liver disease.

CONCLUSION

The nutritional approach to a child with liver disease, irrespective of exact diagnosis, can be generally understood by identifying the predominant pattern of liver malfunction (i.e., cholestasis, acute liver failure, or chronic liver failure) and applying knowledge of the altered pathophysiology. Children with severe jaundice as the major symptom of liver disease will need modification of dietary fat intake and supplementation of fat-soluble vitamins because of the fat maldigestion and malabsorption accompanying cholestasis. Children with liver disease affecting other hepatocyte functions may need glucose supplementation, protein restriction, and sodium restriction. In the acute setting, correction of the metabolic derangements must be as complete as possible. In the chronic setting, other considerations such as palatability of diet and requirements for growth become important.

Gluten-Sensitive Enteropathy

Martin Maksimak

Celiac disease, or gluten-sensitive enteropathy (GSE), is an illness affecting adults and children in which gluten induces diffuse damage to the small intestinal mucosa. This injury is reversed by the withdrawal of the offending agents. Because some individuals are relatively asymptomatic, the true prevalence of GSE is not known. It is estimated to be about 0.03 percent in the United States; in Western Ireland, as many as 1 in 300 people may be affected. Over 80 percent of GSE patients are HLA-B8 positive while only 20 percent of the general population is HLA-B8 positive. HLA-DW3 and IgG allotypes are also associated with the disease [61]. Although only 2 to 5 percent of first degree relatives of patients with GSE are at risk for developing symptoms of GSE, 10 percent of asymptomatic relatives would have an abnormal small bowel biopsy [62]. Thus, the true incidence is undetermined.

PATHOGENESIS

The intestinal lesion and the clinical manifestations of GSE can be induced by the introduction of gluten into the diet of a sensitive patient. The mechanism of injury is unclear but both direct toxicity and immunological mechanisms have been proposed. Gliadin, a component of wheat gluten extractable by alcohol, causes mucosal changes, and even a 1,500-dalton fragment of the peptic-tryptic digest of wheat gliadin is toxic [60]. Wheat, barley, rye, and occasionally oats are toxic to patients; rice and corn do not produce symptoms.

CLINICAL FEATURES

The clinical presentation of GSE is variable; symptoms may be chronic and subtle or acute and life threatening. Although patients usually present symptoms within the first year of life, in some, symptoms may be delayed for decades. The classical presentation to the pediatrician is an irritable infant who has been on a gluten-containing diet for 3 to 9 months with frequent, loose, and foul-smelling bowel movements. Other gastrointestinal symptoms may include occasional vomiting, a distended abdomen, and even constipation. There may be loss of subcutaneous tissue in the proximal limbs and buttocks and a marked slowing of growth (see Fig. 7-8).

The diagnosis may not be apparent in infancy if the symptoms are intermittent and subtle and there is no growth failure. Although symptoms may persist, they often diminish or even disappear completely during adolescence only to recur in the third or fourth decade. A few patients do not have symptoms until middle or old age. It is not known whether or not these patients had asymptomatic gluten intolerance as children.

LABORATORY FINDINGS

Many of the laboratory tests in active celiac disease reflect the severity of malabsorption. Oral tolerance tests have been used to screen for celiac disease, but none is reliable enough to eliminate the disease from consideration. The tests most often used are the D-xylose test, lactose tolerance test, or lactose breath hydrogen test. D-xylose is a pentose sugar that is minimally metabolized and absorbed in the proximal small intestine. A rise in blood xylose of less than 25 mg/dl is suggestive of mucosal injury, although some patients with gluten sensitivity have had an increase of over 28 mg/dl. Normally, 20 percent of the loading dose will be excreted in the urine over 5 hours, but this may be difficult to assess in children. The lactose breath test is based on the premise that lactose not absorbed in the small intestine is metabolized by bacteria in the colon, resulting in the production of H_2, which can be measured in the breath. Finding reducing sugars in the stool after a lactose load also suggests malabsorption. Most patients with GSE will have abnormal tests, but false-negative results can occur. Abnormal results are not specific for GSE and may be seen in other conditions that produce intestinal villus atrophy.

The steatorrhea of GSE is not just a reflection of mucosal injury. It also reflects pancreatic exocrine insufficiency as well as decreased secretion of secretin, pancreozymin, and bile. A Sudan stain of the feces qualitatively identifies fat but the results are often misleading. For more quantitative data, a 2 to 3 gm/kg per day fat intake should be encouraged and the diet should be recorded for 5 days. For the last 3 days, the stool should be collected and the fat extracted. By using the diet history (see Chap. 7), the percentage of fat excreted in the stool can be calculated. Excretion of more than 5 percent ingested fat is abnormal. With steatorrhea, fat-soluble vitamins often will be malabsorbed. This may result in many of the extraintestinal manifestations reported in GSE (Table 8-4). If diarrhea is severe, a metabolic acidosis

Table 8-4. Extraintestinal manifestations of Gluten-Sensitive Enteropathy

Organ System	Manifestation	Probable Cause(s)
Hematopoietic	Anemia	Iron, folate, vitamin B_{12}, or pyridoxine deficiency
	Hemorrhage	Hypoprothrombinemia and, rarely, thrombocytopenia due to folate deficiency
Skeletal	Osteomalacia	Malabsorption of calcium and vitamin D
	Osteoporosis	Malabsorption of amino acids causing negative nitrogen balance
	Pathologic fractures	Osteomalacia and osteoporosis
	Osteoarthropathy	Unknown
Muscular	Atrophy	Malnutrition due to panmalabsorption
	Tetany	Calcium, vitamin D, and/or magnesium malabsorption
	Weakness	Generalized muscle atrophy, hypokalemia
Nervous	Peripheral neuropathy	Vitamin deficiencies such as thiamine and vitamin B_{12}
	Demyelinating central nervous system lesions	Unknown
Endocrine	Secondary hyperparathyroidism	Calcium and vitamin D malabsorption causing hypocalcemia
	Secondary hypopituitarism	Malnutrition due to panmalabsorption
Integumentary	Follicular hyperkeratosis and dermatitis	Vitamin A malabsorption, vitamin B complex malabsorption (?)
	Petechiae and ecchymoses	Hypoprothrombinemia and, rarely, thrombocytopenia
	Edema	Hypoproteinemia
	Dermatitis herpetiformis	Unknown

Source: Trier, J. S. Celiac Sprue Disease. In M. H. Sleiseneger and J. S. Fordtran (Eds.), *Gastrointestinal Disease: Pathophysiology, Diagnosis, Management* (3rd ed.). Philadelphia: Saunders, 1983. P. 1055.

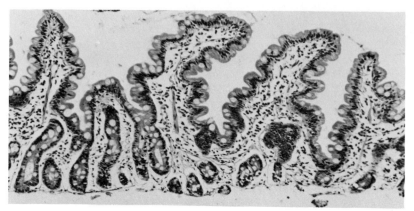

Figure 8-1. Jejunal biopsy from a normal individual. The villi are tall and lined with columnar epithelial cells. There are very few inflammatory cells in the lamina propria.

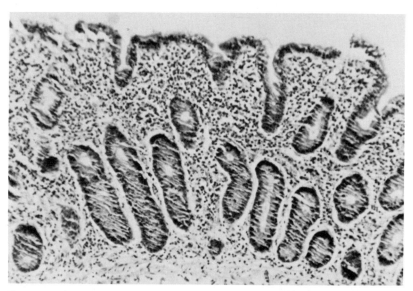

Figure 8-2. Jejunal biopsy from an individual with celiac disease. The villi are blunted. The epithelial lining cells are no longer columnar. Inflammatory cells exist in the epithelium and lamina propria.

and protein-losing enteropathy are common. Despite the low serum proteins, IgA is often elevated.

The radiographic features present after barium contrast are not specific for GSE, and the diagnosis is established by suction jejunal biopsy *while the patient is on a gluten-containing diet*. Trials of gluten-free diets without biopsy evidence of mucosal injury are misleading.

The findings of biopsy include: (1) partial to total villus atrophy; (2) elongated crypts; (3) increased cellularity of the lamina propria consisting of plasma cells and lymphocytes, and occasionally, polymorphonuclear leukocytes; and (4) intraepithelial cytotoxic-suppressor T lymphocytes (Figs. 8-1 and 8-2). Depending upon the severity of the intestinal injury, lactase deficiency and, to a lesser degree, sucrase deficiency may occur and require temporary dietary restriction of these sugars. A flat villus lesion is not unique to GSE, and after the child is thriving on a gluten-free diet, reinjury after a challenge with a small amount of gluten will establish the diagnosis. Once firmly established, the child is restarted on a diet restricting all gluten-containing goods and is supported to maintain this diet throughout life. There is some evidence that patients with GSE have an increased incidence of gastrointestinal lymphoma. The effect of diet on the development of lymphoma is unknown.

TREATMENT
Initially, formulas or foods that contain lactose should be avoided (see Appendix 3). Supplements of fat-soluble vitamins, iron, and folate may need to be prescribed early in treatment. If the diet is adhered to, supplementation need not be continued after the intestinal mucosa has healed.

The treatment of GSE seems simple. However, wheat, oats, barley, and rye, which may be toxic to the GSE patient, are ubiquitous in the American diet and are found as additives in many foods. Thus, to maintain a gluten-free diet, nutrition counseling by a physician and dietician is needed. (Appendix 3 presents a gluten-free diet.)

Infectious Diarrhea
David Perlmutter and Martin Maksimak

Acute infectious gastroenteritis is a common illness in both underdeveloped and modern countries. In Asia, Africa, and Latin America, the morbidity and mortality from diarrhea is significant. Because of the effect on the malnourished host, the prevalence of acute gastroenteritis in underdeveloped nations has serious personal, social, and economic ramifications. Even in industrialized countries such as Great Britain, approximately 400 children die from acute gastroenteritis each year [71].

ETIOLOGY

Only 20 to 30 percent of episodes of acute diarrhea are caused by recognized bacterial agents such as *Salmonella, Shigella, Campylobacter, Yersinia,* and *E. coli* [75]. Parasites, such as *Giardia lamblia,* account for some of the other episodes, but it appears that viruses cause the majority of cases of infectious diarrhea [68]. Rotovirus is the cause of more than 50 percent of the episodes of acute gastroenteritis [70], but in approximately 25 percent of the cases, no known viral, bacterial, or parasitic agent is identified.

The human rotovirus (HRV) is the major cause of acute sporadic viral diarrhea in infants and young children. Most patients affected are between 6 months and 3 years of age, but symptomatic neonatal infections are also common. There is a lower incidence of infection in breast-fed than in bottle-fed infants, presumably due to the transmission of maternal antibody in breast milk. By 3 years of age, circulating rotovirus antibodies are found in the majority of healthy children.

CLINICAL PRESENTATION

Viral-associated diarrhea is generally acquired by the fecal-oral route of transmission. After a 48- to 72-hour incubation period, there is usually fever and upper respiratory symptoms. The diarrhea that follows is generally watery, only occasionally with blood and/or mucus. Vomiting and dehydration are common in rotovirus infections.

The diagnosis of human rotovirus infection has usually been made on the basis of clinical manifestations. It has been necessary in the past to exclude known bacterial and parasitic infections before attributing an episode of diarrhea to viral etiology. The recent development of an enzyme-linked immunoabsorbent assay (ELISA), however, has made it possible to definitively diagnose rotovirus infections. This assay is sensitive and does not require sophisticated equipment or radiation exposure. In the near future, methods for rapid diagnosis of other specific viral pathogens are anticipated.

PATHOLOGY

It appears that clinical manifestations of rotovirus-induced gastroenteritis results from invasion of the intestinal mucosal lining [64]. The majority of pathological findings occur in the small intestine with relative sparing of the stomach and large intestine. Abnormalities include infiltration of the lamina propria with chronic inflammatory cells and a cuboidal appearance as opposed to the normally columnar absorptive cells. The extent of injury varies from patient to patient; some patients even have complete flattening of the intestinal villi. The abnormalities in histology generally revert to normal after 3 to 8 weeks. Intestinal mucosal injury is also reflected in functional impairment, including abnormal D-xylose absorption, depressed mucosal glucose-stimulated sodium transport, depressed activity of the mucosal sodium-potassium-ATP, and low disaccharidase levels. The extent of mucosal abnormalities often determines the severity of clinical manifestations.

OTHER VIRUSES

Although rotovirus is the most commonly known pathogen causing acute infantile diarrhea (especially in the winter months), other viruses have been associated with outbreaks of diarrhea within families or communities. As opposed to rotovirus infections, these outbreaks have chiefly affected school-age children; infants and adults are affected to a lesser extent. The symptoms of nausea, vomiting, diarrhea, abdominal pain, and malaise typically last 24 to 48 hours and rarely require parenteral fluids. The viruses Norwalk and Hawaii appear to be similar to parvoviruses. Adenoviruses have been associated with gastroenteritis after bone marrow transplantation. Other newer viruses suspected in cases of infectious diarrhea include reoviruses, astroviruses, coronaviruses, and caliciviruses, but further studies are necessary to determine the significance of these agents.

PARASITES

Intestinal parasitic infections are common throughout the world. With the advent of rapid, widespread travel, these infections have become more prevalent in the United States [66, 67]. Although many protozoa and helminths can cause diarrhea, this discussion will be limited to *Giardia lamblia*, since it is the most common pathogenic intestinal parasite in this country.

Although many cases of giardiasis have occurred during or after travel abroad, this infection is now often occurring in children and adults who have no history of recent travel. Large-scale water-borne outbreaks have occurred in Colorado, Utah, Oregon, Washington, New Hampshire, Vermont, and New York. Campers, especially in the Rocky Mountain states, have been infected by drinking contaminated mountain stream water. In young children, however, high rates of infection are seen mostly in nurseries or day care centers and appear to result from hand-to-mouth transmission [65].

When giardiasis is associated with clinical symptoms, the onset is usually after an incubation period of 9 to 15 days. There is some evidence that at least 100 cysts are necessary to produce a clinical infection. The severity of symptoms varies widely among individuals. *Giardia* has been found incidentally in some asymptomatic individuals (usually relatives of index cases). In symptomatic patients, the acute manifestations include sudden explosive watery diarrhea, marked abdominal distention, nausea, anorexia, vomiting, and abdominal cramps. Although the acute stage usually lasts only 3 to 4 days, it can last for months and result in severe steatorrhea, weight loss, failure to thrive, and disability. In other individuals, the acute stage is not recognized, and intermittent mild symptoms are noticed over prolonged periods of time. These chronic manifestations include anorexia, nausea, and brief episodes of diarrhea. *Giardia lamblia* is occasionally discovered in infants who are growing poorly but have no obvious intestinal symptoms. Catch-up growth is observed when the *Giardia* is eradicated.

Diagnostic evaluation in children with giardiasis may require examination of as many as three stool specimens. Occasionally *Giardia lamblia* is found on duodenal fluid or small intestinal mucosal examination after thorough examination of three stool specimens has been negative. Therefore, when there is a strong clinical suspicion of giardiasis in a symptomatic child despite negative stool examination, small intestinal biopsy and duodenal fluid aspiration are recommended. In those children who have undergone small intestinal biopsy and evaluation of small intestinal function, a spectrum of observations has been made during *Giardia* infestations. In some children, small intestinal histology is normal. In other individuals, there is a mucosal injury (occasionally complete villous atrophy) associated with varying degrees of fat and carbohydrate malabsorption.

Because there is a dramatic increase in the incidence of *Giardia* infestations in patients with hypogammaglobulinemic and hypochlorhydric disorders [63], immunoglobulin and gastric acid secretion are thought to protect healthy individuals against giardiasis. The almost epidemic prevalence of *Giardia* in healthy populations, however, is evidence that multiple factors are necessary for the host response to this organism. In fact, there is still no widely accepted mechanism for the pathogenesis of giardiasis. On electron microscopic examination, these organisms are observed to attach to the intestinal mucosa through powerful sucking disks. One theory proposes that such action irritates the intestinal villi or even creates a mechanical obstruction to the absorption of nutrients. Occasionally, invasion of the small intestinal mucosa by *Giardia* organisms has been observed, suggesting that direct destruction is the pathogenic mechanism. Other theories have suggested that *Giardia* competes with the host for nutrients such as vitamin B_{12} or causes symptoms by the deconjugation of bile salts.

Most *Giardia* infections will respond to a 7- to 10-day course of Atabrine or metronidazole. If *Giardia* is the reason for poor growth, treatment often results in resumption of weight gain and linear growth. Immunodeficient or hypochlorhydric patients may require several weeks of treatment. The most common cause of treatment failure in children is persistent lactose intolerance while the intestinal mucosa is healing, despite the eradication of the organism.

BACTERIAL AGENTS

Although less common than in previous decades, *Salmonella* and *Shigella* still cause diarrheal illnesses in children. *E. coli* has been associated with diarrhea in children both by enteropathogenic and enterotoxigenic mechanisms. Recently, *Campylobacter* [75], *Yersinia*, and *Clostridium difficile* have been identified as causes of diarrhea in children as well. These infections are more commonly accompanied by blood and mucus in the stools than viral infections. In addition, a history of exposure to contaminated food in cases of salmonellosis, to infected animals in *Campylobacter* infections, or to antibiotic treatment in *Clostridium difficile* toxin-associated infections may distinguish these diarrheal illnesses from viral enteritis. Otherwise, the effect of bacterial enteritis, or enterocolitis, on the infant or young child is similar to that caused by viruses.

EFFECTS OF ENTERITIS

The nutritional effect of infectious diarrhea in infants and children, especially in third world underdeveloped countries, is enormous [76]. Children in these nations are often marginally nourished and thus predisposed to severe malnutrition even after a mild infectious insult. Multiple factors appear to contribute to the nutritional effect of acute gastroenteritis, including inadequate intake, diminished intestinal absorption, and increased metabolic requirements.

As with other infections, acute gastroenteritis is often accompanied by anorexia. In addition, diet is often altered during an acute episode of gastroenteritis to avoid severe vomiting and/or diarrhea. During an acute illness, dietary modification is indicated. Clear fluids are encouraged, and foods high in lactose or fat are discouraged. Often such a diet is used for prolonged periods of time because diarrhea is persistent or intermittent, resulting in pronounced nutritional debilitation.

In addition to decreased or inadequate intake, malabsorption leads to further losses of nutrients. Gastrointestinal infections can lead to malabsorption of carbohydrates, fats, vitamins, and possibly even protein. Because the major sources of calories for infants are lactose-containing maternal or formulated milk, lactose malabsorption secondary to intestinal villous injury is the most serious nutritional effect of gastrointestinal infection. In addition to loss of calories from the gastrointestinal tract, there may be loss of calories, nitrogen, iron, zinc, and ascorbic acid from the urinary system due to the secondary renal effects of acute gastroenteritis. Even with mild subclinical infections, it is estimated that total nitrogen losses are 0.6 to 12.0 gm/kg per day [74].

Finally, gastrointestinal infection may trigger a complex sequence of events that results in increased caloric requirements. Amino acid utilization is increased for the new synthesis of immune response proteins and proteins lost in gastrointestinal secretions. The amino acids are derived from energy-requiring skeletal muscle catabolism and are transported to the liver for energy-requiring protein biosynthesis. Negative nitrogen balance is the result of this increased requirement at a time when there is impairment in gastrointestinal absorption and excess urinary calorie excretion. The physiological stress response that follows any infection can also contribute to negative balance by requiring increased reserves of carbohydrate, fat, potassium, magnesium, phosphates, sulfates, zinc, ascorbic acid, and vitamin A.

With the combination of excessive losses, increased requirement, and anorexia producing inadequate intake of calories, a vicious cycle is established that can easily upset the balance of a marginally nourished infant. It is also possible that these nutritional effects of acute gastroenteritis make the child more susceptible to recurrent gastrointestinal and systemic infections.

TREATMENT

Although there are antibiotics specific for several bacteria that cause acute infectious diarrhea, several effects of these antibiotics should be considered when individual cases arise. Most cases of bacterial gastroenteritis are self-limited, making treatment unnecessary. There is some evidence that antibiotic administration prolongs the carrier state for the *Salmonella* organism. Nevertheless, in infants less than 6 months of age or the moderately ill older child, antibiotics should be considered for *Salmonella* infections to prevent dissemination of the organism. The duration and severity of symptoms caused by *Shigella* infections may be reduced by antibiotic treatment (usually trimethoprimsulfamethoxazole) if given early in the illness. *Clostridia difficile* infections are now being treated with vancomycin or metronidazole. All *Giardia* infestations should be treated, and the parasite should be eradicated with either Atabrine or metronidazole. In most previously well-nourished children, resolution of infectious diarrhea with or without antimicrobial agents will result in regain of weight. Catch-up growth, however, may require as great as 140 percent of maintenance protein and 115 percent of maintenance caloric intake; diets must be adjusted accordingly.

Presently there is no specific treatment for viral gastroenteritis. Thus, supportive measures have become very important. One of the major sequelae of acute gastroenteritis for which supportive measures are vital is secondary lactose malabsorption. Carbohydrate intolerance may affect up to 78 percent of children during the acute stage of gastroenteritis [73] and occasionally lasts for 3 to 4 months [72]. Both fluid and calories are lost with malabsorbed carbohydrate. When lactose is eliminated from the diet in the initial days of infection, diarrhea often decreases (see Appendix 3). As many as 16 percent of these patients also develop monosaccharide intolerance, so that most authorities will recommend a 24-hour period of treatment with glucose-electrolyte solutions for the well-nourished child having acute diarrhea. After 1 day, a dilute proprietary formula that does not contain lactose should be given. If tolerated, the formula should be slowly advanced to full concentration and non-lactose-containing solid foods should be introduced. Generally, within 1 to 2 weeks, lactose can be reintroduced slowly. A similar, although slightly more conservative, approach can be adopted for children with acute diarrhea who require hospitalization for dehydration, inability to handle oral alimentation, or severe nutritional debilitation. If diarrhea reappears when lactose is reintroduced, testing of the fluid fraction of the stool with a Clinitest reagent tablet will determine if the diarrhea is caused by carbohydrate malabsorption. A reaction greater than or equal to ½ percent in this test is indicative of the presence of reducing sugar (usually malabsorbed lactose). In cases of infectious diarrhea that cause more severe intestinal injury, other carbohydrates may not be tolerated. In these patients, stool output is usually greater than 20 gm/kg per day and the stool may be acidic due to the fermentation of malabsorbed carbohydrates. A variation of the Clinitest reagent tablet analysis to detect sucrose malabsorption is useful in these circumstances because it will dictate dietary restriction of sucrose as well as lactose. For detection of sucrose malabsorption, the fluid fraction of the stool is added to an equal volume of 1 N hydrochloric acid, boiled for several seconds, allowed to cool to room temperature, and then applied to the Clinitest reagent tablet. A reaction of ½ percent or greater suggests sucrose malabsorption and necessitates use of an elemental formula (i.e., Pregestimil) or a formula that contains glucose oligosaccharides (i.e., ProSobee) for nutrition. An elemental formula will also be helpful in children who have developed fat malabsorption from acute gastroenteritis [69], since most of the elemental formulas have a higher content of the more readily absorbed medium chain triglycerides.

With use of these general guidelines, prolonged weight loss can be prevented in most children and the need for long-term intravenous nutrition may be avoided.

Short Bowel Syndrome
Martin Maksimak and Jeffrey A. Biller

One of the most challenging nutritional problems in pediatrics is the management of the small infant or young child after an extensive small bowel resection [88]. As late as 1955, Potts stated that newborn infants could not survive with the loss of more than 15 percent of the small bowel [84]. However, with the great progress and advances since that time in neonatal medicine, surgical techniques, anesthesia, and parenteral nutrition, many more infants are surviving the insult of an extensive small bowel resection.

The etiology of the short bowel syndrome in infants and children is somewhat different from that in adults. The most common etiologies in infants and children include volvulus, jejunal, ileal atresia, gastrochesis, omphalocele, and vascular thrombosis [89]. In adults, complication of abdominal trauma, mesenteric thrombosis, inflammatory bowel disease, and atherosclerotic disease are prevalent [89]. The improved survival rate of premature babies after surgery for necrotizing enterocolitis has resulted in its being one of the more prominent causes of short bowel syndrome today. Factors that relate to the ultimate prognosis include: (1) length of the remaining bowel; (2) presence of an ileocecal valve; and (3) degree of intestinal adaptation.

The length of the small bowel from the ligament of Treitz to the ileocecal valve in a full-term newborn is approximately 250 cm [87]. The critical length for survival of small infants without long-term parenteral nutrition seems to be about 40 cm without an ileocecal valve, and at least 15 cm with an ileocecal valve [89].

After small intestinal resection, the remainder of the bowel undergoes a series of morphological and functional changes to allow the organism to remain in homeostasis. This intestinal adaptation occurs to a greater extent in the ileum after a proximal resection than in the jejunum after a distal resection. Morphologically, a hyperplasia of the cells of the villus and crypt occurs allowing a greater absorptive surface. The degree of intestinal hyperplasia is roughly proportional to the extent of intestinal resection. Due to this increased surface area, the specific activity of many of the brush border digestive enzymes is increased when expressed per segment of intestine, although it is somewhat decreased in each epithelial cell lining the villus. Such changes allow the organism to adapt to the shortened bowel length. Many factors have been suggested as being trophic for intestinal adaptation. Intraluminal nutrients appear to have the greatest effect on stimulating intestinal hyperplasia after resection. Pancreatic enzymes as well as enteroglucagon also appear to have trophic effects.

Gastric acid hypersecretion, reported in 50 percent of patients after small bowel removal [82], may cause ulceration of the intestine. The acidic gastric secretions may impair micellar formation, fat lipolysis, and digestion of starch and proteins due to inactivation of pancreatic enzymes [86]. Acid diarrhea may appear with fluid and electrolyte losses leading to metabolic alkalosis and hypokalemia [81]. Although gastric acid hypersecretion may begin within 24 hours after resection, it is usually of short duration, lasting only weeks to months. The amount of acid produced is proportional to the length of small bowel removed. Therapy with cimetidine (20 mg/kg per day divided qid) may be beneficial in controlling hypersecretion.

DUODENAL RESECTION

Absorption of iron and calcium occurs along the entire small bowel but is maximal in the duodenum. Thus, resection of a significant proportion of the duodenum could lead to iron deficiency anemia and/or bone disorders.

JEJUNAL RESECTION

Water-soluble vitamins other than B_{12} are best absorbed in the jejunum but may be well absorbed by the ileum if the jejunum has been resected. In adults with resection of all of the ileum and part of the jejunum, a critical length of 1 to 4 feet of intact jejunum [85] is required to prevent malabsorption of water-soluble vitamins. In children, the length of the small intestine needed to prevent malabsorption of water-soluble vitamins is undetermined.

Removal of large segments of the small bowel decreases total intestinal lactase activity and may significantly decrease other disaccharidases [81]. Normally, when compared to lactase, sucrase is approximately twice as abundant and maltase is 6 to 8 times as abundant. If a resection is large enough, both sucrase and lactase activity may be lower than needed for sugar absorption, but maltase levels may still be adequate. Thus, initial diets should be adapted to take advantage of the greater maltase activity. Elemental formulas in which the carbohydrate concentration can be adjusted are most practical.

ILEAL RESECTION

With ileal resections, vitamin B_{12} and bile salt deficiency can develop. In adults, resections of as little as 50 to 80 cm can result in an abnormal Schilling test [78]. Later, a megaloblastic macrocytic anemia and neurological sequelae may develop from vitamin B_{12} deficiency.

Some passive absorption of bile salts occurs along the upper and mid parts of the small intestine, but the majority reaches the terminal ileum. Here an active transport process efficiently recovers more than 90 percent of the bile acids secreted with a meal. Resections of as little as 25 cm of terminal ileum in an adult may result in bile acid malabsorption [78]. This becomes important because inadequate concentrations of bile salt will eventually cause steatorrhea due to the inability to form micelles.

In normal individuals, the liver synthesis of bile acid is only 10 to 20 percent of its capacity; therefore, the bile acid pool may be restored overnight in people with mild losses. In individuals with limited ileal resections, the bile acid concentration in the small bowel in the morning after a nighttime fast is normal. However, over the day, intraluminal bile acid concentrations decrease with subsequent meals. In developed countries, the meal with the largest fat content is in the evening. If, in addition to the bile acid–absorbing terminal ileum, segments of the duodenum or jejunum have also been removed, greater steatorrhea results due to a loss of absorptive surface area. Feeding larger meals early in the day may improve absorption if bile salt deficiency is a factor.

In patients with short ileal resections, bile acids that are not completely absorbed in the ileum will reach the colon. There they will be converted by bacteria into dihydroxy bile acids, which have been shown to impair absorption of fluids and, if present in high enough concentrations, to cause active fluid secretion. This diarrhea will improve with the administration of the resin cholestyramine, which will bind the bile acids.

In patients with large ileal resections, bile acid synthesis may not be able to compensate for the loss. The intraluminal bile acid concentration will be chronically low, and fat malabsorption will be more severe. The malabsorbed fatty acids that reach the colon can decrease the water and electrolyte absorption of the colon and, thus, diarrhea again results. In this instance, cholestyramine is not helpful because it will exacerbate the steatorrhea. The appropriate treatment would be to decrease the fat intake and change the fat from long chain to medium chain triglycerides, which are absorbed without requiring bile salts [79]. In addition, pancreatic exocrine function may be impaired in some patients with short bowel syndrome and further impair fat absorption. Such patients might benefit from pancreatic enzyme replacements.

Hyperoxaluria and oxalate stones are serious complications of intestinal resection. Oxalates are usually rendered insoluble in the bowel in the form of calcium-oxalate. If calcium is unavailable to bind with oxalate due to its formation of calcium soaps with malabsorbed fatty acids, oxalate is more readily absorbed [77]. In addition, it appears that malabsorbed bile acids may directly render the colon more soluble to oxalates [80].

ILEOCECAL VALVE REMOVAL

If the ileocecal valve is removed, malabsorption may be more severe. The ileocecal valve slows intestinal transit (allowing more time for absorption) and acts as a barrier to colonic bacteria. Bacterial overgrowth of the remaining small bowel further decreases absorption of vitamin B_{12}, carbohydrates, and lipids. In this setting, antibiotic treatment may be necessary.

TREATMENT

The dietary management of patients with small intestinal resection will differ depending on the age of the patient and the extent of surgery. If less than 10 percent of the small bowel length has been resected, the diet can be advanced quickly. Carbohydrate or fat absorption should not be affected significantly. However, the patient should be followed for possible deficiencies that may result in the ensuing months or years. For example, calcium and iron malabsorption from duodenal surgery or vitamin B_{12} deficiency from ileal surgery may appear insidiously.

For patients with more extensive small intestinal resection, initial management involves total parenteral alimentation with the patient initially NPO. The initial parenteral fluid and electrolyte requirements are calculated from the patient's maintenance requirements and ongoing losses. As previously mentioned, enteral feeding is a major trophic factor for intestinal adaptation and should be started once the patient is stable, deficits have been replaced, and the integrity of the remaining bowel is intact. The transition to full enteral feeding may take weeks to months; therefore the patient must, during this period, continue to receive parenteral support. In some patients, frequent small feedings or continuous feedings via nasogastric tube may be better tolerated than large bolus feedings [83].

For a small infant with extensive intestinal resection, the gradual introduction of food may be begun with one of the more elemental formulas such as Ross Modular Formula, Pregestimil, or Portagen. Because patients with short gut often do not tolerate hyperosmolar feedings, the formulas are initially diluted to one-quarter of their full strength. The hydrolyzed casein in Pregestimil and the sodium caseinate in Portagen may be better absorbed because of possible pancreatic insufficiency in these malnourished patients. The loss of absorptive surface following intestinal resection will decrease the total activity of disaccharidases. Because maltase activity is greater than that of lactase or sucrase, the most easily tolerated carbohydrates will utilize maltase activity. The carbohydrates in Pregestimil appropriately are corn syrup solids and modified tapioca starch, while those in Portagen are 75 percent corn syrup solids and 25 percent sucrose. Medium chain triglyceride oil (MCT) is rapidly hydrolyzed and absorbed into the portal venous system without the need for bile salt activity. However, it does not provide a source of essential fatty acids. Thus, some long chain triglycerides (LCT) are needed. The ratio of LCT/MCT in Pregestimil is 3 : 2 and in Portagen 1 : 6.

If the diluted formula is tolerated at a low infusion rate, the concentration of the formula may be gradually increased without changing the formula delivery rate. Criteria that are often used for determination of tolerance include stool volume, stool pH, and the Clinitest reagent tablet test for reducing sugars. The normal stool volume is approximately 20 gm/kg per day to a maximum of 200 gm per day. Stool pH should be greater than or equal to 5.5 to 6.0 and Clinitest reagent tablet results should not be greater than ½ percent.

Once the concentration of formula reaches three-quarters or full-strength concentration, the volume of feedings may be increased slowly via continuous infusion while the parenteral source of calories is decreased. For example, if growth is maintained with an infusion of 30 ml per hour or 90 ml every 3 hours, the 90-ml infusion can be delivered in 2½ hours and then stopped for ½ hour. The time of infusion is shortened by ½ hour each day such that on day 5, 90 ml enters over ½ hour and then is stopped for 2 ½ hours. Bolus feedings of 90 ml can then be given every 3 hours. If oral stimulation is maintained during the continuous infusions and total parenteral nutrition, progression from bolus feedings via tube to oral feedings may be easier. Parenteral nutrition must not be stopped until it is evident that the patient can be maintained in a positive nitrogen balance on enteral feedings alone.

For older children with extensive resections, feedings may start 1 to 2 weeks after surgery. Nasogastric feedings may be necessary with an initially dilute formula. Osmolite and Vital (see Appendix 4) may be used in these patients because the carbohydrate source is mainly corn syrup solids, which require maltase, and the fat composition is 50 percent MCT.

If these formulas are well tolerated, the diet may be advanced to include more table foods. However, concentrated sugars such as table sugar and soft drinks should be restricted. Total fat intake should initially be limited to approximately 50 percent of normal intake, and one-half of that intake should be in the form of MCT. A large proportion of the fat ingested should be given at breakfast, since the intraluminal concentration of bile acid will be greatest after an overnight fast. As adaptation occurs, fat intake may be increased.

Fat-soluble vitamin deficiency can develop in patients with extensive small bowel resections and are most likely related to fat malabsorption due to inadequate surface area, bile salt insufficiency, and possible decreased pancreatic secretion. Thus, vitamins A (5,000 to 10,000 USP units per day) and D (800 to 1,200 USP units per day) are given in aqueous form; aqueous vitamin E is given at 5 IU/kg per day. Vitamin K (5 mg PO twice a week) may be necessary if bleeding abnormalities arise or if a patient is placed on chronic antibiotic therapy. These suggestions are similar to those given to patients with cystic fibrosis.

Water-soluble vitamins (as a standard multivitamin preparation) are usually suggested because cheilosis and tongue changes due to riboflavin deficiency [80] have occurred with the loss of absorptive surface (see Table 7-18). Vitamin B_{12} routinely should be given (1,000 mg IM every 2 months) if there was ileal surgery. Before discontinuing vitamin B_{12} therapy, a Schilling test is needed to confirm adequate absorption.

Calcium and iron absorption are often impaired when the duodenum or proximal jejunum is resected. If iron deficiency anemia develops and oral iron is not effective, intramuscular or intravenous iron may be necessary. In patients with steatorrhea, calcium supplementation is often needed not only to improve serum calcium levels, but also to bind the free oxalate that may be absorbed in the colon. If hyperoxaluria exists, foods such as spinach, rhubarb, and other green leafy vegetables as well as cocoa and chocolate should be avoided. Since ascorbic acid is metabolized to oxalic acid in the body, intake should be restricted to daily requirements. Monitoring the urine for red blood cells and oxalate will indicate the effectiveness of the therapy. Because fatty acids also bind magnesium, their levels should be monitored as well. Parenteral supplementation may be necessary if a deficiency develops that cannot be corrected by oral supplementation.

CONCLUSION

The prognosis for the patient with short bowel syndrome has improved in the past decade. Children who survive infancy may show an initial delay in weight gain during the first year followed by an acceleration in growth to a normal weight for age [86]. If initial nutritional management is successful, most children will develop and grow normally. Because many of the metabolic consequences of the short bowel syndrome present insidiously, the management of these patients requires meticulous long-term follow-up. In order to prevent and correct any nutritional deficiencies, close monitoring becomes a lifetime responsibility for primary care providers.

Cow's Milk Sensitivity and Lactose Intolerance
Martin Maksimak and Harland S. Winter

In the early 1900s, foreign proteins were suspected to be related to the occasional diarrhea, failure to thrive [95], and even anaphylaxis seen in infants fed cow's milk formula. Up until the last few decades, cow's milk allergy was considered rare, but with advances in immunology and pediatric gastroenterology, less severe manifestations have been recognized as common.

Most infants fed cow's milk formula will grow and thrive even though sensitive immunological parameters may suggest a reaction to the foreign cow's milk protein. Only a small minority develop clinical symptoms of cow's milk allergy. Thus, cow's milk sensitivity must be diagnosed on the basis of a clinical reaction to cow's milk and not on the basis of any laboratory tests. There is no definitive immunological test to identify sensitive infants.

PATHOGENESIS

Up to 20 components in cow's milk have been found to be capable of inducing antibody formation. The four most common proteins in cow's milk formulas are beta lactoglobulin, alpha lactalbumin, bovine serum albumin, and casein. Each of these have been found to be allergenic but some are more potent than others. Beta lactoglobulin causes symptoms in 60 to 100 percent of sensitive infants and casein is almost as active. Reactions on challenge tests to alpha lactalbumin and bovine serum proteins are much less common.

In most patients, the immunological reasons for the clinical symptoms cannot be identified. However, there are several immune mechanisms that have been implicated after ingestion of cow's milk in a sensitive infant. In some patients, type I (IgE mediated) reactions cause symptoms within minutes after a challenge. The child may develop an urticarial rash, dyspnea, diarrhea, and cardiovascular collapse. Type 3 (immune complex-complement mediated) reactions have also been implicated but produce effects hours to days after exposure. Gastrointestinal bleeding is thought to be mediated by this mechanism and circulating immune complexes have been identified in some patients.

CLINICAL PRESENTATION

The true incidence of cow's milk allergy is unknown but appears to be increasing. It is highest in children with an underlying allergic diathesis. The age of presentation depends greatly on when cow's milk is introduced. When cow's milk protein is introduced at an early age, most infants who are destined to manifest symptoms will do so within the first month, and 90 percent of the eventually afflicted infants will be symptomatic by the age of 3 months [94]. In a Swedish study in which 45 percent of the infants were entirely breast-fed for 3 months, mean age of symptom onset was later than in previous reports [96].

The symptoms can involve various organ systems, but gastrointestinal involvement is the most common; diarrhea is the most frequent complaint. Its onset may be acute but it often has a more insidious onset. Gross blood in the stool is unusual, but many children have occult blood. Vomiting with colic may lead to dehydration, especially in small infants. With chronic diarrhea, growth may be impaired; weight is usually affected more than height. In some infants colic may be the major symptom.

Atopic dermatitis caused by cow's milk allergy in infants is a controversial subject [99]. Acute urticaria is much less common [98], while angioedema is even more unusual.

Respiratory complaints of idiopathic pulmonary hemosiderosis, rhinitis, and wheezing also have been described. Cow's milk has been implicated in serous otitis media. Other nonspecific symptoms such as irritability, crying, lethargy, and weakness have been described; the mechanism for these symptoms and their relationship to milk remain unclear.

Anaphylaxis is the most serious side effect of cow's milk allergy. Frequently it is accompanied by skin and/or gastrointestinal symptoms. It may be possible to identify children at risk for anaphylaxis by skin tests or radioactive immunoabsorbent tests (RAST) with the putative antigen. Because the reaction is IgE mediated, these tests should identify children at risk if the correct antigen is used.

LABORATORY TESTS
Laboratory findings usually reflect the abnormalities of the gastrointestinal symptoms. Gastrointestinal blood loss may result in iron deficiency anemia. Findings on jejunal biopsy may reveal mild, patchy, or diffusely active inflammation. Sigmoidoscopy and rectal biopsy may demonstrate a nonspecific colitis and there may be polymorphonuclear leukocytes in the stool. Histological abnormalities improve on a diet free of cow's milk and may recur after challenge. Reflecting mucosal injury, disaccharidase levels may be reduced [100] and lactose intolerance is seen in over half the patients [93]. D-Xylose absorption tests also may be abnormal and reflect mucosal injury. These findings improve quickly when cow's milk is eliminated. Other parameters of malabsorption may include hypoproteinemia, steatorrhea, coagulopathy, osteoporosis, and aminoaciduria.

Immunological parameters are of little benefit. RAST shows IgE antibodies to cow's milk in many children with atopic dermatitis as well as cow's milk allergy. However, with the purely intestinal form of cow's milk allergy, the RAST is seldom positive. In addition, some children with no clinical symptoms of cow's milk allergy may have a positive RAST. Scratch tests, like the RAST, are of little diagnostic value.

DIAGNOSIS
Because there is no specific laboratory parameter to establish the diagnosis of cow's milk allergy, the diagnosis rests on the results of clinical withdrawal of cow's milk and an appropriate challenge. With elimination of cow's milk and substitution of another formula such as Pregestimil, Nutramigen, or breast milk, infants respond within 1 to 2 days with a decrease in symptoms. In some children, it may take more than a week to respond, while others may require weeks of intravenous feeding.

If a patient responds to the elimination diet, a challenge with cow's milk is often performed to verify the diagnosis. A challenge should not be performed if life-threatening symptoms occurred. First, skin tests are placed and read for evidence for immediate hypersensitivity reactions. The challenge is best carried out in a clinic or hospital because of the chance of a severe reaction. One way to perform a challenge test is by feeding ½ ounce of cow's milk after a physical examination. For the first 30 minutes and then periodically thereafter, the child is examined for signs of a reaction. If after 24 hours no reactions are noted, the infant is given larger amounts of cow's milk. Many children will have symptoms within one day, but delayed reactions are not unusual. Severe reactions such as shock and anaphylaxis usually occur quickly and need prompt treatment with intravenous fluids and epinephrine.

TREATMENT

The mainstay of treatment is the elimination of the offending antigen. The diet should be nutritionally adequate with respect to calories, protein, carbohydrates, fat, and vitamins. In the young infant, the diet is simple; only a replacement formula needs to be selected. If the mother is able, breast milk may be used with a slow increase in volume (because of secondary lactase deficiency). Pregestimil or Nutramigen may be chosen because they are hypoallergenic. Goat's milk is not used because of the possible crossover reactions to beta lactoglobulin, the suspected offending protein in children with cow's milk allergy. Also, goat's milk is deficient in folic acid. Up to 40 percent of children with cow's milk allergy will also react to soy proteins [102]. Because of the expense of the special formulas and if breast-feeding is not acceptable, a trial of soy formula might be attempted after the child has had a period of good weight gain on a casein hydroxylate formula.

As the infant becomes older, new, simple foods are introduced one at a time every 3 to 7 days. If they are tolerated, they are continued. Foods that tend to cause allergies such as citrus fruits, eggs, nuts, peas, fish, and chocolate should be avoided until approximately 2 years of age. Also, the elimination of gluten-containing cereals should not be recommended unless a prior small bowel biopsy reveals a severe enteropathy.

When the child is 1 year old, we recommend a repeat challenge test. If symptoms recur with cow's milk, elimination is continued until a rechallenge is performed 6 months later.

Disodium cromoglycate has been tried as a treatment for cow's milk allergy with questionable success. Elimination of the allergen is better therapy; medication is best tried when multiple food allergies are present or if it is difficult to identify the specific allergen [101].

In most children, sensitivity to cow's milk disappears by age 1 year [96]. By 2 years of age, most are taking cow's milk without symptoms, but in some the sensitivity persists longer [92]. Children with cow's milk allergies may be at increased risk for developing other allergic tendencies later in life.

PREVENTION

At the present time, the only practical way to prevent cow's milk allergy is to avoid the allergen (e.g., cow's milk, cow's milk–based formulas, and goat's milk in the first few months of life). Breast-feeding should be encouraged, especially in families with an allergic history. However, exposure to the cow's milk protein found in breast milk may cause symptoms. It is not known how long one should avoid cow's milk protein in order to ensure that cow's milk sensitization does not occur.

LACTOSE INTOLERANCE

Lactose intolerance refers to the inability of the infant to hydrolyze the carbohydrate lactose into glucose and galactose. This is accomplished by the brush border enzyme, lactase, found on the surface of the mature enterocyte. Congenital absence of this enzyme is exceedingly rare. Most commonly, lactose intolerance is a consequence of infectious diarrhea and is transient (see section on Infectious Diarrhea). The degrees of intolerance reflect the severity of the injury to the small intestine brush border. This can be diagnosed by clinitest of the stools (e.g., presence of glucose or lactose), the lactose breath hydrogen test [90], or by the lactose tolerance test. In each of these tests, 2 gm/kg of lactose is given after a fast.

In the tolerance test, blood levels of glucose are drawn following the lactose load. A glucose rise of over 20 mg/100 ml from baseline implies normal absorption. The disadvantage of this test is that it requires multiple blood samples.

For the breath test, breath is collected over a 3-hour period and measured for a rise in H_2 content. If the lactose is split and absorbed, there is no rise in breath H_2. However, if the lactose is malabsorbed, it is transported to the colon rapidly as it acts as an osmotic agent, drawing water into the bowel. In the colon, bacteria convert it to lactic acid, releasing H_2 that is then expelled in the breath. Approximately 10 percent of individuals will have bacteria in their colon that produce only methane or other non-H_2 gases [98]; even in the presence of malabsorption, a rise in H_2 will not be detected in these individuals. A rise in H_2 of over 10 ppm from the baseline signifies malabsorption. If the child is under 5 years of age and white or under 3 years of age and black or Oriental, a positive test strongly suggests mucosal injury. In older children, a positive test may be due to genetically determined lactase deficiency alone. For this reason, the breath test is useful as a screening test for mucosal damage in the younger child.

In the older child, malabsorption due to primary enzyme deficiency may result in abdominal pain [91] or diarrhea after eating or drinking foods containing lactose.

TREATMENT

The enzyme may be replaced by adding the commercially available Lactaid to milk prior to drinking, or by taking the capsule, Lactrase, with a lactose-containing meal. The majority of the lactose is split, making it possible for carbohydrate absorption to take place without the brush border enzyme. In the infant, a diagnosis must always be made because small bowel injury is assumed if carbohydrate malabsorption is present.

In the older child and adolescent, mucosal injury is uncommon. If there is mucosal injury, measurements of absorption of another sugar such as sucrose or D-xylose will be abnormal.

The treatment for lactose intolerance is a lactose-free diet (see Appendix 3). Following an acute enteritis, treatment should be limited to a few weeks. *Giardia* is an exception, and even after presumably eradicating the parasite, children may be intolerant of lactose for many months.

Lactose intolerance needs to be distinguished from milk allergy [94]. In infants, lactose intolerance is most often a reflection of intestinal injury that may be caused by an infectious agent, parasite, bacterial overgrowth, or even sensitivity to milk or soy protein. Milk protein sensitivity is a reaction, presumably immunologically mediated, to a protein in milk that is manifested by various symptoms including diarrhea, vomiting, and blood in the stool and colon. This sensitivity has recently been described in breast-fed infants [97]. The true IgE mediated allergy is rarely found. Milk allergy is most often resolved by age 2 years. The clinician needs to separate these two milk-related problems and clarify them diagnostically. If the child becomes ill after drinking milk and the breath test is negative, milk protein sensitivity is suggested. If the breath test is positive, mucosal injury (of which cow's milk sensitivity is but one cause) is likely.

Infantile Colic
Harland S. Winter

Colic refers to a paroxysmal abdominal pain originating in a hollow viscus. Infantile colic is a common problem faced by pediatricians and parents, but the cause of the pain is unknown. Most full-term infants' symptoms begin with unexplained fussy, "colicky" periods between 2 and 3 weeks of age reaching a peak at 6 to 8 weeks of age. In premature infants, colic most frequently begins at 39 to 44 weeks gestational age. Although most children may cry for 90 minutes, some parents have reported "children who never stop crying." Although seemingly unrealistic, it is of no value to the parent, the child, or the physician-family relationship to attempt to validate the observation. Some children appear to be constipated and some will pass flatus, while others draw their legs to their chests, appearing to be in pain. However, children with infantile colic pass appropriate stools for age and gain weight at the normal rate. If a child is passing hard stools, the term colic should not be used unless the crying continues when the stools are soft. Whatever the cause, symptoms abate after 3 months, often with sighs of relief from the family and pediatrician.

Colic is a problem with many causes. Urinary tract infections have been implicated and intra-abdominal partial obstruction can give similar symptoms. In some children, pathological gastroesophageal reflux has been implicated. A urinalysis may be helpful in the child with persistent crying, but x-rays of the abdomen are rarely of benefit unless the infant is failing to thrive or if there is occult or gross blood in the stool.

Recently, cow's milk proteins have been implicated as a cause for colic in breast-fed infants. In the infant who is fed cow's milk, colic has been associated with suspected protein intolerance [104]. This evidence provides a basis for changes in formula that may be beneficial. Because approximately one-third of infants who are intolerant of cow's milk protein will also be intolerant of soy protein, a switch to a soy formula may not be successful. In these situations, a trial of a formula with hydrolyzed protein is worth an attempt.

The explanation for colic in breast-fed infants has been a mystery. Allergies in infants have been attributed to substances that have passed from mother to child in the breast milk [103]. Breast-feeding mothers who have infants with colic have tried eliminating bananas, apples, oranges, strawberries, coffee, or chocolate in an attempt to alleviate the irritability. For an individual mother, it is often difficult to identify the inciting agent. Jakobsson and Lindberg [105] completed a double blind crossover study of the effect of maternally ingested cow's milk protein on the breast-fed baby. Their study suggests that colic was increased when mothers swallowed capsules containing whey protein. The elimination of cow's milk from the maternal diet resulted in the disappearance of colic in over 50 percent of the infants. Although this study implicates cow's milk protein, other protein may also play a role. The mechanism by which ingested proteins cause colic is unclear.

TREATMENT

The treatment of colic should begin with a careful dietary history of both the mother and the baby. In the proper clinical setting, elimination of specific food groups may be beneficial. Above all, the family needs to be reassured that this is a self-limited problem that will not impair the growth and development of the infant.

In addition to dietary manipulations (i.e., formula changes, specific protein elimination from maternal diet), frequent burping, and small feedings may decrease irritability. Movement has been recognized to be of value in treating an attack and many parents have reported that the purchase of a swing has been "lifesaving." Similarly, taking the infant for a ride in the car may cause some relief. Repetitive sounds (i.e., a ticking clock) may calm the infant and also provide some relief.

Colic can be a worrisome problem for a family. Until the crying subsides, the possibility of an undetermined, more serious problem is always present. Living with an inconsolable child frustrates the parents and causes a question regarding the pediatrician's ability to heal. A careful history, physical examination, and frequent reevaluation are important for the ongoing management of the child with colic.

Constipation

Martin Maksimak

Constipation in infancy is a common concern of parents. However, the definition and significance of constipation vary among parents and even physicians. The term may imply that the bowel movements are too infrequent or that the stools are too hard, too small, or too difficult to expel. Attempts at defining the characteristics of constipation are often imprecise. The complaint of hard stool does not seem reliable because this subjective rating varies widely in normal individuals and is dependent on diet. Size may not be an accurate indication because it is determined by the consistency of the stool and the muscular contractions that occur during defecation. Stool weight varies widely between normal individuals and also from day to day in the same individual [110]. Although stooling habits of infants are characterized mainly by frequency, other objective aspects must be considered.

The normal neonate usually will pass the first meconium stool within the first 24 hours of life and almost always by 48 hours. In early infancy, the normal stooling pattern depends on the diet. Nonconstipated, breast-fed infants may have bowel movements that range in frequency from one every feeding to once every 10 days; bottle-fed babies tend to cluster toward the middle of this range. Mildly hyperosmolar feedings may dehydrate feces, producing hard stools that are passed with great effort and grunting. As a child becomes older, the stooling pattern becomes similar to that of an adult. Approximately 95 percent of healthy adults will have bowel movements ranging in frequency from three times a day to once every 3 days [106].

Many factors affect bowel habits, such as exercise, psychosocial influence, and diet. When evaluation for constipation is initiated, many causes should be considered (Table 8-5) [107]. The vast majority of infants will have dietary-related constipation. As an infant's diet is changed from human to cow's milk, stools often become firm, small, and less frequent. At times, straining may be needed to pass such stools. If anal irritation or an anal fissure is present, pain at the time of defecation may result in the development of a withholding pattern [107]. On physical examination, the child with a withholding pattern or encopresis will appear to be thriving and there is often a palpable moveable mass in the lower abdomen without severe abdominal distention. The presence of an anal fissure or firm stool in the rectum is helpful in establishing the diagnosis. Drugs may also induce constipation and should be considered in the evaluation (Table 8-5).

In early infancy, while the child is taking only formula, treatment consists of increasing the free water intake to correct the hyperosmolarity of some formulas. Also, the addition of corn syrup (1 teaspoon for every 4 ounces of formula), is sometimes helpful. Older infants can be encouraged to eat cereal, fruits, vegetables, and to drink fruit juices (especially prune). They should also decrease cow's milk intake.

In the child with severe constipation, two conditions need to be considered. First, the position of the anus in relationship to the pigmented area and the perineum should be noted. The anus should be located in the center of the pigmented area. In children with anterior displacement of the anus, defecation may be more difficult. The vast majority of these individuals will respond to mineral oil. Secondly, Hirschsprung's disease (aganglionosis) is a common cause of intestinal obstruction occurring in 1 in 5,000 newborns [109] and should be considered in infants with constipation. Although Hirschsprung's disease is four times more common in boys than in girls, long segment disease is more common in girls. There is also an association with Down syndrome and other genetic abnormalities in Hirschsprung's disease. The primary defect is the absence of the parasympathetic ganglion cells in the submucosal and myenteric plexuses. In the majority of children, symptoms present within the first week of life. Eighty-three percent develop defecation difficulties in the first month of life and 96 percent have symptoms during the first year [107].

Table 8-5. Causes of Constipation

Diet
    Low in roughage, fiber
    Decrease food intake
    High in refined carbohydrate and/or protein (i.e., cheese)
    Decreased fluid intake
Drugs
    Antacids (calcium and aluminum compounds)
    Anticholinergics
    Anticonvulsants
    Barium sulfate
    Diuretics
    Hematinics (i.e., iron)
    Metal intoxication (arsenic, lead, mercury, phosphorus)
Mechanical Obstruction
    Anorectal stenotic lesions
    Intrinsic and extrinsic tumors
    Crohn's disease
    Necrotizing enterocolitis
Neuromuscular
    Aganglionosis (Hirschsprung's disease)
    Spinal cord lesions
    Amyotonia congenita
    Cerebral palsy
    Poliomyelitis
    Infectious polyneuritis
    Congenital absence of abdominal musculature
Medical/Hormonal
    Infantile renal acidosis
    Diabetes insipidus
    Idiopathic hypercalcemia
    Hypothyroidism
    Hypertonic states

The usual presentation of Hirschsprung's disease is that of a normal-weight newborn who fails to pass meconium. The baby may then develop abdominal distention, refusal of feedings, and bilious vomiting. In others, the passage of meconium may be delayed beyond 24 hours with progressive difficulty in passing stools and abdominal distention. A clinical picture mimicking sepsis may be the sole manifestation.

Older infants with Hirschsprung's disease may have similar symptoms with failure to thrive or even enterocolitis, manifested by forcefully expelled liquid stools, fever, and even perforation, sepsis, and shock. Older children may have intermittent intestinal obstruction from fecal impaction, hypochromic anemia, hypoproteinemia, and failure to thrive. These children usually do not have fecal soiling. The existence of a very short segment of aganglionosis is controversial because the distal rectum normally contains a zone of hypoganglion-osis.

On physical examination, the major finding is abdominal distention with fecal masses palpable in the abdomen. On rectal examination, the anal canal is narrow and the anus and rectum are free of stool. Withdrawing the finger from the anus may produce a gush of flatus and liquid stool. X-ray studies, rectal biopsy, and manometry are frequently used to diagnose Hirschsprung's disease [108]. Rectal manometry is sensitive but not specific, and may be technically difficult in the infant. On barium enema, there is a transition zone located at the junction of the rectum and sigmoid in 80 percent of patients and more proximally in 20 percent of patients. The zone of transition may be less defined in young infants and is often not identified in infants with Hirshsprung's disease who are under 6 weeks of age. In this group of patients, the finding of retained barium 24 hours after the barium enema suggests aganglionosis. Suction rectal biopsies are taken 3 cm from the anal margin to avoid the distal hypoganglionic zone. If no ganglion cells are seen, a full thickness biopsy is necessary to confirm the diagnosis. If no ganglion cells are present, a diverting colostomy is performed to relieve the obstruction. At approximately 1 year of age, a definitive repair may be done. The Soave operation is performed by resecting the aganglionic segment and removing the mucosa from the remaining short rectal segment. The ganglionic bowel is then pulled into the muscular coat of the remaining rectum. The Duhamel operation is performed by bringing the normal colon along side the aganglionic segment, placing two rows of sutures, and incorporating the involved segment into the normal segment that has been pulled through into the anus.

Although surgically correctable causes of constipation need to be considered, constipation will improve in the majority of children after dietary changes have been made. These modifications may be as simple as increasing the intake of water or adding bulk agents or mineral oil to the diet. In the child with encopresis, rectal manipulation—rectal temperatures, enemas, frequent digital examinations—should be avoided. In the vast majority of children, behavior modification, lubricants, and appropriate dietary counseling are sufficient. It remains, however, that constipation is often a chronic problem, and follow-up should continue for many years.

Cystic Fibrosis
Harry Shwachman

Cystic fibrosis is an autosomal recessive disease that occurs primarily in white people affecting approximately 1 in 2,000 live births. It is rare in Orientals and about one-tenth as common in black people as in white people. The gene frequency in the white population is 1 in 20. The enormity of this problem can be seen by the approximate 300 patients admitted each year for the past few years to the Children's Hospital Medical Center and by the over 500 patients seen each year in its clinic. Unfortunately, there is still no method of detecting the carrier of the gene. Other names for this disease include pancreatic cystic fibrosis and mucoviscidosis. It was first described in the United States by Dorothy Andersen in New York and by Blackfan, May, and Wolbach in Boston in 1936 and has since been recognized throughout the world [112]. It occurs equally in both sexes although males afflicted with the disease may have a slightly longer life span. The life expectancy has increased from approximately 2 years in 1940 to over 20 years at the present time. This remarkable advance is due to better recognition of the disease and an easier method of detection, the availability of improved technology, a better understanding of the disease, and improved methods of therapy.

PATHOGENESIS

The disease is a generalized one affecting the mucous secretions and resulting in obstructive lesions in many organs especially in the lungs, liver, pancreas, and gastrointestinal tract. The exocrine pancreas is affected in close to 85 percent of patients with cystic fibrosis and the upper and lower respiratory tract is affected in over 95 percent of patients. The sticky secretions obtained by duodenal drainage and the lack of pancreatic enzymes, trypsin, amylase, and lipase are characteristic of the disease. The pulmonary lesion may begin shortly after birth and is characterized by an obstructive process in the small bronchi

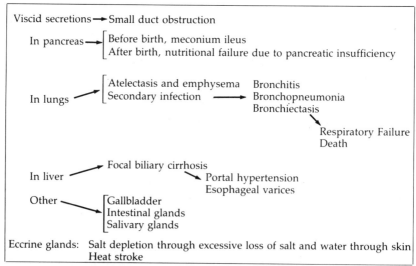

Figure 8-3. The pathogenetic mechanisms in cystic fibrosis.

and bronchioli that soon becomes infected, resulting in bronchiectasis. Few patients escape the pulmonary lesion in childhood.

Figure 8-3 outlines the nature and widespread occurrence of the disease in many organs, while Figure 8-4 illustrates the consequences of the obstructing bronchial secretions. Trapping of air in the lung occurs early in the course of the disease. Bacterial invasion also occurs early and becomes a major issue because the progression of the pulmonary lesions results in pulmonary hypertension and cor pulmonale. The bacteria that initially inhabit the respiratory tract often are replaced by antibiotic resistant bacteria as the patient advances in age. The

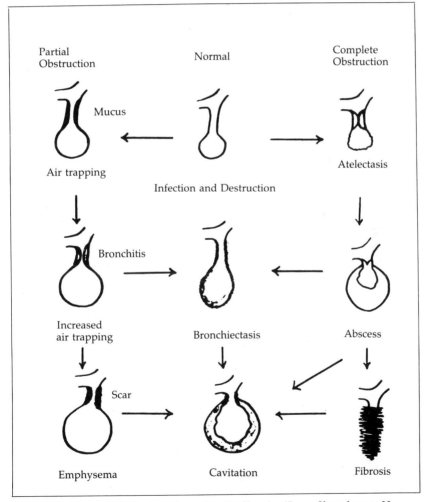

Figure 8-4. The pathologic physiology of cystic fibrosis. (From Shwachman, H. Guide to Diagnostic Management of Cystic Fibrosis. National Cystic Fibrosis Research Foundation, Rockville, Md., 1963.)

great majority of adults with cystic fibrosis are colonized by mucoid strains of *Pseudomonas*. The sinuses are commonly involved and the appearance of nasal polyps may occur at any age (with an increased frequency in adolescents).

CLINICAL FEATURES

The earliest clinical manifestation occurs at birth in the form of intestinal obstruction and meconium ileus. This presentation has been noted in close to 15 percent of all patients with cystic fibrosis. Prior to 1940, this was uniformly fatal. Many advances, both medical and surgical, have altered this situation. Today many infants survive. If they survive the first 6 months of life, the subsequent course will parallel those without this initial complication. Our current roster includes eight patients with cystic fibrosis born with meconium ileus who are over 30 years of age; four had surgery to correct this condition within the first 2 days of life.

One of the early signs of cystic fibrosis is the salty taste of sweat. The exocrine pancreatic insufficiency explains the gastrointestinal symptoms, the abnormal nature of the stool with its foul smell, altered consistency, and increased frequency, and the presence of undigested food and its fatty nature. Many infants have a voracious appetite that many parents fail to recognize as anything unusual. Another serious complaint is recurrent abdominal pain. Failure to grow is a common complaint. Rectal prolapse may occur in over 20 percent of untreated infants.

The pulmonary symptoms, such as rapid respirations and cough, may appear first or simultaneously with the onset of the gastrointestinal complaints in early infancy. The cough may be persistent and infrequent at first, at times almost unnoticed. This is a manifestation of bronchitis and a chest film may show the earliest changes seen in this disease, namely irregular aeration perhaps with a peribronchial cupping. Atelectasis of small segments and, at times, a whole lobe may be involved. Bronchial plugging, pneumonia, abscess formation, and bronchiectasis are subsequent events. Two complications with a serious setback follow, namely pneumothorax and/or massive hemorrhage. Minor degrees of hemoptysis are common and usually subside with rest.

In contrast to the more severe cases, there are some patients with mild to minimal pulmonary involvement who reach early adulthood with no or little interference from the disease. In the past, these individuals were difficult to detect. With increasing diagnostic and clinical experience they are being recognized more frequently. For example, one man who lost a sister to cystic fibrosis was sweat tested and diagnosed 7 years later at age 27. A 40-year-old doctor of electrical engineering was referred for study because of sterility and was found to have cystic fibrosis. He, too, had no obvious symptoms of the disease. It is only within the last decade that unsuspected clinical cases like these have been noted.

DIAGNOSIS

The diagnosis of cystic fibrosis is a clinical one and not a laboratory one [111]. The laboratory tests confirm the impression of the physician. The following features are taken into account: family history, the clinical features relating to pancreatic insufficiency, and pulmonary involvement. The diagnosis is confirmed by a properly conducted pilocarpine iontophoresis sweat test and repeated at least once if positive [113]. The physician should keep in mind that some of the symptoms may be confused with celiac disease, allergy, and a host of other conditions including bronchitis and pneumonia. If the suspicion of cystic fibrosis is high, a sweat test is performed by a proven reliable laboratory.

Table 8-6 suggests conditions that make the performance of a sweat test advisable. Figure 8-5 illustrates the diagnostic range of sodium (Na) and chloride (Cl) in patients with cystic fibrosis (including adults as well as infants and children). No other condition consistently yields

Table 8-6. Indications for Sweat Test

Infants who pass their initial meconium late (i.e., after approximately 30 hours of age) or whose meconium is positive for albumin

Intestinal obstruction in the newborn (to distinguish meconium ileus from other causes)

Infants and children whose sweat tastes salty

All siblings of patients with cystic fibrosis, including the newborn

Failure to thrive in infancy or childhood

All patients suspected of having cystic fibrosis or celiac disease

Infants and children with large, frequent, smelly bowel movements or chronic diarrhea

Infants with rapid respirations and retractions with chronic cough

Infants with diagnosis of asthma

Infants with hypoproteinemia or hypothrombinemia

Infants who show hyperaeration or atelectasis on chest x-ray

Infants and children with rectal prolapse (especially recurrent)

All patients suspected of having disaccharidase intolerance or diagnosed as having celiac disease

Patients with recurrent pneumonia, chronic atelectasis, chronic pulmonary disease, bronchiectasis, or chronic cough

Patients whose sputum cultures show mucoid *Pseudomonas*

Children and adults with nasal polyposis

Children and young patients (nonalcoholic) with cirrhosis of the liver and portal hypertension

Infants of a mother with cystic fibrosis: the obligate heterozygote

Adult males sterile because of aspermia

For any parent who requests a sweat test on his/her child

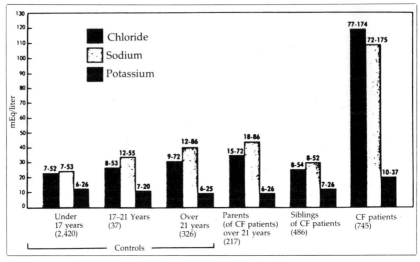

Figure 8-5. Mean sweat electrolyte concentrations. Numbers above bars indicate ranges of results. Numbers of patients in each group appear under headings. Data were collected at The Children's Hospital, Boston, from August 1958 to May 1964. (From Shwachman, H. and Mahmoodian, A. The sweat test and cystic fibrosis. Diagn. Med. 5:68, 1982.)

sweat sodium and chloride levels in a three to fivefold increase over normal. Between 1 and 2 percent of individuals suspected of having cystic fibrosis have sweat values in the borderline range for cystic fibrosis, namely sodium and chloride values between 45 and 65 mEq per liter. These patients are difficult to resolve. We treat them symptomatically and observe them at frequent intervals (about every 4 to 6 months).

The clinical assessment of cystic fibrosis can be aided by the presence of some complications such as nasal polyposis, the presence of mucoid *Pseudomonas* in sputum, azospermia, inguinal hernias, and defects in the vas deferens in the male, and pneumothorax. There is at present no specific laboratory test for cystic fibrosis. Because many patients with cystic fibrosis are diagnosed as having celiac disease, a sweat test is taken whenever the diagnosis of celiac disease is entertained. Unfortunately, some patients have both conditions, although this is very rare.

The degree of elevation of sweat electrolytes is not related to the severity of disease, nor does treatment alter their levels. Carriers of the gene for cystic fibrosis have normal sweat electrolytes. The standard method of diagnosis, the quantitative pilocarpine iontophoresis method, is recommended. The amount of sweat obtained, as well as the concentration of sodium and chloride, should be reported.

TREATMENT

There is no specific therapy for cystic fibrosis because we do not know the nature of the basic defect. Present treatment is empirical, supportive, and prophylactic. Pancreatic enzyme replacement is necessary in most patients. Two most impressive accomplishments concerning therapy were the introduction of an effective oral pancreatic enzyme preparation and the introduction of a broad spectrum antibiotic in the form of Aureomycin in 1948, followed by many other antibiotics including synthetic penicillins and more recently the aminoglycerides that are given intravenously.

NUTRITIONAL THERAPY

Years ago the pancreatic changes that occur with cystic fibrosis were considered consistent with features of vitamin A deficiency. The result of untreated pancreatic insufficiency may result in malnutrition due to the frequent bulky, foul-smelling stools. The exocrine pancreas fails to function in whole or in part in between 80 and 85 percent of patients with cystic fibrosis. Replacement of the missing enzymes with each meal will result in an immediate improvement and hunger will be diminished. There will also be a decrease in the number of stools and some correction of the stool abnormality. Once pancreatic insufficiency is complete, no restoration will occur subsequently. Because oral replacement is satisfactory, the patient will fare better with early recognition of the disease and early treatment. Pancreatic surgery (i.e., transplantation) has no place in cystic fibrosis today.

A high caloric and slightly reduced fat diet is recommended (Table 8-7). In small babies hunger should be satisfied by more frequent feedings. Enzyme replacement is given at the beginning of each meal. Effective pancreatic preparations include Viokase, available in powder and tablet forms. The dose varies with the size and type of meal as well as the age of the patient (Table 8-8). Infants may require from one-quarter to 1 teaspoon of pancreatic preparations given in food such as applesauce. Older children may require up to 5 tablets per meal. More recent preparations include Pancrease and Cotazym-S. These preparations come in capsules filled with microspheruls. Multivitamins are used in double the daily dose. In infants between the ages of 1½ and 2 years, 5 mg of vitamin K is given twice weekly. Vitamin E is administered also (100 to 400 units). Lactose insufficiency is rarely a clinical problem. High caloric supplements such as MCT oil, Polycose, and Sustacal are used as well. We do not advise routine use of intravenous lipids and hyperalimentation.

RESPIRATORY THERAPY

The use of chest physical therapy for the management of the chronic obstructive pulmonary process as practiced at the Brompton St. Clinic

Table 8-7. Daily Nutrient Guidelines for Patients with Cystic Fibrosis

Age	kcal/kg[a]	Protein (gm/kg)[a]	Fat (gm/kg)[b]	
0–1 year	150–200	4	Normal intake	>6.0
			Moderate intake	4.5–6.0
			Low intake	<4.5
1–9	130–180	3	Normal intake	3.0
			Moderate intake	2.0–3.0
			Low intake	1.0–2.0
9–18 years (males)	100–130	2.5–3.0		
9–18 years (females)	80–110	2.5–3.0		

VITAMINS AND MINERALS

Routine Supplementation[c,d]
  Multivitamins
    0–1 year: 0.6 ml bid water miscible
    1–18 years: 0.6 ml water miscible or chewable tablet bid
  Vitamin E
    Asymptomatic patients: 5–10 mg/kg up to 300 mg per day
    Symptomatic patients with severe muscle cramps: 5–10 mg/kg bid until
      remission
  Vitamin K
    Infants to 1 year with prolonged prothrombin time, active bleeding,
      liver cirrhosis: 5 mg 1–5 times per week
  Vitamin A
    Patients with below-normal levels
    Children weighing 20 kg or less: 1,250 IU per day Aquasol A
    Children weighing more than 20 kg: 2,500 IU per day Aquasol A
  Sodium chloride
    Varies depending on amount of sweat, exercise, temperature
      increases: 0.5–2.0 gm tid NaCl given in addition to salt in the diet
Additional Supplementation[d]
  Zinc
    15 mg per day elemental zinc or
    75 mg per day zinc sulfate
  Iron
    Infants: 1–2 mg/kg per day
    Children: 10–18 mg per day elemental iron or
            50–100 mg per day ferrous sulfate
  Selenium
    0.05–0.2 mg per day elemental selenium
    or 0.5 mg per day sodium selenium sulfate
  Vitamin B_{12}
    0.1 μg per day or larger amounts with deficiency states
  Folic acid
    Recommended Dietary Allowance for age (see Appendix 1)
  Linoleic acid
    Essential fatty acid intake should make up 3–5% of caloric intake

Table 8-8. Enzyme Preparations

Name	Dosage	
	Infants and Young Children	Older Children
Cotazym-S	¼–2 packets/meal	1–5 capsules/meal
Viokase	⅓–2 tsp/meal	2–5 tablets/meal
Pancrease	⅓–1 capsule/meal	1–2 capsule/meal

Data from Cystic Fibrosis Clinic. The Children's Hospital, Boston, Ma.

in London was introduced in our clinic in 1968 and is recommended. We also suggest breathing exercises and encourage physical activity and sports. A number of our patients jog, swim, or play tennis. Differing opinions exist concerning the use of mist as well as the benefit of inhalation antibiotics and mucolytic agents such as N-acetyl-L-cysteine. At present very few clinics recommend pulmonary lavage.

CONCLUSION

Because of the complicated nature of cystic fibrosis and the many complications that may occur with the disease, we recommend that patients be followed periodically by a physician experienced with the disease or in a cystic fibrosis clinic/center. There are at least 125 such clinic/centers in the United States and Canada, in small part supported by or affiliated with the National Cystic Fibrosis Foundation, 1600 Executive Blvd., Suite 309, Rockville, MD 20852.

Notes to Table 8-7.

Note: These recommendations should serve only as guidelines owing to the lack of information on nutrient requirements in cystic fibrosis. Patients should be continually monitored for deficiency states.
Source: Compiled by Cynthia Taft Bayerl, M.S., R.D., Cystic Fibrosis Nutrition Consultant, The Children's Hospital, Boston, Ma., 1983 with data from Hubbard V. S. Nutrient Requirements of Patients with Cystic Fibrosis. In *Perspectives in Cystic Fibrosis: Proceedings of the 8th International Congress on Cystic Fibrosis*. Toronto, Canada, 1980, and the following:
[a]*Guide to Diagnosis and Management of Cystic Fibrosis*. Cystic Fibrosis Foundation, 1974.
[b]Cystic Fibrosis Program. The Children's Hospital Medical Center, Boston, Ma., 1983.
[c]Adapted from *Guide to Drug Therapy in Patients with Cystic Fibrosis*. Cystic Fibrosis Foundation, 1974.
[d]Chase, P., et al. Cystic fibrosis and malnutrition. *J. Pediatr*. 95:337, 1979. (Advocates supplementation of these nutrients, but due to the scarcity of data most cystic fibrosis centers do not routinely supplement.)

Iron Deficiency

Martin Maksimak

Iron deficiency is the most common nutritional deficiency in the United States with the highest incidence in children between the ages of 6 months and 3 years. In humans, iron is present in several forms: heme iron (hemoglobin), myoglobin, and iron-dependent tissue enzymes. Iron is absorbed from the diet and lost during bleeding (i.e., menstruation) and during cell turnover. The amount of dietary iron is directly related to the caloric intake, the amount of iron in the diet, the type of iron available for absorption, and the status of the storage pool that, if deficient, can enhance absorption. Iron absorbed from the gastrointestinal tract is transported to the bone marrow for red blood cell synthesis by transferrin. Storage iron exists as ferritin, which is in equilibrium with serum iron, and as hemosiderin, which is not accessible.

Of all the tests for evaluating iron status, the serum ferritin test may be the most precise method. Serum ferritin is high at birth, falls in the first few months of life, and then increases gradually as iron stores become replete. One microgram of ferritin per liter is equivalent to about 140 µg of storage iron per kilogram of body weight. However, when the serum ferritin level is below 8 ng/ml, stores of iron are reduced. A less sensitive but more readily available indicator of iron deficiency is the transferrin saturation (the ratio of serum iron to iron binding capacity). If the transferrin saturation is less than 16 percent, iron deficiency exists.

The diagnosis of iron deficiency is usually initially suspected because of a hemoglobin less than 11 gm/dl and a mean corpuscular volume less than 75 [117]. After checking for blood loss in the stool and urine, a trial of iron therapy is most often prescribed for 3 weeks. When the child fails to respond to oral iron, as determined by an increase in the hemoglobin or the reticulocyte count, poor absorption, ongoing blood loss, or other causes of anemia are considered (See Table 7-18).

MECHANISMS

The development of iron deficiency is determined by four factors: the total body iron present at birth, growth rate, occult blood loss, and iron intake and absorption [121]. Because most iron crosses the placenta to reach the fetus in the third trimester and growth rate is the greatest at this time, total body iron at birth correlates with birth weight and is approximately 60 to 70 mg/kg body weight. A neonate has no tissue iron stores, and all the iron that eventually will be stored is present in circulating red blood cells. Even in premature infants, iron stores can be predicted by weight. Iron deficiency in the mother does not have a significant impact on the infant's ability to accrue iron because the placenta efficiently removes maternal iron [120]. However, infant iron levels can be affected by fetal-maternal transfusion, twin-to-twin transfusions, and blood loss at birth.

It is uncommon to see iron deficiency until the infant's weight becomes 2½ times the birth weight. Earlier development of deficiency suggests ongoing blood loss or a decreased blood volume at birth. Occult blood loss in the stool has been reported most commonly in infants who ingest fresh whole milk but also occurs in children drinking evaporated cow's milk-derived formula or soy formula. The cause for this sensitivity is unclear. Iron deficiency may be the only manifestation of cow's milk protein intolerance.

Iron is absorbed very well in early infancy, but its rate of absorption subsequently decreases [118]. The availability of breast milk iron is much greater than the availability of iron from iron-supplemented cow's milk-derived formula. The factors responsible for this greater absorption are not known. With the introduction of solid foods, the superior bioavailability of iron from human milk decreases. The percentage of iron absorbed also depends on the dose and form of iron. Small doses are better absorbed than large doses; ferrous iron is much better absorbed than ferric iron. Dietary phosphates, pyrolates, and oxalates can also bind inorganic iron into nonabsorbable complexes and decrease iron absorption. Iron is absorbed primarily in the proximal intestine. Chronic enteritis or gluten-sensitive enteropathy that injures the duodenum and upper jejunum are often associated with iron deficiency.

TREATMENT

To replete iron stores, most infants and children with iron deficiency will respond to ferrous sulfate (4 to 5 mg/kg per day divided into three doses for 3 months). Depending on the etiology, a change from cow's milk-derived formula or other dietary alterations may be needed (i.e., weaning a child whose sole source of nourishment is milk or encouraging heme sources of iron in a child's diet. [see Appendix 4]). Occasionally folate and other vitamins will need to be supplemented.

PREVENTION

The Committee on Nutrition of the American Academy of Pediatrics suggests that, after the age of 4 months, breast-fed infants should be supplemented with iron-fortified cereal or 1 mg/kg per day of iron drops in a full-term infant and 2 mg/kg per day in a preterm infant [115]. If iron drops are given, no more than 1 month's supply should be kept in the home because of the possibility of severe toxicity from accidental ingestions. Mothers of bottle-fed infants are encouraged to feed their infants iron-fortified formulas up to age 1 year and to use iron-fortified cereals after age 4 to 6 months. In premature children, if no vitamin E supplementation is given, delayed iron supplementation for 2 to 3 months may be warranted because of the possibility of a hemolytic anemia caused by iron supplementation [116].

Iron deficiency is an important nutritional problem in the growing infant [119]. Its ultimate effect on school performance and overall development is unknown. However, chronic deficiency may result in subtle problems that may be difficult to relate to a long-standing inadequate intake or an excessive loss of iron.

The Premature Infant
Janis Maksimak

Nutritional management of the preterm infant proves to be a difficult dilemma. By definition, this infant arrives early in the world without the nutrient stores of a term infant. After the critical period following birth and once growth begins, this infant has immense nutritional requirements. Precise definition of these nutritional requirements has met with much controversy because investigators cannot agree on what is the optimal rate of growth or how growth should be defined. With the term infant, the thriving breast-fed baby serves as a model system. With the preterm infant, no such model exists. Therefore, for the present, the Committee of Nutrition of the American Academy of Pediatrics suggests that the "optimal diet for the low birth weight infant may be defined as one that supports a rate of growth approximating that of the third trimester of intrauterine life" [123]. This statement itself has been the source of much discussion. The question arises that once the infant is in an extrauterine environment, should the growth rate parallel that of the fetus? Also, some observers equate rate of growth to rate of weight gain without reference to fluid gain or body composition. With these difficulties in mind, some basic nutritional requirements and recommendations will be provided.

ENERGY
The Committee of Nutrition of the American Academy of Pediatrics has recommended an energy intake of 50 to 100 kcal/kg per day for the first week of life, followed by 110 to 150 kcal/kg per day once active growth has begun [123]. However, these caloric recommendations should serve only as a guideline since energy expenditures are influenced by a number of variables including resting metabolic rate, activity, stress, waste, and growth. Also, intestinal absorption, which is influenced by the type of diet, needs to be considered.

By definition, optimal intake is one that provides an adequate rate of growth when compared to a fetus of comparable postconceptional age. This is approximately 20 to 30 gm per day. Once active growth is achieved, catch-up growth may occur that exceeds this expected increment of weight gain. Care should be taken not to become too zealous in the administration of calories. In one study [125], infants were fed up to 182 kcal/kg per day by nasogastric administration, and these high protein and energy intakes resulted in a significant metabolic acidosis and poor growth in some of the infants.

PROTEIN

Much controversy exists about the quality and quantity of protein intake needed for growth in the premature infant. Wide ranges of protein (1.8 to 4.5 gm/kg per day) have been shown to achieve a rate of growth equivalent to that in the third trimester. However, extremes on either end of this recommended range can have adverse effects. Too little protein can produce poor weight gain, low serum protein and albumin, and possibly decreased brain growth. Too much protein can lead to an increased solute load, metabolic acidosis [133], increased blood urea nitrogen levels (BUN), and increased blood ammonia levels. Because breast milk contains low and more variable concentrations of protein (0.7 to 2.0 gm/100 ml) than proprietary formulas (2.2 to 2.4 gm/100 ml), there has been question and conflict about its adequacy for a premature infant. In general, however, very low birth weight infants fed pooled breast milk (mixed milk from a number of women) appear to have slower growth and lower albumin levels, although none of these infants exhibited azotemia, hyperammonemia, or metabolic acidosis. Because milk from mothers of preterm infants has significantly higher amounts of protein (1.5 to 3.84 gm/100 ml) than the pooled breast milk used in these studies, maternal breast milk may indeed be adequate to meet the estimated requirements of the premature infant [124, 127]. Therefore, if breast milk is used as the primary source of nutrients, mother's milk should be used rather than pooled breast milk. The one inconsistency is that there is a wide range in the nutritional composition of the milk among mothers and among samples from the same mother.

The quality of protein also needs to be considered. Cow's milk protein differs qualitatively from human milk protein in that the casein-lactalbumin (whey) ratio is 82:18 and 40:60, respectively [130]. Casein is low in cystine and high in methionine while human milk or whey is high in cystine and taurine and low in methionine, phenylalanine, and tyrosine. Because the fetal liver contains limited amounts of cystathionase, a rate-limiting enzyme used in the conversion of methionine to cystine, the high cystine content of human milk is very important in protein synthesis. Taurine content, which is high in human milk, may also be an important amino acid for the conjugation of bile salts and in the developing retina and brain of the preterm infant [126]. In addition, since premature infants are limited in their ability to metabolize tyrosine, the low levels of tyrosine and phenylalanine in human milk may help to prevent hypertyrosinemia and hyperphenylalaninemia. Investigators have also shown that a high protein formula consisting predominately of casein produces a metabolic acidosis, while a high-protein formula consisting predominately of an equal amount of whey does not [131]. It is possible that the "metabolic price" of the higher protein in casein-rich cow's milk formula may be too high to outweigh the lower protein content of the whey-rich human milk. Because of these findings, two of the formulas specifically designed for premature infants (Special Care, Ross; Enfamil Premature, Mead Johnson) have been formulated to contain a casein-whey ratio similar to breast milk (see Table 5-3).

The use of soybean protein in premature infants has not been adequately investigated and therefore is not recommended. Infants who are thought to have a cow's milk protein allergy should receive either human milk or formula containing casein hydrolysate.

FATS

Fat provides an important source of concentrated calories for the preterm infant. However, premature infants, when compared to term infants, malabsorb more fat, including vegetable oils and breast milk fat. Lower concentrations of intraluminal bile acids [132] and pancreatic lipase [135] in premature infants are thought to be responsible for the malabsorption. Medium chain triglycerides (MCT) should be absorbed better under these conditions, and in practice MCT can be useful in feeding premature infants [132]. Fat absorption is increased and nitrogen balance is improved most likely as a result of the increased calories. Premature infant formulas now contain an increased proportion of their fats as MCT with the remainder as varying amounts of corn or coconut oil (see Table 5-3).

CARBOHYDRATES

Human milk and most formulas provide approximately 30 to 50 percent of their calories as carbohydrate. Lactose is the predominant carbohydrate in human milk and in most standard formulas. When the lactose content in a formula is reduced or excluded, the substituted carbohydrates are usually sucrose or corn syrup solids (glucose polymers derived from the hydrolysis of cornstarch). Lactose is thought to have an advantage over other carbohydrate sources because it enchances absorption of calcium, magnesium, and manganese [129, 134].

Lactose is usually digested well in term infants, but for the premature infant, the selection of a more appropriate carbohydrate may be important. Because the enzyme lactase develops relatively late in gestation, the amount of lactose found in standard proprietary formulas or breast milk may not be easily digested by the premature. Transient lactose intolerance can be found in the infant of less than 32 weeks gestation but is generally self-limited.

In comparison, the enzyme sucrase develops relatively early in gestation and its enzymatic activity is higher than lactase. Therefore, most premature infants can absorb sucrose. Corn syrup solids also appear to be better absorbed than lactose in premature infants. For these reasons, formulas that are specially prepared for low birth weight infants usually contain no more than 50 percent of their carbohydrate content as lactose; the remainder of the carbohydrate source consists of corn syrup solids.

MINERALS

The premature infant is at high risk to develop mineral and trace element deficiencies since these nutrients are usually accumulated late in gestation. Once postnatal growth begins, these limited nutrients can rapidly be depleted. The deficit also may be worsened further by the premature infant's inability to absorb these elements. Although both premature and full-term infants are capable of absorbing iron, a neonate's iron stores are derived from red blood cells present at birth. Thus, with growth, term babies who are not given an adequate placental transfusion and premature infants will have deficient iron stores.

The iron stores usually are sufficient to permit the infant's blood volume and weight to double without allowing the hemoglobin concentration to decrease below 10 gm/dl. This is contingent upon no blood being drawn for laboratory tests. Even without excessive blood loss, "physiologic anemia" usually develops earlier in premature infants between 6 and 10 weeks of age. Premature infants who are supplemented with 2 to 3 mg/kg per day of iron have better hemoglobin levels at 3 months of age than unsupplemented infants. However, premature infants receiving large amounts of iron supplementation may have a decreased hemoglobin concentration if vitamin E (25 IU) is not administered concomitantly. Diets high in linoleic acid and low in selenium may also adversely affect the red cells' susceptibility to iron. Furthermore, the addition of solid food to the diets of infants being breast-fed impairs gastrointestinal iron absorption. Therefore, it is recommended that, in the premature infant, iron supplementation should not exceed 2 to 3 ml/kg per day, and this supplementation should include an adequate amount of vitamin E (25 IU) and a diet not excessive in linoleic acid.

Little is known about the daily requirements for trace minerals in the premature infant. Although low levels of copper and zinc have been described in rapidly growing infants and no guidelines exist for premature infants, the recommendations for trace mineral content in infant formulas from the Committee on Nutrition of the American Academy of Pediatrics are based on amounts required to prevent deficiency states in term infants [128]. In the case of copper, these recommendations appear adequate for premature infants [122]. However, the infant must receive adequate calories to meet these requirements, and if inadequate intake or interruption of feedings occurs for an extended period of time, deficiency states may occur.

When considering human breast milk as an adequate source for minerals, bioavailability, stage of lactation, and maternal nutrition become major issues. In general, it is assumed that breast milk adequately provides these elements for the term infant, but breast milk may not be adequate for the preterm infant.

VITAMINS

With few exceptions, most advisable intakes of vitamins for premature infants are not known and recommended allowances are once again based on the needs of the term infant. However, if a standard infant formula were utilized for nutrition, the average premature infant would not be able to meet these requirements since the premature infant consumes relatively smaller amounts of formula than the larger term infant. Therefore, supplements are necessary. Formulas designed especially for the premature infant tend to have higher concentrations of added vitamins and thereby try to take into account the decreased formula intake.

Some guidelines for premature infants do exist for vitamins E, D, and C and folic acid, and these tend to be higher than those normally accepted for the term infant.

The recommended supplement of vitamin E in premature infants ranges from 15 to 30 mg. However, even with good supplementation, a persistently low serum level of vitamin E may be observed due to a number of factors including impaired absorption of fat, rapid growth, or large quantities of polyunsaturated fats in the diet. Vitamin E acts as a free radical scavenger and antioxidant and is important in preventing hemolytic anemia in the premature infant. Also the role of vitamin E is currently being investigated in the prevention of bronchopulmonary dysplasia and retrolental fibroplasia, but initial results are disappointing.

A vitamin D intake of approximately 600 IU should prevent the development of rickets, which has been observed with lower intakes. Because vitamin D is a fat-soluble vitamin like vitamin E, its absorption may be impaired by other poorly digested fats in the premature infant's diet and the vitamin may be excreted in the stools. Thus, vitamin D recommendations may need to be adjusted if more digestible fats are employed in the diet.

Decreased levels of folic acid are common in premature infants, but megaloblastic anemia is rarely observed. Folic acid is generally absorbed well in the normal premature infant, and between 20 and 50 μg per day is sufficient in preventing folate deficiency. Standard proprietary formulas are capable of providing this. However, if the premature infant is sick with recurrent infection or diarrhea, supplemental folic acid is necessary.

As previously mentioned, transient tyrosinemia may occur in premature infants because of their limited ability to metabolize tyrosine when protein intakes are high. Approximately 60 mg per day of vitamin C may be beneficial in preventing this in the premature infant.

CONCLUSION

Basic guidelines in the rapidly developing field of premature infant nutrition have been recommended. Much controversy exists over even basic definitions, but with further investigation, more precise recommendations hopefully will be formulated. In the interim, careful monitoring of these fragile infants needs to be maintained. Whether breast milk or specially prepared premature infant formulas are used, biochemical and nutritional measurements of energy, protein, fat, carbohydrate, minerals, and vitamins need to be followed closely in order to prevent deficiencies.

Inborn Errors of Metabolism

Frances J. Rohr

Inborn errors of metabolism are hereditary disorders that affect the metabolism of a particular chemical compound. Devastating clinical manifestations and mental retardation often result from untreated inborn errors of metabolism (as in phenylketonuria [PKU] before dietary treatment was devised). Some metabolic diseases are treatable with nutrition therapy, which may consist of a diet restricted in an essential nutrient (i.e., phenylalanine in PKU), a diet where a nonessential nutrient is eliminated (i.e., galactose in galactosemia), or a diet where vitamin supplementation is needed (i.e., vitamin B_{12} in B_{12}-responsive methylmalonic aciduria).

PHENYLKETONURIA

The classic example of a genetic disorder that can be controlled by diet is PKU. The metabolic defect is an absence of the hepatic enzyme, phenylalanine hydroxylase, which normally converts phenylalanine to tyrosine. This defect results in the accumulation of phenylalanine and its metabolites and is associated with mental retardation [143]. PKU occurs in 1 in every 14,000 children born in the United States, and approximately 1 in 60 people is an asymptomatic carrier of the mutant gene. There is no consistent abnormality on neurological examination, but many untreated individuals are hyperactive, hypertonic, or have asocial behavior. They may also have musty odors, fair complexions, or eczema.

The diagnosis of PKU is usually made by routine newborn screening via a filter paper test using a bacterial inhibition assay (Guthrie test). Children who are treated with a special diet may also be monitored with this test. The assay is accurate and should identify essentially all affected infants.

PKU was first described in the 1930s by Fölling [138], and by the 1940s, Jervis had identified almost all the basic biochemical abnormalities associated with the disorder [139]. It was not until the 1950s, however, that Bickel developed the first dietary treatment [137]. The basis of dietary treatment is to restrict the amount of ingested phenylalanine [136]. Special dietary formulas (i.e., Lofenalac and Phenyl-Free [Mead Johnson] and PKU-1 and PKU-2 [Milupa]) that are either very low in or devoid of phenylalanine are used. In order to be nutritionally complete, small amounts of milk or infant formula must be added to supply essential phenylalanine [136]. Complete restriction of phenylalanine causes a phenylalanine deficiency state that can result in failure to thrive, weight loss, negative nitrogen balance, and a change in the concentration of plasma amino acids. Symptoms include skin rash, anemia, and hypoglycemia. The essential amino acid requirements for infants can be seen in Table 8-9. These figures show a wide range in the essential amino acid requirements. Each child's requirement for the offending amino acid should be determined. In PKU, for example, this is done by providing the average amount of phenylalanine tolerated by infants with PKU (approximately 50 mg/kg), monitoring blood levels, and adjusting the amount of dietary phenylalanine until the desired blood phenylalanine level is achieved [136]. By about 1 year of age, the amount of phenylalanine tolerated decreases to 20 to 30 mg/kg.

In well-treated individuals with PKU, normal growth and development can be expected. The special dietary formula is the essential component of the diet; however, the small amounts of milk or infant formula added to supply phenylalanine are gradually decreased with age. When the child is approximately 6 months old, solid foods are introduced and are usually limited to low protein foods such as fruits, vegetables, and grains. The amount of solid food allowed depends on the child's tolerance for phenylalanine. Special low-protein breads,

Table 8-9. Amino Acid Requirements in Infancy

Amino Acid	Age	
(mg/kg)	0–5 months	6–12 months
Phenylalanine	47–90	25–47
Histidine	16–34	16–34
Leucine	76–150	76–150
Isoleucine	70–110	50–75
Valine	65–105	50–80
Methionine	20–45	20–45
Cyst(e)ine	15–50	15–50
Lysine	90–120	90–120
Threonine	45–87	45–87
Tryptophan	13–22	13–22

Data from American Academy of Pediatrics Committee on Nutrition. Special Diets for Infants with Inborn Errors of Amino Acid Metabolism. *Pediatrics* 57:783, 1976.

flours, and pastas are available to facilitate diet management. In addition, foods such as apple juice, apple sauce, hard candies, and oils contain insignificant amounts of phenylalanine and can be used freely.

There has been much discussion as to when the low-phenylalanine diet may safely be terminated. Historically, many individuals treated for PKU were taken off the diet at about age 5 or 6 because it was felt that the brain was developed and high phenylalanine levels could be tolerated. However, on follow-up some children who had been terminated from the diet were found to have learning disabilities, lower IQs, and behavioral problems [144]. Now most clinics recommend that children continue the diet beyond the early childhood years. In addition, women with PKU are at risk for bearing children with problems such as mental retardation, microcephaly, and congenital heart disease. This is believed to be caused by the effects of the mother's high phenylalanine levels on the developing fetus. Therefore, women with PKU are encouraged to follow a low-phenylalanine diet before conception and throughout pregnancy.

In addition to classic PKU, variations in phenylalanine hydroxylase deficiency have been described. Infants with hyperphenylalaninemia may have phenylalanine levels of 12 to 20 mg/dl instead of the levels of greater than 20 mg/dl seen in classical PKU [140]. These infants are said to have "atypical" PKU and also require dietary treatment, although it may not be as restrictive as in classical PKU. Individuals with atypical PKU have about 2 to 5 percent of the normal level of phenylalanine hydroxylase activity, whereas those with classic PKU have no detectable enzyme activity. Individuals with mild, persistent hyperphenylalaninemia whose blood levels range from 2 to 12 mg/dl do not require a phenylalanine-restricted diet, since this appears to

Table 8-10. Examples of Inborn Errors of Amino Acid and Carbohydrate Metabolism

Disorder	Incidence	Biochemical Defect	Biochemical Analysis	
			Blood	Urine
AMINO ACIDS				
Classic phenylketonuria	1 : 12,000	Defective phenylalanine hydroxylase enzyme, which prevents the conversion of phenyl-alanine, an essential amino acid, to tyro-sine, another amino acid	Increased phenylalanine	Increased phenylacids: phenylpyruvic acid, phenylacetic acid, orthohydroxy-phenylacetic acid
Classic homocystinuria	1 : 180,000	Defective cystathionine synthetase enzyme, which prevents the in-teraction between an intermediate product of the amino acid methionine with serine to form cystathionine	Increased methionine and homocysteine	Increased homocysteine
Maple syrup urine disease	1 : 200,000	Defective oxidative de-carboxylase enzymes. Keto acids of the branch chain amino acids (leucine, valine, and isoleucine) are not converted to simple acids	Increased leucine, valine, and isoleucine and their keto acids	Increased leucine, valine, and isoleucine and their keto acids
Hereditary tyrosi-nemia (hepato-renal type)	Not deter-mined	Defect in parahydroxy-phenylpyruvic acid ox-idase and perhaps fu-marylacetoacetase activity	Increased tyrosine and in some cases increased methionine	Increased parahydroxy-phenylpyruvic acid; succinylacetonuria; generalized aminoaci-duria
CARBOHYDRATES				
Classic galactosemia	1 : 100,000	Defective galactose-1-phosphate uridyl transferase. Galactose, a monosaccharide, is not converted to glu-cose	Increased galactose-1-phosphate	Increased galactose; gen-eralized aminoaciduria
Herditary fructose intolerance	More than 40 cases re-ported	Defect in fructose-1-phosphate aldolase. Fructose, a monosac-charide, is not convert-ed to glucose	Increased fructose	Increased fructose

Clinical Symptoms	Treatment	Comment
Infant appears normal at birth, followed by hyperactivity, irritability, persistent musty odor, severe mental retardation, decreased pigmentation, and eczema, if untreated	Phenylalanine-restricted diet: no high-quality protein foods (milk, milk products, meat, fish, poultry, eggs, nuts); controlled amounts of fruits, vegetables, and grain products; special formula, low in phenylalanine, provides protein and is supplemented with vitamins and minerals; treatment monitored with blood phenylalanine levels, growth, and psychological data	Phenylalanine must be provided in amounts sufficient to support growth. There are milder forms that may not require a diet. Also, deficiency of biopterin, a cofactor in conversion of phenylalanine to tyrosine, causes increased phenylalanine but is not responsive to diet
Possible mental retardation; lens dislocation; limb overgrowth; connective tissue defect leading to scoliosis, osteoporosis, vascular thrombosis; fair hair and skin	Methionine-restricted (similar to phenylalanine-restricted) diet, supplemented with cysteine; cysteine, a product of methionine, becomes an essential amino acid when methionine is limited; special low-methionine formula is used, and methionine levels in the blood are monitored, along with growth and psychological functioning	There are other forms of homocystinuria. One is responsive to high doses of pyridoxine (vitamine B_6), a coenzyme of cystathionine synthetase. Another is responsive to vitamin B_{12}, a coenzyme in the remethylation reaction of homocysteine to methionine. Prenatal diagnosis by amniocentesis is possible
Infant appears normal at birth, with symptoms showing in the first few days. Difficulties with sucking and swallowing, irregular respiration, intermittent rigidity and flaccidity, possible grand mal seizures. Urine has the odor of maple syrup. If infant survives, mental retardation is severe if untreated	Diet is restricted in leucine, valine, and isoleucine (similar to phenylalanine-restricted); special formula is prepared; blood leucine, valine and isoleucine are monitored, along with growth and psychological functioning	There is a transient form of the disease, for which treatment is necessary only during times of illness. There is also a thiamine-responsive form. Prenatal diagnosis by amniocentesis is possible
Enlargement of liver and spleen noted early in infancy; abdominal distention, liver and renal damage, vitamin D-resistant rickets	Diet restricted in phenylalanine and tyrosine. The essential amino acid phenylalanine is a precursor of tyrosine; methionine has also been restricted in a few individuals; a special formula is used, and blood phenylalanine, tyrosine, and methionine and growth are monitored	Dietary treatment has not been successful in most cases. Biochemical abnormalities and renal tubular dysfunction have been corrected; however, liver disease is progressive
Infant appears normal at birth with symptoms developing after feedings containing lactose. Symptoms include anorexia, vomiting, occasional diarrhea, lethargy, jaundice, hepatomegaly, increased susceptibility to infection. Later, cataracts and physical and mental retardation develop	Rigid exclusion of lactose and galactose from the diet; hydrolysis of lactose yields glucose and galactose; diet is milk-free, free of milk products; lactose-free formula is used. If children do not accept formula, diet will need nutrient supplementation	Nonclassic forms include galactokinase and epimerase deficiency. The clinical features are not the same in all three forms. Prenatal diagnosis by amniocentesis is possible
For infants, symptoms include anorexia, vomiting, failure to thrive, hypoglycemic convulsions, dysfunction of the liver and kidney. For older children, spontaneous hypoglycemia and vomiting occur after the ingestion of fructose	Elimination of fructose and sucrose from the diet; hydrolysis of sucrose yields glucose and fructose	Differentiate from transient neonatal tyrosinemia

Adapted with permission from Howard, R. B., and Herbold, N. H. (Eds.). *Nutrition in Clinical Care* (2nd ed.). New York: McGraw-Hill, 1982.

be a benign condition. A related disorder in phenylalanine metabolism due to a deficiency of biopterin (cofactor in the conversion of phenylalanine to tyrosine) presents with elevated blood phenylalanine and causes progressive neurological deterioration; it is not responsive to diet.

GALACTOSEMIA

Galactosemia is the most commonly occurring inborn error of carbohydrate metabolism with an incidence of approximately 1 in 60,000 newborns [141]. Galactosemia, like PKU, can be detected through routine newborn screening. There are three enzyme defects that can cause galactosemia, the most common of which is a deficiency of galactose-1-phosphate uridyl transferase. In the presence of uridine diphosphoglucose, this enzyme converts galactose-1-phosphate to uridine diphosphogalactose and glucose.

A deficiency of the transferase enzyme causes galactose to accumulate in the blood and urine and galactitol to accumulate in the urine and ocular lenses [142]. In untreated galactosemia, these biochemical abnormalities result in the development of cataracts, mental retardation, and cirrhosis of the liver. The newborn with galactosemia usually has hepatomegaly, jaundice, and failure to thrive, symptoms that develop shortly after exposure to milk feedings.

A galactose-free diet should be instituted as soon as the infant is diagnosed as having galactosemia. Because galactose is one of the monosaccharides found in lactose, milk and milk products must be avoided [136]. In infancy, lactose-free formulas, such as Isomil (Ross) and ProSobee (Mead Johnson) are used (see Table 5-3). When the child begins to eat solid foods, parents must learn to read ingredient labels carefully and avoid such substances as whey, casein, lactose, nonfat dry milk, and milk solids. Parents must be aware that lactose is used widely in food processing and is present in many pharmaceutical products as well (see Appendix 3). Organ meats must also be avoided because galactose is stored in the liver, the pancreas, and the brain [136]. If properly planned and monitored, the galactose-free diet is nutritionally complete and is effective in preventing mental retardation, cataracts, and liver disease.

Other examples of inborn errors of metabolism and their treatments are presented in Table 8-10.

SUMMARY

This section is intended as an overview of two of the most common inborn errors of metabolism. Because these conditions often present as feeding difficulties or failure to thrive in the newborn period, the nutritional and medical care of individuals with phenylketonuria or galactosemia should be carried out by specialists.

Conclusion

In this chapter, the importance of nutrition in illness becomes obvious. As seen in some conditions, such as cow's milk protein allergy and celiac disease, proper dietary management is itself the treatment. In other disease states, appropriate nutritional management can greatly enhance medical therapy. The optimal use of nutrition in medical therapeutic regimens can have a tremendous impact on the health and well-being of sick children and should be integrated into clinical management.

REFERENCES

CONGENITAL HEART DISEASE
1. Report of the New England Regional Infant Cardiac Program. *Pediatrics* 65(4 Suppl.) part 2, 1980.
2. Sondheimer, J. M., and Hamilton, J. R. Intestinal function in infants with severe congenital heart disease. *J. Pediatr.* 92:572, 1978.
3. Vanderhof, J. A., et al. Continuous enteral feedings. *Am. J. Dis. Child.* 136:825, 1982.
4. Winter, H. Personal communication. The Children's Hospital, Boston, Ma., 1983.

RENAL DISEASE
5. Alvestrand, A., Ahlberg, M., Furst, P., and Bergstrom, J. Clinical experience with amino acid and keto acid diets. *Am. J. Clin. Nutr.* 33:1654, 1980.
6. Alvestrand, A., Bergstrom, J., Furst, P., Germainis, G., and Widstam, U. Effect of essential amino acid supplementation on muscle and plasma free amino acids in chronic uremia. *Kidney Int.* 14:323, 1978.
7. Arnold, W. C., Erhard, D., Ramirez, J., and Holliday, M. A. Effects of calorie supplementation in uremic children. *Clin. Res.* 25:194A, 1977.
8. Aronson, A. S., Furst, P., Kuylenstierna, B., and Nyberg, G. Essential amino acids in the treatment of advanced uremia: Twenty-two months experience in a five year old girl. *Pediatrics* 56:538, 1975.
9. Baxter, J. H., Goodman, H. C., Allen, J. C. Effects of infusions of serum albumin on serum lipids and lipoproteins in nephrosis. *J. Clin. Invest.* 40:490, 1961.
10. Berger, M., James, G. P., Davis, E. R., et al. Hyperlipidemia in uremic children. Response to peritoneal dialysis and hemodialysis. *Clin. Nephrol.* 1:19, 1978.
11. Betts, P., and Magrath, G. Growth pattern and dietary intake of children with chronic renal insufficiency. *Br. Med. J.* [Clin. Res.] 2:189, 1974.
12. Betts, P. R., Magrath, G., and White, H. R. Role of dietary energy supplementation in growth of children with chronic renal insufficiency. *Br. Med. J.* [Clin. Res.] 1:416, 1977.
13. Chan, J. C., Kodroff, M. B., and Landuehr, D. M. Effect of 1,25-dihydroxyvitamin D_3 on renal function, mineral balance and growth in children with severe chronic renal failure. *Pediatrics* 68:559, 1981.

14. Chantler, C., and Holliday, M. A. Growth in children with renal disease with particular reference to the effects of calorie malnutrition. *Clin. Nephrol.* 1:229, 1973.
15. Chantler, C., El-Bishti, M., and Counahan, R. Nutritional therapy in children with chronic renal failure. *Am. J. Clin. Nutr.* 33:1682, 1980.
16. Chesney, R. W., Rosen, J. F., Hamstra, A. J., et al. Serum 1,25-dihydroxyvitamin D levels in normal children and in vitamin D disorders. *Am. J. Dis. Child.* 134:135, 1980.
17. Chopra, J. S., Mallick, N. P., and Stone, M. C. Hyperlipoproteinemias in nephrotic syndrome. *Lancet* 1:317, 1971.
18. Ciechanover, M., Peresechenschi, G., Aviram, A., et al. Mal-recognition of taste in uremia. *Nephron* 26:20, 1980.
19. Cohen, B. D. Disturbances of Nitrogen, Carbohydrate, and Lipid Metabolism. In C. M. Edelmann Jr. (Ed.), Pediatric Kidney Disease. Boston: Little, Brown, 1978. P. 432–442.
20. Cohen, B. D., Patel, H., and Kornhauser, R. S. Proteins in atherogenesis. *Diabetes* 26:392, 1977.
21. Coleman, A. J., Arias, M., Carter, N. W., et al. The mechanism of salt wastage in chronic renal disease. *J. Clin. Invest.* 45:116, 1966.
22. Conley, S. B., Rose, G. M., Robson, A. M., and Bier, D. M. Effects of dietary intake and hemodialysis on protein turnover in uremic children. *Kidney Int.* 17:837, 1980.
23. Counahan, R., El-Bishti, M., and Chantler, C. Oral essential amino acids in children on regular hemodialysis. *Clin. Nephrol.* 9:11, 1975.
24. DeFronzo, R. A., Alvestrand, A., Smith, D., et al. Insulin resistance in uremia. *J. Clin. Invest.* 67:563, 1981.
25. El-Bishti, M., Barke, J., Jones, W., et al. Body composition in children on regular hemodialysis. *Clin. Nephrol.* 15:43, 1981.
26. El-Bishti, M., Counahan, R., Bloom, S. R., et al. Hormonal and metabolic responses to intravenous glucose in children on hemodialysis. *Am. J. Clin. Nutr.* 31:1865, 1978.
27. Feldman, H. A., and Singer, I. Endocrinology and metabolism in uremia. *Medicine* (Baltimore) 54:351, 1975.
28. Flinn, R. B., Merrill, J. P., and Welzart, W. R. Treatment of the oliguric patient with a new sodium-exchange resin and sorbitol. *N. Engl. J. Med.* 264:111, 1961.
29. Giordano, C. Use of exogenous and endogenous urea for protein synthesis in normal and uremic subjects. *J. Lab. Clin. Med.* 62:231, 1963.
30. Giovannetti, S., and Maggiore, Q. A low-nitrogen diet with proteins of high biological value for severe chronic uremia. *Lancet* 1:1000, 1964.
31. Grupe, W. E. Nutritional Considerations in the Prognosis and Treatment of Children with Renal Disease. In R. M. Suskind, (Ed.). *Textbook of Pediatric Nutrition.* New York: Raven, 1981. Pp. 527–535.
32. Grupe, W. E. Minimal change disease. *Semin. Nephrol.* 2:241, 1982.
33. Grupe, W. E., Harmon, W., and Spinozzi, N. S. Protein and energy requirements in children receiving chronic hemodialysis. *Kidney Int.,* in press.
34. Grupe, W. E., Spinozzi, N. S., and Harmon, W. E. Protein balance more dependent on protein intake than on energy intake in hemodialyzed children. *Kidney Int.* 23:149, 1983.
35. Harvey, R. M., Enson, Y., Lewis, M. L., et al. Hemodynamic effects of dehydration and metabolic acidosis. *Trans. Assoc. Am. Physicians* 79:177, 1966.

36. Holliday, M. A. Calorie deficiency in children with uremia: Effect upon growth. *Pediatrics* 50:590, 1972.
37. Holliday, M. A., Arnold, W. C., and Wassner, S. J. Characteristics of renal insufficiency in children. *Kidney Int.* 14:306, 1978.
38. Holliday, M. A. and Chantler, C. Metabolic and nutritional factors in children with renal insufficiency. *Kidney Int.* 14:306, 1978.
39. Holliday, M., Richardson, K., and Portale, A. Nutritional management of chronic renal disease. *Med. Clin. North Am.* 63:5, 1979.
40. Johnson, W. J., Haggine, W. W., Wagoner, R. O., et al. Effects of urea loading in patients with far advanced renal failure. *Mayo Clin. Proc.* 47:21, 1972.
41. Jones, R. W. A., Dalton, N., Start, K., El-Bishti, M. M., and Chantler, C. Oral essential amino acid supplements in children with advanced chronic renal failure. *Am. J. Clin. Nutr.* 33:1696, 1980.
42. Kleinknecht, C., Broyer, M., Gagnadoux, M., et al. Growth in Children Treated with Longterm Dialysis. A Study of 76 Patients. In J. Hamburger, J. Crosnier, J. P. Grunfeld, et al. (Eds.), *Advances in Nephrology 19* Chicago: Year Book, 1980. Pp. 133–163.
43. Kopple, J. D. Dietary Requirements. In S. G. Massry and A. L. Sellers (Eds.), *Clinical Aspects of Uremia and Dialysis.* Springfield: Thomas, 1976. Pp. 353–489.
44. Kopple, J. D. Abnormal amino acid and protein metabolism in uremia. *Kidney Int.* 14:340, 1978.
45. McKenzie, I. F. C. and Nester, P. J. Studies on the turnover of triglyceride and esterified cholesterol in subjects with the nephrotic syndrome. *J. Clin. Invest.* 47:1685, 1968.
46. Pennisi, A. J., Heuser, E. T., Mickey, M. R., et al. Hyperlipidemia in pediatric hemodialysis and renal transplant patients. *Am. J. Dis. Child.* 130:957, 1976.
47. Reaven, G. M., Weisinger, J. R., and Swensen, R. S. Insulin and glucose metabolism in renal insufficiency. *Kidney Int.* 6:563, 1974.
48. Schoeneman, M. Dietary and Pharmacologic Treatment of Chronic Renal Failure. In C. M. Edelman (Ed.), *Pediatric Kidney Disease.* Boston: Little, Brown, 1978. Pp. 475–487.
49. Simmons, J. M., Wilson, C. J., Potter, D. E., and Holliday, M. A. Relation of calorie deficiency to growth failure in children on hemodialysis and the growth response to calorie supplementation. *N. Engl. J. Med.* 285:653, 1971.
50. Slatopolsky, E., and Bricker, N. S. The role of phosphorus restriction in the prevention of secondary hyperparathyroidism in chronic renal disease. *Kidney Int.* 4:141, 1973.
51. Spinozzi, N. S., Murray, C. L., and Grupe, W. E. Altered taste acuity in children with end-stage renal disease. *Pediatr. Res.* 12:442, 1978.
52. Walser, M., Mitch, W. E., and Collier, V. U. The effect of nutritional therapy on the course of chronic renal failure. *Clin. Nephrol.* 11:66, 1979.
53. Wassner, S. J. The role of nutrition in the case of children with renal insufficiency. *Pediatr. Clin. North Am.* 29:973, 1982.
54. West, C. D., and Smith, W. C. An attempt to elucidate the cause of growth retardation in renal disease. *Am. J. Dis. Child.* 91:460, 1956.

LIVER DISEASE

55. Andres, J. M., et al. Liver disease in infants. I. Developmental history and mechanisms of liver function. *J. Pediatr.* 90:686, 1977.

56. Daum, F., et al. Hydroxy-cholecalciferol in the management of rickets associated with extra hepatic biliary atresia. *J. Pediatr.* 88:1041, 1976.
57. Heubi, J. E., et al. 1,25-Di-hydroxy vitamin D_3 in childhood hepatitis osteodystrophy. *J. Pediatr.* 94:977, 1979.
58. Ponchon, G., et al. "Activation" of vitamin D by the liver. *J. Clin. Invest.* 48:2032, 1969.
59. Watkins, J. B. Mechanisms of fat absorption and the development of gastrointestinal function. *Pediatr. Clin. North Am.* 22:721, 1975.

GLUTEN-SENSITIVE ENTEROPATHY

60. Falchuk, Z. M. Update on gluten-sensitive enteropathy. *Am. J. Med.* 67:1085, 1979.
61. Kagnoff, M. F., et al. Immunoglobin allotype markers in gluten sensitive enteropathy. *Lancet* 1:952, 1983.
62. Lebenthal, E. Childhood celiac disease—a reappraisal. *J. Pediatr.* 98:681, 1981.

INFECTIOUS DIARRHEA

63. Ament, M. E., and Rubin, C. E. Relation of giardiasis in abnormal intestinal structure and function in gastrointestinal immunodeficiency syndromes. *Gastroenterology* 62:217, 1972.
64. Bishop, R. F., et al. Virus particles in epithelial cells of duodenal mucosa from children with acute non-bacterial gastroenteritis. *Lancet* 2:1281, 1973.
65. Black, R. E., et al. Giardiasis in day-care centers: Evidence of person to person transmission. *Pediatrics* 60:486, 1977.
66. Brasitus, T. A. Parasites and malabsorption. *Am. J. Med.* 67:1058, 1979.
67. Centers for Disease Control: Intestinal parasite surveillance. *Annual Summary,* 1976.
68. Davidson, G. P., et al. Importance of new virus in acute sporadic enteritis in children. *Lancet* 1:242, 1975.
69. Jonas, A., et al. Disturbed fat absorption following infectious gastroenteritis in children. *J. Pediatr.* 95:366, 1979.
70. Kapikian, A. Z., Kim, H. W., Wyatt, R. G., et al. Human reovirus-like agent as the major pathogen associated with "winter" gastroenteritis in hospitalized infants and young children. *N. Engl. J. Med.* 294:965, 1976.
71. Kuzemko, J. A. Gastroenteritis in infancy. *Postgrad. Med. J.* 45:732, 1969.
72. Lifshitz, F., et al. Monosaccharide intolerance and hypoglycemia in infants with diarrhea. I. Clinical course of 23 infants. *Pediatrics* 77:595, 1970.
73. Lifshitz, F., et al. Carbohydrate intolerance in infants with diarrhea. *J. Pediatr.* 79:760, 1971.
74. Powanda, M. C. Changes in body balances of nitrogen and other key nutrients: description and underlying mechanisms. *Am. J. Clin. Nutr.* 30:1254, 1977.
75. Rettig, P. J. *Campylobacter* infections in human beings. *J. Pediatr.* 94:855, 1979.
76. Scrimshaw, N. S. (1977) In Symposium on Impact of Infection on Nutritional Status of the Host. W. R. Beisel (Ed.). [Reprinted from *Am. J. Clin. Nutr.* 30:1536, 1977.]

SHORT BOWEL SYNDROME

77. Dabbins, J. W., and Bundes, H. J. Importance of the colon in enteric hyperoxaluria. *N. Engl. J. Med.* 296:298, 1977.

78. Fromm, H., Thomas, P. J., and Hoffmann, A. F. Sensitivity and specificity in tests of distal ileal function: Prospective comparison of bile acid and vitamin B_{12} absorption in ileal resection patients. *Gastroenterology* 64:1077, 1973.
79. Hoffman, A. F., and Poley, J. R. Role of bile acid malabsorption in pathogenesis of diarrhea and steatorrhea in patients with ileal resection. *Gastroenterology* 62:918, 1972.
80. Hoffman, A. F., et al. Complex pathogenesis of hypooxaluria after jejunal bypass surgery. *Gastroenterology* 84:293, 1983.
81. Klish, W. J. The short gut. *Am. J. Dis. Child.* 135:1056, 1981.
82. Murphy, J. P., King, D. R., and Dubois, A. Treatment of gastric hypersecretion with cimetidine in short bowel syndrome. *N. Engl. J. Med.* 300:80, 1978.
83. Parker, P., Stroop, S., and Greene, H. A controlled comparison of continuous versus intermittent feeding in the treatment of infants with intestinal disease. *J. Pediatr.* 99:360, 1981.
84. Potts, W. J. Pediatric surgery. *J.A.M.A.* 157:627, 1955.
85. Scheimer, E., Shih, M. E., and Vouamell, P. Malabsorption following massive intestinal resection. *Am. J. Clin. Nutr.* 17:64, 1965.
86. Seal, A. M., Debos, H. T., Reynolds, C., et al. Gastric and pancreatic hyposecretion following massive small-bowel resection. *Dig. Dis. Sci.* 27:117, 1982.
87. Siebert, J. R. Small-intestine length in infants and children. *Am. J. Dis. Child.* 134:593, 1980.
88. Weser, E. The management of patients after small bowel resection. *Gastroenterology* 71:146, 1976.
89. Wilmore, D. W. Factors correlating with a successful outcome following extensive intestinal resection in newborn infants. *J. Pediatr.* 80:88, 1972.

COW'S MILK SENSITIVITY AND LACTOSE INTOLERANCE

90. Barr, R. G., Perma, J. A., Schoeller, D. A., and Watkins, J. B. Breath tests in pediatric gastrointestinal disorders: New diagnostic opportunities. *Pediatrics* 62:393, 1978.
91. Barr, R., et al. Recurrent abdominal pain of childhood due to lactose intolerance: A prospective study. *N. Engl. J. Med.* 300:1449, 1979.
92. Bock, S. A., et al. Studies of hypersensitivity reactions to foods in infants and children. *J. Allergy Clin. Immunol.* 62:327, 1978.
93. Boey, C. G., Prathap, M. C. K., Yadar, M., Lam, S. K., and Puthucheary, M. D. Acquired carbohydrate intolerance and cow's milk protein-sensitive enteropathy in young infants. *J. Pediatr.* 95:373, 1979.
94. Gerrard, J. W., MacKenzie, J. W., et al. Cow's milk allergy: Prevalence and manifestations in an unselected series of newborns. *Acta Paediatr. Scand. [Suppl.]* 234:1, 1973.
95. Hamburger, F. Biologisches uber die Eiweisokorper der Kuhmilch und uber sauglingsernahrung. *Wien. Klin. Wochenschr.* 14:1202, 1901.
96. Jakobsson, I., and Lindberg, T. A prospective study of cow's milk protein intolerance in Swedish infants. *Acta Paediatr. Scand.* 68:853, 1979.
97. Lake, A. M., Whitington, P. F., and Hamilton, S. R. Dietary protein-induced colitis in breast fed infants. *J. Pediatr.* 101:906, 1982.
98. McCalla, R., Savilahti, E., Perkkio, M., Kuitunen, P., and Backman, A. Morphology of the jejunum in children with eczema due to food allergy. *Allergy* 35:563, 1980.
99. Rajka, G. *Atopic Dermatitis,* Pp. 46–104, Philadelphia: Saunders, 1975.

100. Walker-Smith, J., Harrison, M., Kilby, A., Phillips, A., and France, N. Cow's milk sensitive enteropathy. *Arch. Dis. Child.* 53:375, 1978.
101. Watson, J. B., and Timmins, J. Food allergy-response to treatment with sodium cromoglycate. *Arch. Dis. Child.* 54:77, 1979.
102. Whitington, P. F., and Gibson, R. Soy protein intolerance: Four patients with concomitant cow's milk intolerance. *Pediatrics* 59:730, 1977.

COLIC

103. Gerrard, J. W. Allergy in breast fed babies to ingredients in breast milk. *Ann. Allergy* 42:69, 1979.
104. Jakobsson, I., and Lindberg, T. A prospective study of cow's milk protein intolerance in Swedish infants. *Acta Paediatr. Scand.* 68:853, 1979.
105. Jakobsson, I., and Lindberg, T. Cow's milk protein causes infantile colic in breast fed infants: A double-blind crossover study. *Pediatrics* 71:268, 1983.

CONSTIPATION

106. Drossman, D. A., et al. Bowel patterns among subjects not seeking health care. Use of a questionnaire to identify a population with bowel dysfunction. *Gastroenterology* 83:529, 1982.
107. Fitzgerald, J. F. Difficulties with defecation and elimination in children. *Clin. Gastroenterol.* 6:283, 1977.
108. Mahboubi, S., and Schnaufer, L. The barium-enema examination and rectal manometry in Hirschsprung's disease. *Radiology* 130:643, 1979.
109. Passarge, E. Genetics of Common Gastrointestinal Malformations and the Heterogeneity of Hirschsprung's Disease. In J. I. Rotter, I. M. Samloff, and D. L. Rimoin, (Eds.), *The Genetics and Heterogenicity of Common Gastrointestinal Disorders.* New York: Academic Press, 1980. P. 441.
110. Rendtorff, R. C., et al. Stool patterns of healthy adult males. *Dis. Colon Rectum* 10:222, 1967.

CYSTIC FIBROSIS

111. Shwachman, H. Guide to diagnosis and management of cystic fibrosis. *National Cystic Fibrosis Research Foundation.* Prepared by Professional Education Committee, Shwachman, H., Chairman. Rockville, Maryland, 1973.
112. Shwachman, H. Nutritional Considerations in the Treatment of Children with Cystic Fibrosis. In R. M. Suskind (Ed.), *Textbook of Pediatric Nutrition.* New York: Raven Press, 1980.
113. Shwachman, H., and Mahmoodian, A. The sweat test and cystic fibrosis. *Diagn. Med.* 5:61, 1982.
114. Shwachman, H., Mahmoodian, A., and Neff, P. K. The sweat test. Sodium and chloride values. *J. Pediatr.* 98:576, 1981.

IRON DEFICIENCY

115. Committee on Nutrition of the American Academy of Pediatrics. Iron supplementation for infants. *Pediatrics* 58:765, 1976.
116. Dallman, P. R. Iron, vitamin E, and folate in the preterm infant. *J. Pediatr.* 85:742, 1974.
117. Dallman, P. R., et al. Diagnosis of iron deficiency: The limitations of laboratory tests in predicting response to iron treatment in 1-year-old infants. *J. Pediatr.* 98:376, 1981.

118. Garby, L., and Sjolin, S. Absorption of labelled iron in infants less than three months old. *Acta Paediatr. Scand.* (Suppl. 117):24, 1959.
119. Lozoff, B., et al. Developmental deficits in iron-deficient infants: Effects of age and severity of iron lack. *J. Pediatr.* 101:948, 1982.
120. Rios, E., et al. Relationship of maternal and infant iron stores as assessed by determination of plasma ferritin. *Pediatrics* 55:694, 1975.
121. Woodruff, C. W. Iron deficiency in infancy and childhood. *Pediatr. Clin. North Am.* 24:85, 1977.

THE PREMATURE INFANT

122. American Academy of Pediatics Committee on Nutrition. Commentary on breast-feeding and infant formulas, including proposed standards for formulas. *Pediatrics* 57:278, 1976.
123. American Academy of Pediatrics Committee on Nutrition. Nutritional needs of low-birth-weight infants. *Pediatrics* 60:519, 1977.
124. Atkinson, S., et al. Human milk feeding in premature infants: Protein, fat and carbohydrate balances in the first two weeks of life. *J. Pediatr.* 99:617, 1981.
125. Brooke, O., et al. Energy retention, energy expenditures, and growth in healthy immature infants. *Pediatr. Res.* 13:215, 1979.
126. Gaull, G., et al. Milk protein quantity and quality in low-birth-weight infants. III. Effects on sulfur amino acids in plasma and wine. *J. Pediatr.* 90:348, 1977.
127. Gross, S., et al. Composition of breast milk from mothers of preterm infants. *Pediatrics* 68:490, 1981.
128. Hillman, L., et al. Effect of oral copper supplementation on serum copper and ceruloplasmin concentration in premature infants. *J. Pediatr.* 98:311, 1981.
129. Koboyashi, A., et al. Effects of dietary lactose and lactase preparation on the intestinal absorption of calcium and magnesium in normal infants. *Am. J. Clin. Nutr.* 28:681, 1975.
130. Raiha, N., et al. Biochemical basis for nutritional management of preterm infants. *Pediatrics* 53:147, 1974.
131. Raiha, N., et al. Milk protein quantity and quality in low-birthweight infants: I. Metabolic responses and effects on growth. *Pediatrics* 57:659, 1976.
132. Roy, C., et al. Correction of the malabsorption of the preterm infant with a medium chain triglyceride formula. *J. Pediatr.* 86:446, 1975.
133. Svenniengsen, N., et al. Incidence of metabolic acidosis in term, preterm and small for gestational age infants in relation to dietary protein intake. *Acta Paediatr. Scand.* 62:1, 1973.
134. Ziegler, E., et al. Lactose and mineral absorption in infancy. *Pediatr. Res.* 14:513, 1980.
135. Zoppi, G., et al. Exocrine pancreas function in premature and full-term neonates. *Pediatr. Res.* 6:880, 1972.

INBORN ERRORS OF METABOLISM

136. Acosta, P., and Elsas, L. *Dietary Management of Inherited Metabolic Disease: Phenylketonuria, Galactosemia, Tyrosinemia, Homocystinuria, and Maple Syrup Urine Disease.* Atlanta, Georgia: ACELMU Publishers, 1975.
137. Bickel, H., et al. Influence of phenylalanine intake on phenylketonuria. *Lancet* 2:812, 1953.

138. Folling, A. Uber assuheidung von Phenylbrenztraubensauere in den Harn als Stoffwechselanomalie in verbindung mit Imbezillitat. *Z. Physikal. Chem.* 227:169, 1934.

139. Jervis, G. Metabolic investigations on a case of phenylpyruvic oligophrenia. *J. Biol. Chem.* 126:305, 1938.

140. Levy, H. L. Treatment of Phenylketonuria. In C. S. Bartsocas and C. J. Papadatos (Eds.), *Management of Genetic Disorders: Proceedings*. New York: A. Liss, 1979. Pp. 171–182.

141. Levy, H. L. and Hammersen, G. Newborn screening for galactosemia and other galactose metabolic defects. *J. Pediatr.* 92:871, 1978.

142. Segal, S. Disorders of Galactose Metabolism. In J. B. Stanbury, J. B. Wyngaarden, D. S. Frederickson, J. L. Goldstein, and M. S. Brown, (Eds.), *The Metabolic Basis of Inherited Disease* (5th ed.). New York: McGraw Hill, 1982. P. 167.

143. Tourian, A. Phenylketonuria and Hyperphenylalaninemias. In J. B. Stanbury, J. B. Wyngaarden, D. S. Fredrickson, J. L. Goldstein, and M. S. Brown (Eds.), *The Metabolic Basis of Inherited Disease* (5th ed.). New York: McGraw Hill, 1982. P. 270.

144. Waisbren, S., Schnell, R., and Levy, H. Diet termination in children with phenylketonuria: A review of psychological assessments to determine outcome. *J. Inherit. Metab. Dis.* 3:149, 1980.

9. The Child Who Fails to Thrive

William G. Bithoney

Failure to thrive (FTT) is a growth disorder with multiple etiologies. Virtually every serious medical disease of childhood eventually can, and does, manifest itself as organic failure to grow and gain weight [5]. So-called nonorganic failure to thrive is defined as failure of growth without any diagnosable medical etiology. As a generic diagnosis, organic and nonorganic FTT account for fully 1 percent of all pediatric hospitalizations [2]; 80 percent of the time these patients present before age 18 months [4]. Mitchell and colleagues [17] found that 10 percent of a rural outpatient population suffered from FTT. None of their patients, selected from a primary care setting, had an organic cause for their disorders. While the diagnostic criteria for FTT vary somewhat, the term is routinely used to describe children whose weight is persistently below the third percentile for age on appropriately standardized growth charts (e.g., National Center for Health Statistics charts) [19] (see Appendix 2). Other criteria, such as weight less than 85 percent of the mean, fiftieth percentile weight for age, or a rapid decrement of 2 or more major percentiles in a previously well child, are also used to make the diagnosis of FTT.

Recently, a number of authors have questioned the adequacy of the dichotomous (organic/nonorganic) view of FTT etiology described above, suggesting instead that at least three categories are necessary to describe etiology in FTT: (1) organic, (2) nonorganic, and (3) mixed [12]. In their study, Homer and Ludwig [12] demonstrated that more than one-quarter of all FTT cases can present with a mixed etiology, including both organic and nonorganic concomitants that are potentially the cause of FTT. Sameroff and Chandler [26] have suggested that there exists a continuum of reproductive (organic) and caretaking (nonorganic) causality in "psychosomatic" diseases such as FTT and other pediatric social illnesses. This approach to understanding FTT etiology is a fruitful one. For example, children with obvious temperamental aberrations (felt to be the nonorganic etiology of their FTT) may be suffering from a purely medical disease, malnutrition. Thus, their FTT would be organic rather than nonorganic. Unless and until such children are offered and retain adequate calories, they continue to manifest the organically determined irritability, temperamental disturbances, and altered feeding interactions described in children suffering from malnutrition per se [21, 29].

Such pure organic temperamental disturbances are often virtually impossible to differentiate from inherent or innate temperamental problems. Thus, the treatment of malnutrition with the provision of adequate calories is the physician's first responsibility. Often, behavioral problems will improve as nutritional requirements are met.

If interactional problems exist between caretaker and child, these must be addressed at the outset. Similarly, parental psychological problems associated with child neglect and abuse must be faced and actively treated. Above all, the physician must treat nonorganic causes of FTT with the same concern he or she treats organic causes. Previous medical studies of children who fail to thrive have focused on extensive laboratory workups treating nonorganic FTT as a diagnosis of exclusion, entertained only after all possible organic diseases have been ruled out [2, 4, 5, 11]. Such an approach to FTT is not only highly cost ineffective and potentially harmful to the child but also often misleading to the physician [5]. For example, if a child is hospitalized and given multiple laboratory tests that require prolonged fasting or invasive procedures such as esophagoscopy, it is highly unlikely that his failure to gain weight in the hospital can be used as a helpful diagnostic clue of the presence or absence of organic medical disease. Furthermore, evaluation of caretaker-child interaction, temperament, and child development will be difficult and misleading if conducted in a hospital setting with concomitant invasive testing.

The knowledgeable physician is aware that the overwhelming majority of outpatient FTT cases are without diagnosable organic causes [17]. The organic and nonorganic risk factors are identified by medical and nutritional assessments (see Chap. 7) as well as by social, temperamental, and developmental evaluations. Thus, the full range of potential causes of FTT is considered, and useless hospitalizations and fruitless or misleading laboratory evaluations are prevented.

ORGANIC RISK FACTORS

FTT is best considered as a combination of organic and nonorganic risk factors [12]. In general, the organic risk factors to be evaluated are minor congenital anomalies, prenatal malnutrition, prematurity, and any ongoing, chronic medical illness. A comprehensive (but not exhaustive) list of causes of growth failure is presented in Table 7-16.

MINOR CONGENITAL ANOMALIES

Multiple, miscellaneous patterns of deformity are documented as routinely being associated with both short stature and depressed weight [20]. Typical cosmetic deformities known to be associated with FTT when catalogued into identifiable syndromes are anteverted nostrils, abnormal interpupillary distance, and low set ears. Obviously, such abnormalities should be looked for and noted in all cases of FTT. An attempt should be made to categorize anomalies as belonging to identifiable syndromes known to be associated with both intrauterine growth retardation and subsequent FTT (such as fetal alcohol syndrome) [18]. Interestingly, a number of authors have noted an association between FTT and a high incidence of alcohol use in FTT families [9, 16, 20, 23]. Such children, prior to the description of fetal alcohol syndrome in the literature, may have been diagnosed as suffering from nonorganic FTT.

PRENATAL MALNUTRITION

Infants who suffer intrauterine growth retardation due to inadequate maternal nutrition during gestation, congenital infection, or inadequate placental function of any kind are usually small for gestational age (SGA) at birth. In one of the most informative studies of the effect of prenatal malnutrition on later growth of the affected child, Fitzharding and Steven followed 96 SGA infants for 4 years. They found that one-third of them were below the third percentile for both weight and height when evaluated in early childhood [10]. Fitzharding and Steven also noted that infants from the lowest socioeconomic group have the poorest outcome in growth and that their parents did not provide enough stimulation for them. However, the effects of intrauterine growth retardation were clear-cut and significant in all socioeconomic strata. These children are usually diagnosed as having nonorganic FTT when they present with delayed growth. They often have no diagnosable organic medical disease but clearly have suffered an intrauterine organic insult. Als and Brazelton [1] have observed that such children are significantly more likely to suffer from other pediatric social illnesses, such as child abuse and neglect. They also demonstrate a markedly aberrant repertoire of behaviors compared to controls, reacting hypersensitivily and emotionally to most stimuli [8].

PREMATURITY

Prematurity per se may also predispose children to FTT. While the incidence of low birth weight (LBW) in the population-at-large is 10 percent, reports of the incidence of LBW in children suffering from FTT range from a minimal estimate of 10 percent to as high as 40 percent [9, 17, 24]. Data in LBW children are somewhat complicated because of the need to differentiate between SGA premature infants and appropriate-for-gestational age premature infants. The high incidence of FTT in LBW infants may be due to perinatal morbidity unrelated to prematurity per se. Mitchell and colleagues have reported that there is a two-fold increase in perinatal complications in FTT infants versus controls [17]. Such perinatal complications, if associated with even mild cerebral anoxia, may result in subtle neural damage that is subsequently associated with aberrations in growth and cognition. These aberrations may be incorrectly diagnosed as nonorganic in children with temperamental and behavioral problems who do not have definitive clinical evidence of medical illness.

NONORGANIC RISK FACTORS IN FTT

TEMPERAMENTAL AND BEHAVIORAL ALTERATIONS IN FTT

Recent studies of FTT have described a number of behavioral variations that differentiate nonorganic FTT infants and their families from organic FTT infants. Bithoney and colleagues [6] noted that FTT infants were markedly developmentally delayed when compared to control infants.

The FTT infant is described as being highly reactive with an extremely variable tempo of play and a limited repertoire of reactions to external stimuli. The most striking finding of this study was the maternal perception of the child with nonorganic FTT as being extremely ill. Pollitt [22] also describes similar behavioral changes and developmental immaturity in FTT children. In addition, the mothers of FTT infants are described by Bithoney and associates [6] as being socially isolated and emotionally overwhelmed. It is not clear from any of the studies of FTT whether the temperamental/behavioral aberrations seen in FTT children are the cause of FTT or merely its effect. Furthermore, it is not clear whether the sense of social isolation and depression experienced by FTT mothers is the cause of their children's disease or whether such maternal emotion is engendered by the experience of raising a sickly, behaviorally difficult child. These studies found an increased family density in FTT families suggesting that having many children, especially if they are close in age or temperamentally difficult, predisposes to FTT.

Feeding interactions in FTT children are frequently described as disordered [6, 17, 21, 22]. Not surprisingly, these children also demonstrate deficits in their nonfeeding interactions with caretakers. There appear to be a number of potential risk factors that may interact to cause nonorganic FTT. Socially isolated, stressed caretakers confronted with a difficult child and many siblings (also demanding attention) may be unable to effectively care for their infant. As malnutrition progresses, the child may become more and more difficult to nurture with a temperament worsened by malnutrition and an increasingly stressful feeding interaction.

EVALUATION OF FTT

Differential diagnosis of FTT is complex and anxiety provoking and spans the entire range of general pediatric expertise. The clinician is aware that virtually every serious medical illness of childhood can manifest itself as FTT. Yet, it is imperative for clinicians to remember that in the outpatient, nontertiary care setting, most FTT will be without purely medical etiology. The medical history and physical examination repeatedly have been shown to be the best ways of screening for organic disease. Indeed, the medically oriented studies of FTT demonstrate that lab tests are rarely, if ever, positive, unless there is a specific indication for obtaining the test [2, 4, 5, 24, 27]. Thus, after the clinician has performed a thorough history and physical examination and ruled out organic causes, he or she can feel quite confident in actively pursuing nonorganic areas of risk without performing multiple laboratory tests. Using a stepwise approach to carefully analyze each area of potential clinical risk, the clinician can be assured of adequately diagnosing the etiology of FTT.

MEDICAL AND NUTRITIONAL ASSESSMENT

The evaluation of FTT should begin with a growth data analysis. Is the child failing to thrive on appropriately standardized growth charts? The National Center for Health Statistics charts [19] (see Appendix 2) are standardized for all races of children in the United States, whereas the Boston charts currently in use in many centers are standardized on only 100 white, middle class children of Northern European ancestry.

If the child's weight truly is below the third percentile, an assessment of mid-parental height (average height of both parents) should be performed. Tanner and coworkers [28] have developed charts that make adjustments for the effect of height and growth variations among the offspring of short parents. Use of this chart will prevent the unnecessary workup of children who are constitutionally small (Fig. 9-1). Unfortunately, such charts are not useful prior to age 2 because the correlation of mid-parental height with the growth parameters of their children is not yet strong enough to be useful clinically [28].

DIET HISTORY AND FEEDING OBSERVATION

Once it is determined that the child is indeed failing to thrive given his genetic growth potential, the most helpful diagnostic test one can perform is a 3-day nutrition history [7] (see Table 7-6).

The history is used to obtain a calorie count that will inform the medical provider whether or not the child is being offered and retaining adequate nutrients. The aid of a trained nutritionist as a member of the evaluation team is invaluable in this analysis. The next step in FTT diagnosis should be a feeding observation. The trained clinician should characterize aberrant or dysfunctional feeding patterns that may be treatable (see Table 11-2). These observations may also be used to verify diet history. If the child is hospitalized, feeding assessments as well as other developmental assessments should be undertaken only during periods that are relatively free of intensive or invasive medical procedures. Otherwise, any observations made may be misleading.

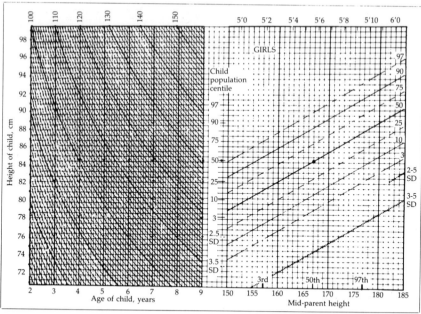

Figure 9-1. Standards for height for girls age 2 to 9 allowing for mid-parental height. In order to use the chart, first find the child's height and subsequently follow the curve until the child's age is reached. Next, place a ruler horizontally from this point to the right side of the chart. The point where the horizontal line crosses the vertical line of the mean parental height is noted and the percentile of the child's height is recorded. (From Tanner, J., Goldstein, H., and Whitehouse, R. Standards for children's height at ages 2–9 years allowing for height of parents. Arch. Dis. Child. 45:755, 1970.)

MEDICAL HISTORY

After obtaining the diet history and feeding evaluations, a comprehensive, detailed history of the present illness should be obtained. It is imperative to emphasize known organic and nonorganic risk factors for FTT in the history. The review of systems should be no different than the standard systematic review given to all medical patients with attention to the gastrointestinal, neurological, and endocrine systems, which are most frequently abnormal in organic FTT (Table 9-1). The past history must include a neonatal history emphasizing the presence of prematurity or deviations from normal gestational weight. Also, any and all past hospitalizations should be understood in detail. All chronic or recurrent symptoms of any kind must be evaluated. The family history should include organic medical illnesses with genetic implications as well as a history of FTT either in the parents or other siblings.

Table 9-1. Studies of Ultimate Diagnoses in Failure to Thrive

Findings	English (1978)	Sills (1978)	Hannaway (1970)	Riley et al. (1968)	Shaheen et al. (1968)	Ambuel and Harris (1963)
Number of cases	77[a]	185[a]	100[a]	83[a]	287[a]	100[b]
Diagnoses (%)						
Organic	53	18	49	48	85	68
Gastrointestinal[c]	19	8	12	14	15	9
Neurologic	14	4	18	12	18	10
Genitourinary	4	0	5	5	5	4
Endocrine	4	1	5	1	4	5
Cardiac	7	1	4	2	13	31
Other	5	5	5	13	29	9
Environmental	38	55	39	31	15	NR
No cause (or constitutional) (%)	9	26	12	20	NR	32

Source: Used by permission from Berwick, D. Nonorganic failure-to-thrive. *Pediatr. Rev.* 1:266, Copyright American Academy of Pediatrics 1980.
[a]Children hospitalized to diagnose FTT
[b]Survey of all children in hospital who have FTT
[c]Includes cystic fibrosis
NR = Not reported

PHYSICAL EXAMINATION

A comprehensive, standard physical examination should be performed on all children with minor dysmorphic features and/or with more major congenital anomalies, abnormalities of muscular tone, fine motor delays, and abnormal posture [3, 15]. One must be especially vigilant for signs of child neglect or abuse, such as bruises, fractures, and burns. Children who suffer from both FTT and child abuse may be at extremely high risk: Hufton and Oates [13] as well as Koel [14] have described a surprisingly high mortality in such cases in small samples. In their reports, the mortality was due to ongoing physical abuse rather than malnutrition.

LABORATORY EVALUATION

Laboratory evaluation must be precise, goal-oriented, and initiated only after the history and physical examination have been performed [2, 4, 5]. A few screening lab tests, however, are appropriate for all children with FTT. These tests are shown in Table 9-2.

DEVELOPMENTAL ASSESSMENT

The majority of children seen with FTT suffer from gross motor delays and cognitive delays, specifically expressive and receptive language delays. There is usually a relative sparing of fine motor development [5]. On follow-up evaluation, anywhere from 50 to 70 percent of FTT children will suffer from some form of intellectual impairment [5]. Thus, all children should receive appropriate developmental testing, and most will require specific developmental stimulation either in the home under active pediatric supervision or by referral to infant stimulation programs.

Table 9-2. Routine Laboratory Tests in FTT

Complete blood count (CBC)
Urinalysis
Urine culture
Urine for reducing substances
Blood urea nitrogen (BUN) or creatinine
Tuberculin test
Free erythrocyte protoporphyrin (FEP/Pb)
Stool for pH, reducing substances, occult blood, ova and parasites*
Sweat test
Albumin (in severe FTT only)
Chest x-ray

*Useful in recent immigrant children (e.g., Hispanics and in children from areas where *Giardia* is endemic).
Modified from Berwick, D. Nonorganic failure to thrive. *Pediatr. Rev.* 1:265, 1980.

SOCIAL EVALUATION

The standard medical history taken in FTT cases should include a social history that allows the clinician to understand the internal structure and functioning of the family. Such an understanding can be diagnostic in cases of nonorganic growth failure. An obvious example is the situation in which a child begins failing to grow immediately after a severe family stress (i.e., divorce or when taken care of by members of the extended family). The elucidation of such dynamics can result in relatively straightforward prescriptions that can immediately alleviate growth failure.

INTERACTIVE EVALUATION

Children suffering from FTT are classically described as suffering from interactive disorders. Rosenn and associates [25] showed that nonorganic FTT infants could be distinguished from organically ill, malnourished infants using their preference for interacting at a distance. Nonorganic FTT children preferred to remain aloof with little physical contact, while organically ill children demonstrated a strong preference for close, warm, physical interactions with caregivers.

Pollitt [22] as well as Bithoney [6] have noted difficult feeding interaction as an important factor in discriminating FTT children from controls. The evaluation of interaction between caretaker and child by the clinician in both feeding and nonfeeding situations can result in concrete recommendations to improve interaction. For example, the mother and child that manifest little play and relatively impoverished interaction obviously require counseling. The mother can be instructed in en face feeding techniques and encouraged by the child's responsiveness to appropriate verbal and nonverbal cues. Some caretakers may require referrral to parenting centers for more intensive guidance.

THERAPEUTIC INTERVENTION

Upon completing the initial evaluation of FTT, the physician must decide the best mode of intervention and treatment. While the overwhelming majority of FTT cases should be managed on an outpatient basis, some children require immediate hospitalization with inpatient evaluation of medical, developmental, and social functioning. Three groups of patients should be routinely hospitalized:

1. The *seriously ill* child with severe protein-calorie malnutrition and/ or dehydration must be hospitalized immediately and medically stabilized.
2. *Children suffering from child abuse or neglect* should also be hospitalized and immediately protected. In the United States, most mortality

in FTT children is related to abuse and neglect rather than overwhelming dehydration, malnutrition, and secondary infection.

3. *Children who fail outpatient management* obviously require closer observation and intervention in order to alleviate FTT that is intractable to outpatient therapy.

If at all possible, the treatment of FTT is best undertaken by a treatment team consisting of a pediatrician/clinician, nutritionist, and social worker. The first phase of treatment must include ongoing nutritional counseling and intervention. All children who suffer from FTT (whether organically or nonorganically induced) require adequate nutrient intake before any amelioration can begin. Concrete and specific recommendations must be given. Infants who are eligible should be placed on the WIC (Women's, Infant's, and Children's) supplemental nutrition program (see Appendix 9). The use of high-caloric food supplements (see Tables 5-2 and 6-7) such as Polycose and medium chain triglycerides may also be helpful.

After initiation of adequate nutritional and medical support to alleviate acute problems, social and psychological intervention should begin. The assistance of a trained social worker in identifying resources that may be helpful to the child with FTT is usually required. Social workers can work with the family to coordinate ongoing services such as visiting nurses, infant stimulation programs, and psychological counseling services. Also, in cases of child abuse and neglect, their assistance in dealing with distressed parents and child protective service agencies is invaluable for the protection of the child.

CONCLUSION

The involvement of the pediatrician as the primary medical caregiver and as a consistent resource is perhaps the single most important aspect of care for children with FTT. It is the responsibility of the pediatrician to follow the child for the long haul, coordinating and observing progress in all aspects of FTT. Sustained weight gain in FTT children is the ultimate indication that treatment has been successful.

ACKNOWLEDGMENT

The author would like to thank Donald Berwick, Debra Frank, and Jennifer Rathburn, who have helped in the evolution of his clinical approach to FTT.

REFERENCES

1. Als, H., and Brazelton, T. B. Behavior of the full term but underweight newborn infant. *Dev. Med. Child Neurol.* 18:580, 1976.
2. Ambuel, J. P., and Harris, B. Failure to thrive. *Ohio State Med. J.* 59:997, 1963.
3. Barbero, C. J., and Shaheen, E. Environmental failure-to-thrive: A clinical review. *J. Pediatr.* 71:639, 1967.
4. Berwick, D. Non-organic failure-to-thrive. *Pediatr. Rev.* 1:9, 1980.

5. Berwick, D., Levy, J., and Kleinerman, R. Failure to thrive: Diagnostic yield of hospitalization. *Arch. Dis. Child.* 57:347, 1982.
6. Bithoney, W. G., et al. Non-organic FTT. Developmental and familial characteristics. *Pediatr. Res.* 16(4):84, 1982.
7. Bithoney, W. G., and Rathburn, J. Failure to Thrive. In M. Levine, et al. (Eds.). *Developmental and Behavioral Pediatrics.* Philadelphia: Saunders, 1983.
8. Brazelton, T. B. Nutrition During Early Infancy. In R. M. Suskind (Ed.). *Textbook of Pediatric Nutrition.* New York: Raven, 1981.
9. Elmer, E. Failure to thrive: Role of the mother. *Pediatrics* 25(10):717, 1960.
10. Fitzharding, P., and Steven, E. The small-for-date infant. I. Later Growth Patterns. *Pediatrics* 49:671, 1972.
11. Hannaway, P. Failure to thrive: A study of 100 infants and children. *Clin. Pediatr.* 9(2):96, 1970.
12. Homer, C., and Ludwig, S. Categorization of etiology of failure to thrive. *Am. J. Dis. Child.* 135:848, 1981.
13. Hufton, I., and Oates, R. Non-organic failure to thrive: A long term follow-up. *Pediatrics* 59(1):73, 1977.
14. Koel, B. S. Failure to thrive and fatal injury as a continuum. *Am. J. Dis. Child.* 118:565, 1979.
15. Krieger, I., and Sargent, D. A. A postural sign in the sensory deprivation syndrome in infants. *J. Pediatr.* 70:332, 1967.
16. Leonard, M. Failure to thrive in infants. *Am. J. Dis. Child.* 3:600, 1966.
17. Mitchell, W., Correll, R., and Greenberg, R. Failure to thrive: A study in a primary care setting. *Pediatrics* 65(5):971, 1980.
18. McMillan, J., Nieburg, P., and Oski, F. *The Whole Pediatrician Catalog: A Compendium of Clues to Diagnosis and Management.* Philadelphia: Saunders, 1977, Pp. 89–92.
19. NCHS Percentiles. Adapted from Hamill, P. V., et al. Physical growth: National Center for Health Statistics percentiles. *Am. J. Clin. Nutr.* 32:607, 1979.
20. Patterns of Malformations. In V. C. Vaughn, R. J. McKay and R. E. Behrman, (Eds.), *Nelson Textbook of Pediatrics* (11th ed.). Philadelphia: Saunders, 1979. P. 2035.
21. Pollitt, E., and Thompson, C. Protein-calorie malnutrition and behavior: A view from psychology. *Nutrition and the Brain* 2, 1977.
22. Pollitt, E. Failure to thrive: Socioeconomic, dietary intake, and mother-child interaction data. *Fed. Proc.* 34:1593, 1975.
23. Pollitt, E., et al. Psychosocial development and behavior of mothers of failure-to-thrive children. *Am. J. Orthopsychiatry* 45:4, 1975.
24. Riley, R. L., et al. Failure to thrive: An analysis of 83 cases. *California Med.* 108:32, 1968.
25. Rosenn, D., et al. Differentiation of organic from non-organic failure to thrive syndrome in infancy. *Pediatrics* 66:689, 1980.
26. Sameroff, A. J., and Chandler, M. J. Reproductive Risk and the Continuum of Caretaking Casualty. In P. D. Horowitz (Ed.), *Review of Child Development Research.* Chicago: Univ. of Chicago Press, 1975. P. 187.
27. Sills, R. H. Failure to thrive: The role of clinical and laboratory evaluation. *Am. J. Dis. Child.* 132:967, 1978.
28. Tanner, J. M., et al. Standards for children's height at age 2–9 years allowing for height of parents. *Arch. Dis. Child.* 45:755, 1970.
29. Whitten, C., Pettit, M., and Fischoff, J. Evidence that growth failure from maternal deprivation is secondary to undereating. *J.A.M.A.,* 209:1675, 1969.

10. Obesity in Infancy

William H. Dietz, Jr.

Since the report that 36 percent of infants with weights greater than the ninetieth percentile before 6 months of age became obese adults [4], concern has focused on the risk of excessive fatness in young children for later obesity. Based on other epidemiological studies, the risk of obesity in adulthood appears more strongly affected by onset of obesity in later childhood and by severity than by obesity of infantile onset [6]. In this chapter we will address the assessment of fatness, the factors affecting obesity in infancy, and the influences that promote the persistence of excessive fatness.

ASSESSMENT

Body Composition

The principal methods used to assess body composition in humans are potassium-40 (^{40}K) counting, underwater weighing (body density), neutron activation, measurement of total body water with stable or radioactive isotopes of hydrogen or oxygen [6, 15], and EMME (electronic meat-measuring equipment). Because of the limited availability of ^{40}K measurements in infants, the technical difficulties of underwater weighing or measuring residual air in the lungs, and the unjustifiable exposure of infants to radiation, the most accessible of these methods is the measurement of total body water with stable isotopes of hydrogen or oxygen. The EMME method [20] is also a noninvasive method but has not yet been compared with other more common measures of body composition.

Studies of total body water are based on the dilution principle. Baseline measurements of the enrichment of body water with ^{2}H or ^{18}O are compared with the enrichment following a measured dose of isotope to calculate the space in which the isotope is diluted. Because the ratio of water to lean tissue mass in older subjects is constant, lean body mass may be calculated. However, the assumption that the water:mass ratio is constant may not apply in infants, particularly because extracellular water is increased in infancy [16].

These suppositions were confirmed in an early study of total body water in infants [17]. Body water as a percent of body weight in premature and term infants ranged from 70 to 80 percent of body weight. Assuming the normal ratio of water to solids in humans, these data indicate that over 100 percent of the newborn's mass is lean tissue, which is clearly wrong. Although indirect, Fomon's calculations [12] suggest that approximately 25 percent of body weight in the 4-month-old male reference infant is fat. Fomon's calculations also suggest that female infants are fatter in infancy than at any other time until adolescence, and that males are fatter in infancy than at any other time until middle adulthood.

ANTHROPOMETRIC MEASUREMENTS

The validity of anthropometric measurements to assess fatness depends on the strength of the correlation between the measure and body fatness measured by one of the techniques used to measure body composition. Because of the alterations in body composition discussed previously, as well as the paucity of body composition studies in this age group, no reliable anthropometric measurement of total body fat has yet been developed for infants. However, because most fat is distributed subcutaneously, assessments of fatness can be based on the measurement of multiple skinfolds such as the triceps, biceps, subscapular, and abdominal. Although this technique has been applied to investigations of factors affecting fatness in early life, the measurement of multiple skinfolds is not a technique adapted easily to the assessment of normal infants and therefore is of limited utility in more routine clinical assessments.

Almost by default, weight for height remains the most readily determined, and probably most widely used, index of adiposity. Because of the lack of reliable measures of body composition against which weight for height as an index of adiposity can be compared, a direct relationship between weight for height and fatness cannot be assumed. Nonetheless, cautious use of a weight in excess of 120 percent of the weight expected for height is probably justified as an index of excessive fatness, but only when the diagnosis is confirmed by inspection of the infant. If the diagnosis of obesity on these grounds is questionable, measures of skinfolds are essential. Reference standards that include standard deviations have been published [12, 34]. In borderline cases, it is prudent to measure skinfolds rather than to label an infant obese using a measure that has received no validation.

NATURAL HISTORY

Obesity should constitute a pathological diagnosis rather than a diagnosis designating an infant with fatness greater than the norm expected for age. No consistent studies associate excessive fatness in infancy with pathological consequences at this age. Although it is becoming increasingly clear that excessive fatness in later childhood has pathological consequences, these consequences occur with low prevalence. In addition, as discussed later, there is virtually no correlation of fatness or excessive fatness at birth with fatness at later ages. Therefore, it is not at all clear that obesity as a pathological diagnosis has any validity in infancy. However, because obesity in later childhood and adolescence has a significant morbidity, including a higher likelihood of persistence into adulthood [6], identification of infants at high risk for the persistence of obesity is a matter of considerable clinical importance.

FATNESS AT BIRTH

The duration of gestation, maternal weight, and maternal weight gain during pregnancy appear to be the principal factors affecting fatness at birth.

The last trimester of pregnancy is accompanied by the rapid growth of fetal adipose tissue, which accounts for approximately 1 percent of body weight at 26 weeks of gestation and 16 percent of body weight at term [15]. Clearly, premature infants will have a reduced fat mass.

Obese mothers and their infants form a particularly high risk group. Obese mothers demonstrate a significantly increased prevalence of eclampsia, gestational diabetes, wound or episiotomy infections, and surprisingly, inadequate weight gain [9]. In a 10-year survey of maternal mortality [26], severe obesity occurred six times more frequently in mothers who died than in a control group. Most deaths were due to pulmonary embolism or hemorrhage.

Pregnancy also constitutes a period of high risk for the development of obesity in women. Although no good prospective data document the incidence of obesity during pregnancy, retrospective data suggest that 30 to 50 percent of persisting obesity in women began during pregnancy or postpartum [1, 30]. Maternal obesity may reflect serial transmission through successive generations; significantly more obese mothers also had mothers who became obese during their pregnancy.

Both prepregnancy obesity and excessive weight gain of women during pregnancy has been associated with greater average birth weights and increased adiposity of infants [35, 36]. The effect of these variables persists even when maternal populations are controlled for parity, smoking, blood pressure, or a family history of diabetes. Abnormal glucose metabolism is frequent among the obese, and there is a positive correlation of maternal blood glucose levels and neonatal adiposity [37]. Therefore, at least part of the effect of maternal obesity on neonatal adiposity might be attributable to the effect of adiposity on maternal glucose metabolism.

NATURAL HISTORY OF ADIPOSITY IN INFANTS

Growth of fat during the first 12 months of life is associated with an increase in fat cell size; from 12 to 18 months, increases in fat are due primarily to an increase in fat cell number [19, 23]. Based on these observations, a relationship between excessive fatness in the second year of life and the risk of persisting obesity might be expected. However, only a small proportion of obese adolescents were obese in early childhood. Remission rates for excessive fatness are highest in early life and fall with advancing age [6].

The risk posed by excessive fatness in infancy for the persistence

Table 10-1. The Persistence of Obesity in Infants

Study	Age in Months								
	0	3	6	12	24	36	48	60	72
Fisch, 1975 [11]	100%						26%*		19%
Mack, 1974 [25]		100%			38%		26%		
Huenemann, 1974 [22]			100%				25%		
Asher, 1966 [2]			100%				44%		
Sveger, 1975 [32]				100%	50%				

*Percentage of infants originally obese who remained obese at the follow-up examination.

of obesity in adolescence or adulthood remains controversial. However, as shown in Table 10-1, there is a high frequency of spontaneous remission of obesity in affected infants. In a large population of infants of low income families in Philadelphia, weight for height at birth accounted for only 3 percent of the variance in weight for height at 4 months of age [25]. Similarly, no significant correlation was shown between skinfold thickness at birth and 1 year of age [38], nor was there any significant difference in the sum of four skinfolds at 1 year of age in the fattest and thinnest groups of infants at birth [10]. It therefore appears likely that the canalization of fatness occurs later in childhood.

Nonetheless, several sources of data suggest that a disproportionate share of later obesity may have its origins in infancy or very early childhood. For example, 36 percent of infants exceeding the ninetieth percentile of weight at least once in the first 6 months of life became overweight adults, compared to 14 percent of average and lightweight infants [4]. Furthermore, the influence of the infant's weight on adult weight appeared independent of the presence or absence of parental obesity. However, neither the potentially confounding influences of parental obesity nor socioeconomic class on adult weight were separated from the influence of infant weight in a statistically satisfactory fashion.

The more important variable affecting the risk of persistence of fatness in infancy may be the severity of obesity. Although no data are available for infants, data from older children indicate that the greater the severity of obesity, the lower the likelihood of remission [3].

These data offer reassurance to pediatricians and nurse practitioners. The finding of rapid growth or mild degrees of excessive fatness in infants should not occasion undue alarm. The majority of these cases are likely to remit spontaneously. However, weight in excess of 120 percent of ideal weight in infants who clearly appear excessively fat, particularly those in whom fatness is associated with other epidemiological risk factors (discussed later), should prompt efforts to apprise parents of the risks of later obesity and provide counseling aimed at achieving weight maintenance.

ENERGY BALANCE

Excessive fatness can only result from an energy intake in excess of expenditure. In infancy, attention should rightfully focus on factors affecting energy intake, the principal determinants of energy expenditure, and the epidemiological factors that serve to identify infants at high risk for the development of obesity.

ENERGY INTAKE

Because infants appear able to regulate food intake appropriately over a wide range of caloric density [12], attention has focused on the mode of feeding and the time of introduction of solids (over which the infant has no control). The principal assumption underlying these investigations is that breast-fed infants will feed to satiety because mothers are unable to regulate the quantity of breast milk taken by infants, whereas bottle-fed infants may overfeed because parents persuade them to finish bottles, even after satiety has been achieved.

Despite an abundant literature on the effect of bottle- or breast-feeding on infant growth, firm evidence that breast-feeding reduced the prevalence of obesity is still lacking. Virtually all of the published studies that assert that differences do exist contain significant methodological problems. The more important of these are failure to include a control group, bias in the selection of a control group, failure to define breast-feeding or its duration, inadequate verification of reported information in retrospective surveys, and use of weight rather than direct measures of fatness. Birth weight doubling time is significantly faster in bottle-fed infants [28], but whether the increased weights among bottle-fed infants is associated with increased fatness remains unclear. In the few instances where breast-feeding and its duration have been carefully specified, no significant differences in weight [33] or fatness [10] have been observed, nor could differences in feeding patterns between obese and nonobese infants be demonstrated [8]. Nonetheless, in at least two of these investigations [8, 10] the populations studied were small, raising the possibility of Type II error.

Although retrospective in nature, one of the most careful studies revealed an effect of breast-feeding on obesity in adolescents, with a small but significant inverse correlation between the duration of breast-feeding and relative weight [24]. However, the significant methodological difficulties accompanying these and the remainder of the studies to date leave the protective effects of breast-feeding unproven.

Concern about the effect of the addition of solid food to the diet on the prevalence of obesity was initially raised by the observation that solid foods appeared to provide additional calories to infant diets, rather than to replace foods already being consumed. In contrast to the literature regarding breast-feeding, somewhat more uniform data suggest that the early addition of solids has little effect on weight gain. For example, rates of weight and length gain over a 3-month period did not differ significantly among infants fed formula, formula and solids started before age 6 weeks, or formula and solids started between ages 6 weeks and 3 months [5]. Although infants fed formula with solids before age 2 months were found to have larger fat folds at age 3 months, by age 5 months no significant differences in skinfolds existed between breast-fed or formula-fed infants with or without supplemental solids [10]. The type of food therefore appears to have little effect.

Infants also appear capable of regulating caloric intake within a narrow range, regardless of the caloric density of the formula [12]. Furthermore, the distribution of calories as fat or carbohydrate appears to exert little effect on either energy intakes or rates of gain in length or weight [13].

ENERGY EXPENDITURE

Few data are available regarding energy balance in obese and nonobese infants. Although energy intake can be determined more reliably in infancy than at later ages, few techniques are available to measure energy expenditure in this age group.

Daily energy requirements in infancy are approximately 120 kcal/kg of body weight in the first 3 months of life and fall to approximately 105 kcal/kg by 1 year of age [14]. The daily energy cost of maintenance has been estimated at 1½ times the basal metabolic rate or approximately 80 kcal/kg [14]. Assuming that the reference 3.5 kg infant doubles his or her birth weight in 4 months and that the energy cost of growth is 5 kcal/gm of new tissue [29, 31], calculations indicate that 20 kcal/kg per day of energy intake will be utilized for growth, and only 20 kcal/kg per day will remain for activity. With age, the energy requirement for growth decreases, and the energy available for activity will progressively increase [29]. These estimates are consistent with the gradual increase in activity that accompanies development in the first year of life.

An alternative argument is also consistent with the notion that muscular activity plays a minor role in energy expenditure in infancy [21]. Basal metabolic rate per kilogram is highest in infancy and falls progressively with age. Over the same period, the percent of body weight contributed by the high energy producing organs (the liver, kidneys, lungs, brain, and heart) decreases, whereas the less active tissue mass of muscle increases. Therefore, the greatest proportion of metabolic rate in infants is contributed by the sum of metabolic activity of the high-energy-producing organs, whereas a significantly greater proportion in adults is contributed by muscle [21]. Together with the data on the compartmentalization of energy requirements, these data suggest that the contribution of muscle to metabolic rate in infancy must be small.

Careful studies of energy balance in obese and nonobese infants and children have not been performed. The essential questions such studies must address is whether the impaired regulation of energy balance that results in obesity is endogenous or environmental in origin. Endogenous factors might include an increased efficiency in the deposition of fat, a reduced capacity to dissipate excess energy intake as heat, or a reduction in the energy cost of activity. Any of these mechanisms would explain the findings of comparable energy intakes among obese and nonobese infants. Adequate methodologies to evaluate these possibilities are not currently available.

An equally difficult methodological problem lies in the comparison of energy intakes. Dietary histories are of limited reliability and are probably too inaccurate to detect the small differences capable of producing obesity. For example, an excess energy intake of 50 kcal per day will produce 5 pounds of excess fat per year (1 lb of fat = 3,500 kcal). Furthermore, caloric intake, as well as growth, may vary widely from week to week. These data suggest that the origins of obesity are not likely to be demonstrated in the near future.

EPIDEMIOLOGICAL ASSOCIATIONS

Obesity in children is associated with a number of epidemiological variables. The most important of these appear to be family characteristics [7]. It is now well recognized that the prevalence of obesity is increased in families in which one or both parents are obese. Although this association suggests the possibility of a genetic causality, heredity does not explain the resemblance in fatness of spouses [18], nor the association of obesity in pet dogs and their owners [27]. Obesity occurs with an increased frequency among children in single parent families and among children of older parents. The prevalence of obesity in children also is inversely affected by family size; prevalence is greatest among single children and declines as family size increases.

Surprisingly, the behaviors within families have been given little attention. Interviews with mothers of both fat and lean infants [22] indicated that mothers of overweight infants were less knowledgeable about infant diets and were less likely to withhold desserts if the child did not finish a meal. Households of overweight infants were more likely unconventional and there existed a high likelihood that mothers of obese infants were obese themselves.

In contrast, another study [8] has suggested that mothers of obese infants showed a comparable sensitivity to infant cues regarding feeding when compared to mothers of control infants. Both groups of mothers relied equally on external cues for feeding, such as time of day or prepared portion size, rather than infant signals to begin or end feedings. Likewise, comparable numbers of mothers in both groups tried to feed more food than their infants seemed to want and did not differ with respect to offering food to stop their baby's crying. Mothers of a subgroup of severely obese infants recognized their infant's obesity as a problem; in this group, mothers appeared somewhat more capricious than other mothers with respect to over- or under-feeding their infants. However, these differences were not statistically significant.

The major problem with these observations is that they are derived from self-reported rather than observed practices. Although the significant associations with family variables suggest an impact of attitudes and family dynamics on the energy balance of infants, the mechanisms by which these interactions generate their effect is unknown. Such data are essential for effective prevention and treatment of affected infants. Nonetheless, the family associations of obesity should serve to identify infants at high risk for the development of obesity and should alert pediatricians and nurse practitioners to the need for careful preventive counseling and early intervention should excessive gains in fat occur.

PREVENTION

Efforts directed at preventing the development of obesity during infancy should begin at birth and should be directed primarily at high-risk infants. These are best identified by the epidemiological characteristics associated with childhood obesity: parental obesity, older or single parents, single children, or children in small families. The prevalence of obesity in families in which either parent is obese is the same, regardless of the sex of the parent or the child. These data suggest that obesity is not simply a consequence of poor mothering and that counseling should be directed at both parents. The principal goal of these early discussions should be to make obesity a legitimate topic for discussion at a time when parents are most receptive to information from pediatricians or nurse practitioners.

Educational efforts should include discussions regarding the mode of infant feeding, clues as to infant satiety, and the appropriate times to introduce solids. Although clear evidence regarding the protective effect of breast-feeding is lacking, this mode of feeding should be encouraged for all infants. However, parents should not be told to breast-feed in order to prevent obesity. Parents should be apprised of the risks of obesity in later childhood, especially the psychosocial difficulties regarding obesity. This may be a particularly effective technique if obese parents can recall their own childhood difficulties related to fatness.

TREATMENT

Given the natural history of obesity in infants, treatment of obesity should only be undertaken for infants whose weight is in excess of 120 percent of ideal weight for height, but only if excessive fatness is confirmed visually or, preferably, by skinfold measurements.

As with prevention, efforts at treatment should begin with the whole family, rather than just with the mother. Although mothers frequently assume the major responsibility in the selection, purchase, and preparation of food, fathers have at least an equal influence on these decisions. Furthermore, practices within the home are usually a consequence of tacit agreements between parents; these undoubtedly apply to infant feeding. Additional family members such as grandparents may either have direct responsibility for child care or a highly significant impact on parental decisions; these family members should also be included in early sessions aimed at treating obesity.

Our experience with families of young obese children suggests that their parents are often dominated by their infant's perceived needs and tend to be overresponsive to cues regarding hunger. Such parents are frequently overanxious and feel guilty when they say no to their infants, because they believe that this may imply rejection or lack of love for the infant. Resolution of this problem is crucial to the management of obesity, because it is essential that parents set reasonable and consistent limits on their infant's food intake. Likewise, conflict between spouses or in-laws regarding the correct approach must be successfully resolved; otherwise, the potential for sabotage or unresolved conflicts about the child's weight is increased.

In infants and young children, weight maintenance or below-normal weight gain, rather than weight loss, should be the goal of therapy. Because infants may vary considerably in energy requirements, weekly or biweekly adjustments of the diet may be necessary before the maintenance of energy requirement is established for the obese infant. During the period of weight maintenance, it is essential to maintain protein intake at maintenance levels. This is best achieved by delivering maintenance calories as formula in which the calorie-protein ratio is constant. Dilute formulas should be avoided; small stomach volumes may make it impossible for infants to ingest the quantities of a dilute formula necessary to supply maintenance nutrients. Solid foods should be substituted for foods already in the diet to maintain the same level of caloric and protein intake. In many cases, excess calories can be controlled by substituting water for juice and by eliminating added fat and sugar (see Table 6-12).

Frequent meetings with both parents at the outset of therapy may be essential for adequate compliance and dietary safety. Anxiety regarding the effect of calorie restriction on infant growth may be reduced by weekly weigh-ins and discussions. A review of infant behavior may disclose that normal behaviors such as finger or thumb sucking are being misinterpreted as evidence of a ravenous appetite. Parents must be made to understand that their preoccupation with food may be projected onto the infant. Finally, parents need empathetic support and frequent reassurances to alleviate the guilt they may feel at withholding food from an obese infant.

CONCLUSION

Pediatricians and nurse practitioners are ideally suited for the task of early recognition and intervention in obesity of infants and young children. During this period there are frequent contacts between infants, parents, and professionals that directly affect attitudes and practices in health and disease. Furthermore, with the continuing decline of extended families, pediatricians and nurse practitioners are assuming a more important role as a source of information and direction for parents with regard to child rearing.

Obesity is currently the major nutritional problem of children in the United States. Although the prevalence of infantile-onset obesity in obese adults is controversial, efforts at treating and preventing obesity in infants and young children may meet with greater success than the treatment of affected children and adolescents. The family associations of childhood obesity not only serve as risk factors for the development of the disease but emphasize the crucial need for efforts directed at therapy and prevention.

REFERENCES

1. Angel, J. L. Constitution in female obesity. *Am. J. Phys. Anthropol.* 7:433, 1949.
2. Asher, P. Fat babies and fat children. *Arch. Dis. Child.* 41:672, 1966.
3. Borjeson, M. Overweight children. *Acta Paediatr. Scand.* 51:[Suppl.] 132, 1962.
4. Charney, E., et al. Childhood antecedents of adult obesity. *N. Engl. J. Med.* 295:6, 1976.
5. Davies, D. P., et al. Effects of solid foods on growth of bottle-fed infants in the first three months of life. *Br. Med. J.* 2:7, 1977.
6. Dietz, W. H., Jr. Obesity in infants, children and adolescents in the United States. I. Identification, natural history, and aftereffects. *Nutr. Res.* 1:117, 1981.
7. Dietz, W. H., Jr. Obesity in infants, children and adolescents in the United States. II. Causality. *Nutr. Res.* 1:193, 1981.
8. Dubois, S., et al. An examination of factors believed to be associated with infantile obesity. *Am. J. Clin. Nutr.* 32:1997, 1979.
9. Edwards, L. E., et al. Pregnancy in the massively obese: Course, outcome, and obesity prognosis of the infant. *Am. J. Obstet. Gynecol.* 131:479, 1978.
10. Ferris, A. G., et al. The effect of feeding on fat deposition in early infancy. *Pediatrics* 64:397, 1979.
11. Fisch, R. O., et al. Obesity and leanness at birth and their relationship to body variations in later childhood. *Pediatrics* 56:521, 1975.
12. Fomon, S. J. *Infant Nutrition* (2nd ed.). Philadelphia: Saunders, 1974.

13. Fomon, S. J., et al. Influence of fat and carbohydrate content of diet on food intake and growth in male infants. *Acta Paediatr. Scand.* 65:136, 1976.
14. Food and Agriculture Organization of the United Nations and World Health Organization Expert Committee Report. *Energy and Protein Requirements.* Geneva, Switzerland: World Health Organization, 1973.
15. Forbes, G. B. Methods for determining composition of the human body. *Pediatrics* 29:477, 1962.
16. Friis-Hansen, B. J. The extracellular fluid volume in infants and children. *Acta Paediatr. Scand.* 43:444, 1954.
17. Friis-Hansen, B. J., et al. Total body water in children. *Pediatrics* 7:321, 1951.
18. Garn, S. M., et al. Synchronous fat changes in husbands and wives. *Am. J. Clin. Nutr.* 32:2375, 1979.
19. Hager, A., et al. Body fat and adipose tissue cellularity in infants: Longitudinal study. *Metabolism* 26:607, 1977.
20. Harrison, G. G., and Van Itallie, T. B. Estimation of body composition: A new approach based on electromagnetic principles. *Am. J. Clin. Nutr.* 35:1176, 1982.
21. Holliday, M. A. Metabolic rate and organ size during growth from infancy to maturity and during late gestation and early infancy. *Pediatrics* 47:169, 1971.
22. Huenemann, R. L. Environmental factors associated with preschool obesity. *J. Am. Diet. Assoc.* 64:480, 1974.
23. Knittle, J. L., et al. The growth of adipose tissue in children and adolescents. *J. Clin. Invest.* 63:239, 1979.
24. Kramer, M. S. Do breast-feeding and delayed introduction of solid foods protect against subsequent obesity. *J. Pediatr.* 6:883, 1981.
25. Mack, R. W., and Ipsen, J. The height-weight relationship in early childhood. *Hum. Biol.* 46:21, 1974.
26. Maeder, E. C., et al. Obesity: A maternal high risk factor. *Obstet. Gynecol.* 45:669, 1975.
27. Mason, E. Obesity in pet dogs. *Vet. Rec.* 86:612, 1976.
28. Neumann, C. G., and Alpaugh, N. Birth weight doubling time: A fresh look. *Pediatrics* 57:469, 1976.
29. Payne, P. R., and Waterlow, J. C. Relative energy requirements for maintenance, growth and physical activity. *Lancet* 2:210, 1971.
30. Sheldon, J. H. Maternal obesity. *Lancet* 2:869, 1949.
31. Spady, D. W., et al. Energy balance during recovery from malnutrition. *Am. J. Clin. Nutr.* 29:1073, 1976.
32. Sveger, T., et al. Nutrition, overnutrition and obesity in the first year of life in Malmo, Sweden, *Acta Paediatr. Scand.* 64:635, 1975.
33. Swiet, M. de, et al. Effect of feeding habit on weight in infancy. *Lancet* 1:892, 1977.
34. Tanner, J. M., and Whitehouse, R. H. Revised standards for triceps and subscapular skinfolds in British children. *Arch. Dis. Child.* 50:142, 1975.
35. Udall, J. N., et al. Interaction of maternal and neonatal obesity. *Pediatrics* 62:17, 1978.
36. Whitelaw, A. G. L. Influences of maternal obesity on subcutaneous fat in the newborn. *Br. Med. J.* 1:985, 1976.
37. Whitelaw, A. G. L. Subcutaneous fat in newborns of diabetic mothers: An indication of quality of diabetic control. *Lancet* 1:15, 1977.
38. Whitelaw, A. G. L. Infant feeding and subcutaneous fat at birth and at one year. *Lancet* 2:1098, 1977.

11. The Child with Special Feeding Needs

Dorothy M. MacDonald

The need for special feeding techniques is determined by the type of anomaly (i.e., cleft lip, cleft palate, Pierre Robin syndrome) and the child's oral ability. For infants on hyperalimentation or nasogastric or gastrostomy feedings, the techniques are complex, while in others the techniques require only a thickening of the formula and/or a special nipple. However, in all instances, when special feeding methods are introduced, both the parents and the infant need the support of trained personnel.

After the birth of a child with anomalies, parents must deal with the perceived loss of a normal baby and any guilt they might feel about causing the defect. Thus, before special feeding techniques are introduced, the practitioner must help parents deal with these and other issues that might interfere with bonding. Parents need a complete understanding of the anomaly, the expected feeding behaviors, and the effects of the condition on growth and development. They need continuous support and the opportunity to ventilate their feelings in order to establish a healthy parent-child relationship.

To enhance the parent-child relationship, parents may need help focusing on their child's positive attributes such as hair, eyes, or social responsiveness versus the anomaly or feeding failures. Personal experience has demonstrated that a supportive environment that encourages parent-child interaction (i.e., holding the child, singing, talking) can help ameliorate adjustment problems. Many children with oral-facial anomalies are deprived of "normal" feedings. While a positive feeding experience can enhance development, the emphasis is better placed on the establishment of a meaningful parent-child relationship rather than on feeding.

Children with oral-facial anomalies need an opportunity to exert some control during feeding and to establish their own feeding patterns (See Chap. 2). Adaptation to specialized feeding techniques will occur when parents are comfortable with the technique and support systems are operational. This chapter gives practitioners the basic information needed to provide a supportive role for these children. While the complexities of care usually require follow-up in medical centers, informed local health care providers can provide a more personal and long-term commitment to the family.

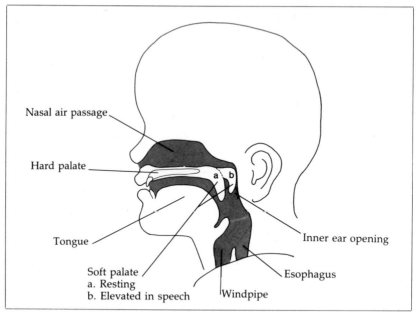

Figure 11-1. Normal physiology of the oropharynx. (Reprinted with permission from Howard, R. B., and Herbold, N. H. [Eds.]. Nutrition in Clinical Care [2nd ed.]. New York: McGraw-Hill, 1982.)

FEEDING EVALUATION

For infants and children with oral-facial anomalies or alimentary canal malformations, assessments of their feeding ability should take place in the neonatal period (Fig. 11-1). Careful note should be made of the primitive feeding reflexes (Table 11-1), oral ability, and coordination of breathing with sucking and swallowing. Table 11-2 details all of the factors to be considered in a feeding assessment. Although not as relevant in the newborn period, all factors in the child's environment must be considered as possible influences on feeding ability. Signs of neurological dysfunction including poor suck, prolonged feeding time, small amounts per feeding, gagging, drooling, aspiration (including change of color), and choking should be carefully noted.

Feeding evaluations are best accomplished by interdisciplinary teams that depend upon available professional resources. Some feeding teams may comprise pediatric nurses, nutritionists, physical therapists, speech pathologists, dentists, and psychologists, while other teams may rely upon only the nurse and pediatrician. The timing of the observation period is critical. Feeding evaluations are best made when the infant/child is hungry and appropriate feeding equipment (i.e., nipples, feeders) is available (Fig. 11-2 and Table 11-3). Both the child's

Table 11-1. Primitive Reflexes in Feeding

Reflex	Description
Moro reflex	A proprioceptive response elicitied by dropping the head back suddenly; the response includes a rapid extention and abduction of the limbs, followed by flexion and adduction of the limbs
Asymmetrical tonic neck reflex	A proprioceptive response elicited by turning the head from side to side; increased extention is seen in the limbs on the face side and increased flexion is seen in the opposite limbs
Hand grasp	A stimulus to the palm of the hand (from the ulnar side) elicits finger flexing and grasping of the object; normal occurrence: birth to 3 or 4 months; retention produces fisted hands, difficulty in opening hands; interferes with holding utensils
Suckle-swallow	A stimulus introduced into the mouth elicits vigorous sucking followed by a swallow if liquid is present; normal occurrence: 1 or 2 days after birth to 3–5 months; retention produces suckling response to any oral stimuli; interferes with taking food from spoon with lips, cup drinking, chewing
Rooting	A stimulus to the oral area (corners of the mouth, upper and lower lip) causes lips, tongue, and finally head to turn toward the stimulus; normal occurrence: birth to 3–5 months; retention produces asymmetrical oral response to stimuli, head turning to oral stimuli; interferes with maintaining head position for appropriate feeding
Gag	A stimulus to the posterior tongue or soft palate causes constriction of the posterior oral musculature to bring stimulating substance forward; normal occurrence: birth to adulthood; retention produces increased oral sensitivity; interferes with hyperactive gag (food is constantly pushed forward and out of the mouth), hypoactive gag (food can passively enter the esophagus or trachea)
Bite	Pressure on the gums elicits a phasic bite and release; Normal occurrence: birth to 3–5 months; retention produces biting all objects placed in mouth; interferes with mouthing activities, ingesting food, more mature biting, chewing

Source: Howard, R. B., and Herbold, N. H. (Eds.). *Nutrition in Clinical Care* (2nd ed.). New York: McGraw-Hill, 1982.

Table 11-2. Feeding Evaluation Observations

Oral ability
 Sucking
 Oral prehension
 Swallowing
 Breathing, swallowing
  coordinated
 Drooling
 Lips
 Tongue size
 Tongue thrust
 Tongue mobility
 Bite
 Munching
 Chewing
 Drinking
Oral structure
 Occlusion
 Teeth
 Caries
 Gingiva
 Oral hygiene
 Palate
 Pain on examination
 Hypersensitivity
 Teething stage
Body position
 Head control
 Sitting balance
 Placement of feet
 Usual feeding position
Hand use
 Palmar grasp
 Pincer grasp
 Opposition finger/thumb
 Hand-to-mouth control
Developmental feeding
 Breast ___ bottle ___ weaned ___
 Baby food ___ junior food ___
 Mashed table food ___
 Minced foods ___
 Cut table foods ___
 Regular table foods ___
 Closes hands in on bottle
 Hand to mouth/sucks on fingers
 Teething biscuit/holds and brings
  to mouth

Finger feeds
Opposes lips to rim of cup
Attempts to grasp spoon
Grasps spoon
Dips spoon in dish
Brings spoon to mouth
Holds bottle and drinks
 independently
Grasps cup
Raises cup to mouth
Cup-lifting, drinking, replacing
Scoops well with spoon
Feeds independently with spoon
Straw drinking
Spears with fork
Spreads with knife
Feeding environment
 Time of feeding (note how long
  feeding takes)
 Atmosphere of feedings (tense,
  pleasant, unpleasant)
 Person responsible for feeding
 Parental and/or caretaker's
  attitude toward feeding
 Past successful and unsuccessful
  methods
 Identify positive and negative
  reinforcing behaviors
Usual food intake
 24-hour recall and/or 1- or 3-day
  food diaries, depending on the
  situation:
Total fluid intake
Medications
 Type
 Dosage
 Time given
Bowel concerns
 Regular
 Constipation
 Diarrhea
Anthropometric data
Clinical data
Laboratory findings

Data courtesy of Feeding Team, Developmental Evaluation Clinic, The Children's Hospital, Boston, Ma.

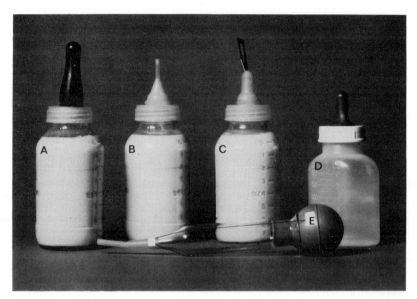

Figure 11-2. Variety of nipples and feeders: (A) lamb's nipple, (B) Ross nipple, (C) nipple with razor inserted to show technique for enlarging the nipple, (D) Mead Johnson feeder, and (E) Breck feeder.

Table 11-3. Variety of Nipples for Infant Feeding

Nipple	Technique
Lamb's	1. Can be obtained from a feed and grain store
	2. Prepare infant
	3. Place nipple over the neck of appropriate size bottle or adapt a regular cap nipple by using the rim of a nipple as a washer
	4. Slowly insert nipple into the infant's mouth on top of tongue until infant finds a comfortable position on the nipple
	5. Feed in an upright position watching the infant's cues
Ross	1. Can be adapted to any standard infant bottle
	2. Prepare infant
	3. The flow on this nipple is easily controlled
	4. Use only for infants with very weak sucks
Cross-cut	1. Standard yellow nipple (use a sharp blade to cut a cross in the nipple)
	2. When the bottle is tipped upside down, milk should drip out easily
	3. Prepare infant
	4. Place nipple over tongue and hold bottle in such a way that one finger is free to place under the infant's chin
	5. As infant sucks, place gentle pressure under the chin
	6. Follow infant cues

Note: These nipples are used with Breck feeder or Mead Johnson feeder.

Table 11-4. Feeding Methods for Congenital Anomalies

Anomaly	Method
Oral-facial	Breck feeder, Ross or Mead Johnson feeder, cross-cut nipple, lamb's nipple, breast
Alimentary canal	Gastrostomy, gavage, nasal duodenal, hyperalimentation

and the parents' response to feeding is noted. In addition to the feeding style, the type and the amount of the feedings is monitored.

Careful anthropometric measurements (i.e., height, weight, head circumference) and biochemical indices may be used to determine nutritional status (see Chap. 7). In some instances, when swallowing ability cannot be evaluated clinically, a barium swallow with cinefluoroscopy may be necessary.

FEEDING TECHNIQUES

The optimal method of feeding will be determined by the type of anomaly and the child's oral ability (Table 11-4). Volume limitations may necessitate using energy-dense formulas (see Table 5-3) or nutritional supplements. Children who do not have oral ability may require tube feedings. This may be accomplished by orogastric, nasogastric or nasoduodenal instillation. Tables 11-5, 11-6, and 11-7 describe different feeding techniques. Diets and tube feedings need constant revision because needs change with age and growth.

The infant should be weighed weekly and increments in formula and changes in strength should be made appropriately. The amount of intake per 24-hour period is more important than the amount of each feeding. If there is any question about intake, fluid intake should be recorded and the infant watched carefully for signs of dehydration (i.e., blood urea nitrogen, urine specific gravity, number of wet diapers, dry oral mucosa, thick ropey saliva).

During and after feedings, infants are held, stroked, and periodically burped. The feeding time is limited to a 20- or 30-minute period because prolonged feeding often stresses both the child and the feeder. After feeding, infants may be placed on their right side or in a sitting position to facilitate gastric emptying.

At least three people should learn the feeding technique in order to provide some relief for the primary caretaker. Good communication is essential for consistency between those involved in feeding.

ORAL-FACIAL MALFORMATIONS

Children with oral-facial defects require specialized care by professionals who are able to overlook the disfigurement and establish a

Table 11-5. Gavage Feeding

General information
   Gavage feedings may be given by orogastric or nasogastric method
1. Orogastric: Neonates are obligatory mouth breathers because their nasal passages are not large enough to allow air flow
2. Nasogastric: Infants pass the mouth breathing stage at 3 to 4 months of age

Purpose
1. To ensure proper and adequate nourishment when an alternative feeding method is impossible or contraindicated
2. To instill fluids, feeding, and medication safely and efficiently
3. To prevent aspiration or abdominal distention
4. To maintain proper fluid and electrolyte balance
5. To conserve calories in a premature infant and to decrease stress and fatigue

Resources needed by caretaker
1. Feeding tube, number 5 or 8 French
2. Nasogastric tube or double lumen tube (if double lumen tube is used, tie off side lumen)
3. Syringe
4. Stethoscope
5. Feeding fluid
6. Tape (adhesive and paper)
7. Restraint
8. Appropriate feeding apparatus/gavage set

Technique
1. Select appropriate fluid (should be at room temperature)
2. Insert tube and test for placement. The proper insertion and anchoring of the tube is required prior to instillation to prevent aspiration of fluid into trachea. Measure from the xyphoid process to the tip of the nose to the middle of the ear lobe with the feeding tube
3. Restrain the child comfortably with head and shoulders elevated at a 30-degree angle. This will promote more efficient emptying of the stomach
4. Aspirate tube to check for placement in stomach and for presence of residual gastric contents. If aspirate is half or more of total feeding, hold feeding
5. For most infants, the amount of gastric residual secretions aspirated is refed and subtracted from total volume to be administered unless feeding volume is to be advanced, aspirate contains evidence of blood and excessive mucus, or inappropriate amount of previous feeding is retained. Water should not be added to the formula during feeding to thin it out, since this will increase the volume
6. Attach feeding apparatus to feeding tube. If medication is to be administered in conjunction with feeding, it should be poured into feeding set first. Pour small amount of fluid into syringe to begin gravity flow; height of feeding set may need to be increased. If the child is crying or restless, stomach musculature may contract, which can also stop the fluid flow. In this instance, the infant will need to be cuddled

Table 11-5 (Continued)

7. The usual feeding time is approximately 20 minutes. The rate of flow is slow to prevent gastric distention (rate depends on lumen of feeding tube and consistency of fluid)
8. Assess respiratory rate, chest excursion, activity level, and skin color during feeding. If child coughs or gags, pinch off tube and stop the feeding until episode subsides
9. After feeding, flush tubing with small amont of water or air to clear the tubing
10. Cap or clamp the feeding tube if it is to remain indwelling
11. To remove the tube (if gavage feeding is being done intermittently), pinch the tube off and withdraw it at a steady, moderate pace to prevent entry of fluid into trachea during withdrawal of feeding tube. This pace will help to avoid vomiting and/or trauma
12. Monitor child's activity level following the feeding. Subdued activity will help to ensure proper absorption
13. Document volume and appearance of residual aspirate as well as type and amount of fluid absorbed on proper documentation form(s)
14. Note child's response to feeding and medication. Monitor intake, output, and daily weight. Assess fluid and electrolyte balance

Data from *Nursing Policy and Procedure Manual*, The Children's Hospital, Boston, Ma.

Table 11-6. Gastrostomy Feeding

General Information
1. A gastrostomy tube is placed through the abdominal wall into the stomach and anchored with a purse-string suture during surgery
2. Postoperatively, the area should be kept clean and dry and covered with a dry, sterile dressing
3. The dressing should be secured with an anchoring piece of tape to prevent excessive movement of the tube

Purpose
1. To promote absorption of fluids through the stomach by avoiding esophageal reflux and vomiting/aspiration
2. To promote fluid and electrolyte balance
3. To promote weight gain

Resources needed by caretaker
1. Gastrostomy feeding apparatus
2. Feeding or medication at room temperature
3. Syringe adapter or catheter-tip syringe
4. 10–60 ml syringe

Technique
1. Feeding should be at room temperature
2. Position child comfortably with head and shoulders elevated at 30-degree angle. This prevents reflux of fluid
3. Aspirate gastrostomy tube prior to feeding. This ensures proper placement of tube in stomach and determines the amount absorbed from prior feeding

Table 11-6 (Continued)

4. Refeed or discard aspirate depending on individual needs. Residual amount is indicative of ability to tolerate type and amount of feeding. Maintenance of adequate fluid and electrolyte levels is ensured by refeeding aspirate
5. Offer pacifier to infant if appropriate. The pacifier is used to help the infant associate oral gratification with hunger
6. Connect gastrostomy feeding apparatus or syringe to tube. The syringe adapter or catheter-tip syringe is used to obtain a tight fit between tube and syringe to permit feeding to flow and prevent leakage of fluid
7. If medication is to be administered in conjunction with feeding, medication should be poured into feeding set first. This ensures that the entire medication is administered
8. Regulate rate of feeding by monitoring drip of gastrostomy set or noting speed with which syringe is emptying. The height of the feeding apparatus above the infant's stomach determines the rate of flow. Clamping or pinching the tube will prevent fluid from entering the stomach rapidly. The length of feeding time should be equivalent to the time required for oral feeding
9. Assess patient for respiratory or gastrointestinal distress. Close observation is vital during feeding
10. Flush tube with small amount of water or air at completion of feeding. This ensures patency of the tube and delivery of the entire feeding
11. At completion of feeding, leave the apparatus attached if the gastric tube is to remain open. If the tube is to be clamped, remove the feeding apparatus. An open gastrostomy tube will permit reflux and prevent distention
12. Record amount and character of aspirate as well as the amount and type of fluid given on the appropriate documention form(s). Note and record activity level and manner with which fluid was accepted
13. Monitor output and weight daily

Data from *Nursing Policy and Procedure Manual*, The Children's Hospital, Boston, Ma.

Table 11-7. Nasoduodenal Feeding

General information
A method of feeding to infuse nutrients continuously into the pylorus when the infant is unable to tolerate intermittent gastric feedings or is having difficulty with aspirations or gastric feedings
Purpose
1. To ensure proper and adequate nourishment when an alternative feeding method is impossible or contraindicated
2. To instill fluids and feeding
Resources needed by caretaker
1. Silastic feeding tube
2. Number 5 French feeding tube

Table 11-7 (Continued)

3. Measuring tape
4. Syringe
5. Three-way stopcock
6. Male Luer-Lok
7. Sterile water
8. Formula or breast milk
9. Infusion pump

Technique
1. Follow steps for gavage feeding implementation
2. When determining the length of the tube to be inserted, first mark the length to be inserted into the stomach
3. To determine the additional length needed to reach the duodenum, place the tip of the catheter between the infant's eyebrows and extend the catheter down to the outstretched heel
4. Attach a 3-way stopcock to feeding tube. Place syringe and Luer-Lok cap in stopcock parts
5. Set the rate of flow on the infusion pump
6. Note infant's response to feeding, monitoring intake, output, and daily weight. Assess fluid and electrolyte balance

Data from *Nursing Policy and Procedure Manual*, The Children's Hospital, Boston, Ma.

helping relationship that is individualized to the needs of the parents and the child. An understanding of the defect and knowledge of the required feeding equipment gives parents the confidence to master feeding techniques.

CLEFT LIP AND CLEFT PALATE

There are four types of cleft lips (Fig. 11-3): (1) unilateral complete, (2) unilateral incomplete, (3) bilateral complete, and (4) bilateral incomplete. Cleft lips may occur in isolation or in conjunction with a cleft palate. The defect occurs in the sixth to eighth week of gestation and the incidence is 1 in 850 live births.

The feeding problem results from the cleft not allowing the lip to form a seal around the feeding device. Feeding methods vary with the preference of the plastic surgeon because the type of feeding device can interfere with surgical correction. The infant usually will learn to feed by any method that is started early and provided consistently.

A cleft palate can occur with or without a cleft lip and occurs about the eleventh or twelfth week of gestation. The incidence is also approximately 1 in 850 live births.

The hard, or primary, palate consists of the premaxilla, maxilla, and palatine bone. The soft, or secondary, palate is a fibromuscular structure that divides the nasal from the oral pharynx. It is constantly modified in shape and position by palatal musculature. The incisive foramen (with a bilateral suture extending to the interproximal space

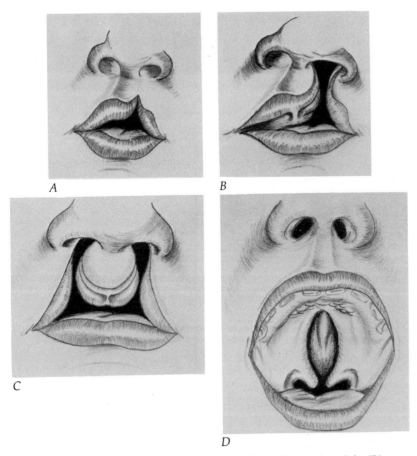

Figure 11-3. Defects of the lip and palate: (A) unilateral incomplete cleft, (B) unilateral complete cleft, (C) bilateral complete cleft, and (D) cleft palate. (Illustration courtesy of John B. Mulliken, M.D., Division of Plastic Surgery, The Children's Hospital, Boston, Ma.)

between the maxillary lateral incisor and canine) is the dividing line between the primary and secondary palate (see Fig. 11-3).

A cleft in the palate can occur unilaterally, bilaterally, only in the soft palate, or in the soft palate with an extension into the hard palate. Clefts also vary in severity from a slight indentation to a wide gap.

When the cleft occurs only in the soft palate, most infants can eat successfully after minor adjustments have been made in the feeding method. However, if the cleft is in the hard palate, the infant may have a normal sucking motion, but there will be no suction; special techniques will be needed with feeding. As the infant sucks, the caretaker should gently pulsate the bulb on the Breck feeder or squeeze the bottle when using a Mead Johnson feeder. Suggestions for using the Breck and Mead Johnson feeders are summarized in Tables 11-8 and 11-9. When a standard nipple is used with bottle-feeding, a cross

Table 11-8. Technique with Breck Feeder

1. Use a bulb-type glass or plastic syringe with a rubber tip on the end
2. The rubber tip should be firmly attached to the glass and extend 1 inch from the glass
3. Prepare the infant for feeding (i.e., change diapers, wrap in blanket)
4. Newborn's arms should be wrapped in an enclosure
5. Prepare formula at room temperature or slightly warmer; also prepare a small amount of water
6. Choose a comfortable chair or rocker and have equipment within reach
7. Hold the infant in a comfortable upright position
8. Fill syringe with formula
9. Insert the tip of the syringe in the infant's mouth (at least ⅓ to ½ way back on the tongue)
10. Leave the syringe in place until the infant starts to suck
11. Observe the infant's sucking motion
12. Gently use your thumb to put pressure on the bulb
13. As the infant sucks, pulsate the bulb to coordinate with the infant's sucking
14. Watch the infant closely for sucking and pause phases.
15. Only remove the syringe from the infant's mouth when it is empty or the infant has disengaged
16. Bubble the infant well
17. Insert syringe and begin to feed again. Only remove the syringe from the infant's mouth when it is empty or the infant has disengaged
18. When the formula is finished, rinse the syringe and give the infant a small amount of water to rinse the mouth
19. Clean the syringes with soap and water, rinse well, and boil for 5 minutes

Table 11-9. Technique with Mead Johnson Feeder

1. Use a bulb-type glass or plastic syringe with a rubber tip on the end
2. The rubber tip should be firmly attached to the glass and extend 1 in from the glass
3. Prepare the infant for feeding (i.e., change diapers, wrap in blanket)
4. Newborn's arms should be wrapped in an enclosure
5. Prepare formula at room temperature or slightly warmer; also prepare a small amount of water
6. Choose a comfortable chair or rocker and have equipment within reach
7. Hold the infant in a comfortable upright position
8. The nipple already has a cross cut, but you may find it necessary to enlarge it
9. Place the nipple on the top of the infant's tongue
10. Stimulate sucking by stroking the cheeks
11. As sucking begins, gentle squeeze the plastic bottle
12. Pressure on the bottle should be coordinated with the infant's sucking and swallowing
13. Allow for sucking and pause phase
14. Do not remove the nipple from mouth unless infant disengages
15. These feeders can be reused

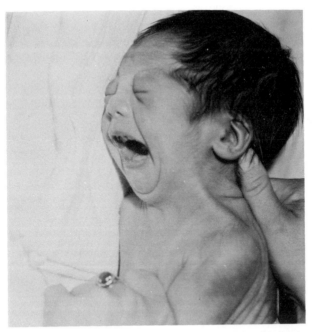

Figure 11-4. Infant with Pierre Robin syndrome (note retrognathic jaw).

cut on the top of the nipple facilitates flow. When breast-feeding, the mother may need to apply gentle pressure to her breast and hold her breast in a V shape to keep the nipple extended.

If the feeder is noting the infant's cries, pauses, and disengagements, a rhythm will develop that will promote the coordination of sucking and swallowing (See Chap. 2). Incoordination of these movements results in milk being regurgitated from the nose and subsequent choking. Holding the infant's head higher than the chest may minimize these problems. The feeding should take 20 to 30 minutes.

Pierre Robin Syndrome

Pierre Robin syndrome is associated with a retrognathic jaw (Fig. 11-4) and tongue as well as a U-shaped cleft that extends into the primary palate. The most dangerous aspect of this anomaly is the obstruction of the airway by the tongue, which may present a difficult problem when feeding.

The degree of airway obstruction and the presence of tongue-tie determine the feeding approach. If there is tongue-tie, the infant usually will maintain an airway only with proper positioning. When there is airway obstruction, a nasopharyngeal endotracheal tube must be passed to keep the tongue forward. The infant must be prone at all times with a blanket roll under the chest or hips to keep the mandible forward (Fig. 11-5). Alternatively, the infant can be held in an upright

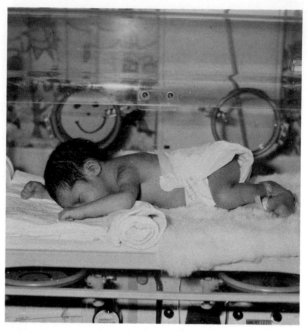

Figure 11-5. Positioning for infant with Pierre Robin syndrome (note blanket roll under chest to keep jaw forward).

position with the caretaker holding the back of the head and positioning his or her thumb and middle finger behind the mandible. Signs of respiratory distress during the feeding include nasal flaring, circumoral cyanosis, and increased contractions of the chest.

During the first 2 weeks of life, feeding is often very difficult and it may be necessary to pass a nasogastric tube. Once the infant begins to coordinate breathing and swallowing, a nipple or Breck feeder may be introduced (see Table 11-8).

If the tongue is severely retrognathic, the Breck feeder is desirable because the tubing can be placed far enough back on the tongue to avoid obstruction (Fig. 11-6). As the infant starts to suck, coordinated pulsation on the bulb should commence. If, after adequate trial, the infant's respiratory status is compromised with feedings, a gastrostomy or tracheostomy is indicated.

HEMIFACIAL MICROSOMIA

Hemifacial microsomia is a unilateral deformity and involves the structures of the first and second brachial arches (Fig. 11-7). The incidence is 1 in 5,600 live births. In this syndrome, underdevelopment of any or all of the structures of the first brachial arch (zygoma, maxilla, mandible, muscles of mastication, trigeminal nerve, upper part of external ear, and parotid gland) and second brachial arch (temporal bone,

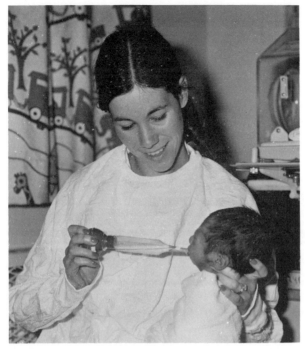

Figure 11-6. Feeding position for infant being fed with Breck Feeder.

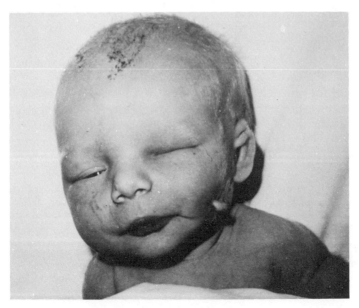

Figure 11-7. Newborn with hemifacial microsomia.

external and middle ear, facial nerve, and muscles of facial expression) exist. Macrostomia, a cleft at the corner of the mouth, is often present in conjunction with an abnormal upward tilting of the occlusal plane on the affected side [8]. Because of cranial nerve involvement, many children with hemifacial microsomia demonstrate neurodysfunction of the palate. They lack motion and sensation of the palate and subsequently have difficulty with liquids. This can be determined simply by placing a finger in the child's mouth and assessing the sucking ability and gag.

Until the macrostomia is surgically corrected, feeding is difficult because the infant is unable to create a seal around the feeding device causing formula to drool from the side of the mouth.

When feeding, the infant is best held in a face forward, semi-upright position, preferably leaning on the caretaker's crossed knee. The feeding device is held in one of the caretaker's hands while the other hand holds the affected side of the mouth and cheek upward. Infants can better control the flow of formula with a lamb's nipple because its length allows it to extend over the first half of the tongue (see Fig. 11-2 and Table 11-3). When lamb's nipples are not available, a cross-cut nipple or a Mead Johnson feeder are recommended.

PARTIAL AIRWAY OBSTRUCTION

Obstruction of the naso-oral airway is usually noted at birth or within the first month of life. The three conditions requiring specialized feeding are choanal atresia, congenital nasal obstructions, and macroglossia. Frequently, the placement of a tracheostomy for an airway and/or a gastrostomy for feeding is necessary.

Choanal Atresia

Choanal atresia is a blockage of the nasal airway due to a unilateral or bilateral overgrowth of nasal cartilage. This causes a significant problem for newborns because they are obligate nose breathers for the first 3 to 4 months of life. Until surgical correction, maintenance of an airway during feeding is critical. A plastic airway may be placed through a nipple for the infant to suck without compromising air exchange (Fig. 11-8). Bilateral obstruction necessitates the use of gavage-feeding until surgical correction (see Table 11-5). However, with a unilateral choanal atresia, if the nasal passage is kept clear of mucous and the infant is fed in an upright position, standard nipples may be used.

Congenital Nasal Obstructions

Dermoids, hemangiomas, or encephaloceles growing along the nasal pharynx may cause partial airway obstruction. Diagnosis is established by direct examination and x-ray. Until surgical correction, the feeding method is identical to that outlined for choanal atresia.

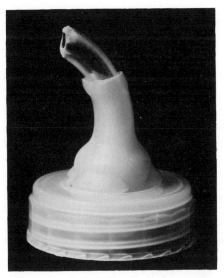

Figure 11-8. Nipple airway developed by Donna Morash, R.N., The Children's Hospital, Boston, Ma.

Macroglossia

Macroglossia is an enlarged tongue (Fig. 11-9) caused by either vascular malformation or endocrine disorder (e.g, cretinism, Beckwith-Wiedemann syndrome). The tongue may be so large that oral feedings are not possible and a gastrostomy is needed. If sucking and swallowing can be coordinated without aspiration, feeding can be attempted. The longer lamb's nipple is placed toward the back of the tongue with the infant in an upright position (see Table 11-3). The caretaker's hand that is holding the bottle can help to close the infant's mouth. Water should be given after feeding and the tongue may be washed with glycerine and lemon swabs to maintain oral hygiene.

ESOPHAGEAL ATRESIA/TRACHEOESOPHAGEAL FISTULA

Many gastrointestinal anomalies occur in the first 3 months of gestation. One of the most common is esophageal atresia with or without tracheoesophageal fistula. The incidence of these malformations is 1 in 3,000 live births [4]. Surgery is required soon after birth to divide the fistula and/or repair and restore the continuity of the esophagus. The most common malformation is a proximal esophageal pouch with a tracheoesophageal fistula to the distal esophageal pouch (Fig. 11-10A). A fistula to the upper pouch (Fig. 11-10B) or two fistulas from the trachea to each esophageal pouch (Fig. 11-10C) are very rare. Esophageal atresia (Fig. 11-10D) and tracheoesophageal fistula (Fig. 11-10E) occur infrequently as isolated entities.

Most children with esophageal malformations require a gastrostomy

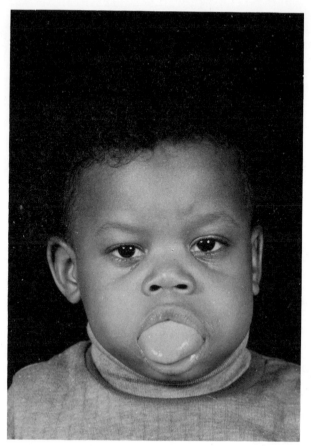

Figure 11-9. Child with macroglossia.

Figure 11-10. (A) Esophageal atresia with distal tracheoesophageal fistula. The upper part of the esophagus communicates with the trachea. This is the most common malformation. (B) Esophageal atresia with proximal tracheoesophageal fistula. A fistula from the proximal esophageal pouch to the trachea. (C) Esophageal atresia with both proximal and distal tracheoesophageal fistula. There is a fistula to the trachea with the esophagus ending blindly. (D) Esophageal atresia. The upper esophageal pouch ends blindly and has no connection to the trachea. There is no connection to the stomach and the distal esophageal section is quite short. (E) Tracheoesophageal fistula without esophageal atresia. The esophagus is connected to the stomach but has a fistula to the trachea. (Photographs courtesy of Holder, T. M., and Ashcraft, K. W. Pediatric Surgery, Philadelphia: Saunders, 1980.)

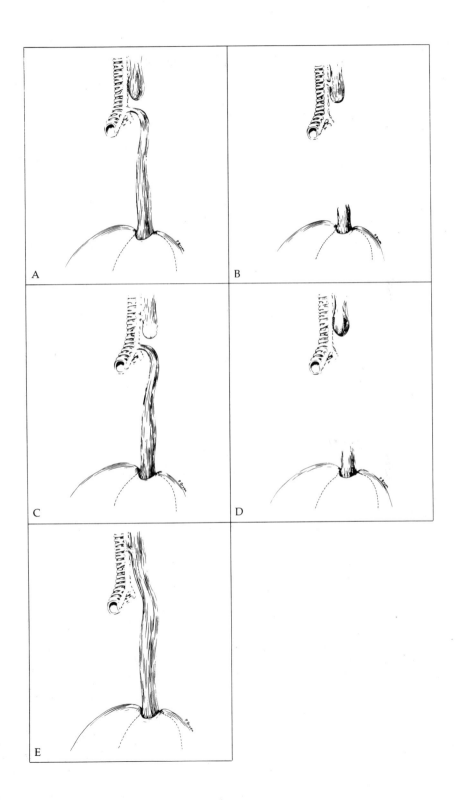

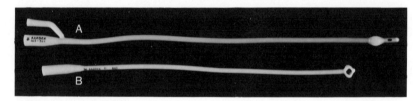

Figure 11-11. Gastrostomy tubes: (A) Foley catheter—preferred for temporary placement, and (B) Malencot tube—preferred type of tube.

to decompress the stomach pre- and postoperatively and to permit enteral feedings (Fig. 11-11). Prior to primary closure, infants were maintained by gastrostomy feedings until they weighed enough for complete surgical repair [11] (see Table 11-6). At one time, this was not done until the infant was 6 months to 1 year of age. To prevent tracheal aspirations, a fistula or cervical esophagostomy was created in the neck to allow secretions to be removed. To prevent oral aversion to food, sham feedings were introduced in which small amounts of food were given by mouth during a gastrostomy feeding. The masticated food was expelled through the fistula in the neck. Dressings or small fistular pouches were used to collect the feeding and saliva. Recently, with the ability to close atretic segments and the use of total parenteral nutrition, oral feedings can be started 10 to 14 days postoperatively.

The goal of postoperative management of children with esophageal atresia is to reestablish oral intake. After a few weeks, gastrostomy feedings are tapered and oral intake is begun. Feedings always start slowly, and frequent regurgitation and incoordination of the swallowing mechanism are common.

All children with esophageal malformations, have an abnormality in the motility of the esophagus. There is no consistent pattern, and the intrinsic motor disturbance does not resolve over time. Although this dysmotility may cause some difficulty in oral feeding and swallowing, it is rarely a problem that cannot be overcome by drinking and eating slowly. If not approached carefully, it can lead to food aversion and food phobias. In children with complicated postoperative courses, feeding problems may persist. Encouragement and small feedings accompanied by thickened liquids are often beneficial in alleviating the problem. As the child matures and takes more responsibility for the feeding, the motility disorder usually becomes less of a problem. However, in some children, the feeding difficulties are enhanced because of gastroesophageal reflux and delayed acid clearance from the esophagus. It is not uncommon for children to develop narrowing at the anastomotic site in the esophagus. This narrowing may be related to the primary surgery, but more recently, it has been shown that persistent narrowing in the anastomosis may be related

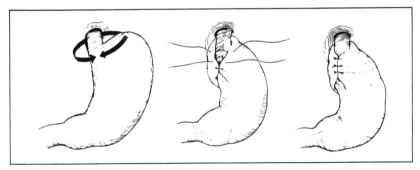

Figure 11-12. Nissen fundoplication. (From Schatzlein, M., et al. Gastroesophageal reflux in infants and children. Arch. Surg. 114:505, 1979. Copyright 1979, American Medical Association.)

to gastroesophageal reflux [10]. The sphincter pressure and the normal number of acid refluxes in a 24-hour period tends to be normal in children with esophageal atresia with or without tracheoesophageal fistula. Their motility disorder contributes to the delayed clearance in acid from the distal esophagus, which places them at an increased risk for the development of esophagitis. This may cause discomfort with swallowing and, in infants, may affect caloric intake. After appropriate evaluation, including pH probe studies, esophageal manometry, and endoscopy with esophageal biopsy, therapeutic intervention may include antacids and possibly cimetidine. In children with esophagitis and reflux who cannot be controlled medically, a fundoplication (Fig. 11-12) may be necessary [9]. However, the fundoplication can potentially further delay esophageal emptying and enhance the esophageal acid injury. Nevertheless, in a limited number of patients with intractable symptoms and acid reflux, this may be the only recourse.

Other problems associated with esophageal atresia/tracheoesophageal fistula are aspiration and pneumonia. They can be due to pharyngeal dysmotility, gastroesophageal reflux, stricture, or recurrent tracheoesophageal fistula. A diagnostic evaluation should differentiate these various possibilities.

GASTROESOPHAGEAL REFLUX

Regurgitation of feedings occurs in as many as 40 percent of normal newborn infants but frequently resolves by 15 months of age. It is usually nonbilious and effortless and can be noted on barium swallow in as many as 50 percent of otherwise normal newborns. Vomiting may be caused by pyloric stenosis, gastroenteritis, protein intolerance, or malrotation, but these conditions are found infrequently. The mechanism for regurgitation in most situations is unclear but most likely relates to the inability of the lower esophageal sphincter and

Table 11-10. Technique for Thickening Feeding

1. During the first 3 months of life, rice, or barley cereal are used to thicken formula feedings (rice cereal is more constipating than barley cereal; therefore, the infant's stools should be noted for consistency when selecting the cereal)
2. Start with ½ tsp cereal per ounce of formula
3. Gradually mix formula with cereal to a smooth consistency in a small bowl
4. Formula is best mixed at room temperature because the heated mixture tends to separate more easily
5. Continue to add cereal until consistency is like heavy cream
6. Place a large cross cut in a regular nipple
7. Continue to shake the formula after the infant disengages from the nipple
8. If constipation is a problem, increase the osmolarity by adding strained fruit or dark Karo syrup

gastroesophageal junction to provide a competent barrier for acid reflux. The infant with nonbilious, recurrent regurgitation who is thriving, not having recurrent pulmonary problems, and having no evidence of gastrointestinal blood loss either by anemia or occult blood in the stool does not need to be evaluated unless the symptoms persist after 15 months of age.

Conservative management and reassurance are often most helpful in managing these children. Thickening the feeding by adding ½ teaspoon of rice cereal to each ounce of formula may dramatically decrease the regurgitation. Some infants may require very thick formula containing as much as 1 tablespoon per ounce. This necessitates crosscutting the nipple or making a hole to allow the mixture to flow. Care must be taken to avoid too rapid feedings and choking. Breast-fed infants appear to have a much lower incidence of regurgitation as compared with those who are bottle-fed. If a breast-fed baby requires thickened feedings, the cereal can be introduced with a spoon, or if not tolerated, expressed breast milk may be thickened in a bottle with rice cereal (Table 11-10). It is not unusual for infants to have difficulty coordinating their swallowing mechanism for solid-liquid mixtures until 2 to 3 months of age.

In addition to dietary management, positioning during and after feeding may be beneficial. During feedings, the child should be held upright with his or her back straight and jaw forward. Frequent burping and an upright position for 30 to 60 minutes after feeding enhance gastric emptying. The use of an infant seat or placement of blocks under the head of the crib can be used to maintain the upright position. If regurgitation occurs during sleep, it is of more concern. These infants may not respond as well to conservative therapy, and referral for evaluation is indicated early. Elevation of the head of the bed or crib mattress and restricting feedings 1 to 2 hours before sleep may help to improve mild cases.

The mechanism by which this conservative therapy is successful is unknown. It may be related to effects on gastric motility or the smaller thickened volume may put less of a stress on the gastroesophageal junction. For some reason, most children respond to conservative therapy, but if there is a failure to gain weight, pulmonary problems, or gastrointestinal blood loss, a diagnostic workup is indicated. Many methods have been employed to define the cause of the reflux. They include upper gastrointestinal x-rays, nuclear medicine scans, esophageal manometry, continuous intraesophageal pH probe monitoring, and esophageal biopsies.

The continuous pH probe study is the most sensitive test to define the presence of pathological reflux or delayed acid clearance from the esophagus and also identifies the time when the reflux is occurring. Reflux at night is related to pulmonary disease, and postprandial reflux occurs when the lower esophageal sphincter is weak.

The severity and duration of reflux are best assessed by esophageal biopsy. If inflammatory changes are present, it is highly suggestive that there is ongoing acid reflux with delayed clearance. The patient with esophagitis needs initial medical therapy with antacids and possibly cimetidine. Cimetidine and antacids should not be given together because antacids inhibit the absorption of cimetidine.

Esophageal motility studies provide information on motility in the body of the esophagus as well as information on the pressure of the lower esophageal sphincter. It was initially thought that patients with pathological reflux had a decreased lower esophageal sphincter pressure, but only 30 percent of children with pathological reflux have diminished sphincter pressure. Thus, this test is of little clinical value in the initial assessment of reflux in children. But, if surgery is contemplated, a motility study should be performed in order to rule out a primary motility disorder.

Bethanechol, a parasympathomimetic agent, has been used to increase lower esophageal sphincter pressure and prevent gastroesophageal acid reflux in infants [1]. It is contraindicated in children with pulmonary disease because it also causes contraction of the bronchial smooth muscle.

Nuclear medicine scans in which technetium-99m is swallowed with milk or water are beneficial in defining the rate of gastric emptying. Delayed gastric emptying is one possible cause for reflux in infants and it is enticing to hypothesize that the reason for the success of thickened feedings is that the rate of gastric emptying is enhanced. The drug metoclopramide increases antral motility and thereby enhances gastric emptying. It also increases the lower esophageal sphincter pressure and promises to be a useful therapy in the future for pathological reflux. Unlike bethanechol, it does not act on bronchial smooth muscle and, therefore, can be used in asthmatics.

The barium swallow is the test most often requested in infants with regurgitation. It is the least sensitive for identifying pathological reflux, and there is a poor correlation between reflux on a barium swallow and the continuous intraesophageal pH probe study. Nevertheless, if an anatomical abnormality is suspected, a barium swallow should be performed, and if normal, more invasive studies can be delayed pending failure of conservative management.

Infants with neurological disease, muscular problems, and dysautonomia have an increased incidence of pathological gastroesophageal reflux that may eventually result in stricture. These problems need to be identified early and preventive measures taken. The relationship of reflux to apnea and sudden infant death syndrome remains unclear. Although suspected as being a cause, the temporal relationship between the pulmonary and the esophageal events is uncertain [2].

Children without medical complications who respond to initial conservative therapy do well without any known long-term sequelae. However, children with reflux often have an increased oral intake that compensates for what is lost with regurgitation. These children can become accustomed to overeating, which, as the condition resolves, can lead to obesity. Therefore, the caloric intake must be adjusted to the child's changing needs.

Children with pathological reflux and esophagitis present difficult feeding issues. They may refuse feeds and develop an aversive type of feeding behavior. With medical therapy this may improve, but close observation is needed because the symptoms can insidiously reappear after many years. The multifactorial aspects of the feeding problem need to be considered in these children (see Table 11-2).

NEUROMUSCULAR DISORDERS AND FEEDING TECHNIQUES

Damage to the central nervous system can occur at any time. Disorders can be caused by known genetic abnormalities or there can be insults during embryogenesis (e.g., myelodysplasia), pregnancy, at birth (e.g., cerebral palsy), or during early childhood. These insults can affect the motor centers of the brain, causing the persistence of primitive reflexes and abnormal muscle tone or causing damage to the nerves controlling sucking, swallowing, or lip closure. This may be clinically manifested by dysphagia, choking, gagging, or vomiting. Because poor oral motor ability causes food and fluid losses and antiseizure medications inhibit nutrients (see Appendix 6), these children are nutritionally at risk and require close nutritional supervision [5]. Furthermore, it is often difficult to determine whether poor growth is related to their underlying condition or malnutrition. Pryor and

Thelander [7] relate the degree of growth impairment in a population of mentally retarded children to the time in development at which the insult occurred. For example, in Down syndrome caused by chromosomal aberrations, growth is most seriously affected. The next group most affected were children who suffered insults during embryogenesis. The growth deficits are less in children with cerebral palsy, many of whom have injuries during birth. While growth potential is often difficult to determine in children with neuromuscular disorders, their nutritional status must not be overlooked as a contributing factor for failure to thrive.

Growth increments can be plotted on the standard NCHS charts or growth charts appropriate to the condition (see Appendix 2). For many children in the Down syndrome population, the norm will be closer to the fifth percentile. Plotting the relationship of the child's height for age to weight for age will give the clinician only some information on the appropriateness of growth. More useful is to determine height and weight for age and to monitor the child's own growth curve.

CEREBRAL PALSY

Cerebral palsy is a nonprogressive central nervous system disorder caused by perinatal or intrauterine damage to the motor centers. Physical and cognitive handicaps range from mild to severe. The neuromuscular problems of cerebral palsy include spasticity (hyperactive muscle stretch reflexes), choreoathetosis (involuntary movements), or flaccidity (decreased muscle tone). Both the degree of involvement and the type of neuromuscular problem determine the severity of the feeding problem. Children who lack mouth, head, or trunk control, sitting balance, and hip flexion will have the most feeding difficulty. Oral motor control is particularly difficult for children in whom primitive reflexes persist. This is manifested by tongue thrusting, an exaggerated bite, easy startle, poor sitting balance, or incoordinated hand-to-mouth activities as occur with the persistence of the asymmetrical tonic neck reflex. Because of these complex neurological problems, individualized feeding techniques must be designed by physical and occupational therapists who consider the need for positioning or techniques that inhibit primitive reflexes and enhance oral motor ability.*

The infant with spasticity presents a particular challenge to the feeder. Positioning provides body control and facilitates feeding. The newborn may be wrapped in a blanket (papoose style) and the child's body is prevented from hyperextending by supporting the head and back in an upright position. A firm nipple with an extra cross cut is

*For a more detailed discussion of methods, the reader is referred to: Finnie, N. R. *Handling the Young Cerebral Palsied Child at Home.* New York: Dutton, 1975.

placed in the infant's mouth; with the same hand that holds the bottle, pressure is placed under the chin with a finger. Observing the child's feeding pattern, the infant is fed in synchrony with the burst-pause sucking pattern (see Chaps. 2 and 3). Liquid feedings may need to be thickened with cereal or fruit to aid swallowing (see Table 11-10). Overstimulation of the mouth by stroking the cheeks and/or excessive wiping of the mouth should be avoided because they can cause hypersensitivity around the oral region.

If tongue control and gagging are a problem, the infant should be placed facing the caretaker in a lightweight infant seat or against a foam wedge or firm pillow. The infant is kept from hyperextending by placing a hand firmly on his or her chest [3]. Occasionally both hands are needed to control the jaw, and this necessitates using the forearm to support the infant's chest.

In order to control the tongue, the head is positioned slightly forward with the hand firmly holding the mandible and the cheeks. If the child is held from the side, the feeder's thumb is placed on the jaw point, the index finger is placed between the chin and lower lip, and the middle finger applies constant pressure behind the chin. When the infant is facing the caretaker, the thumb is placed between the chin and lower lip, the index finger is placed on the jaw point, and the middle finger applies pressure behind the chin. As the infant grows older, techniques and positions must be adapted for the introduction of solid food. When the child is not receiving sufficient volume, energy-dense foods and formulas can be used (see Tables 5-2, 6-7, and Appendix 3).

MYELODYSPLASIA

Myelodysplasia is a developmental defect of the spinal column that occurs near the fourth week of gestation. This condition occurs with varying severity and, depending on the level of the lesion, can cause loss of function from the neck to the sacrum. In some children, hydrocephalus occurs and a shunt is required.

Feeding difficulties are common, but may be a sign of either shunt failure or increasing hydrocephalus. Signs and symptoms include vomiting, increased gagging, irritability or lethargy, and lack of appetite. Another problem sometimes confused with symptoms of shunt malfunction is excessive gagging and choking. This may be caused from spinal cord compression causing dysfunctional sucking and swallowing. Many children with myelodysplasia have oral ability, good upper extremity motor control, and are free from feeding problems. Because of inactivity, obesity may be the major concern as they get older.

The infant experiencing feeding difficulties should be held in an upright position with the head slightly forward. If there are problems sucking, a cross cut is made in the nipple and the feedings may be thickened with cereal. When the nipple is placed in the child's mouth, the feeder's middle finger is placed under the chin to provide jaw control. If the infant starts to gag, the nipple should be removed immediately, but the pressure under the jaw should be maintained. After the gagging subsides, the nipple may be reinserted to resume feeding. To enhance gastric emptying and minimize gastroesophageal reflux, the infant should be kept in an upright position for a minimum of 30 minutes after feeding is completed.

Feeding problems tend to improve after the first 3 months of life, but if they continue after the first year, a multidisciplinary feeding evaluation is needed, to differentiate the behavioral aspects from the organic aspects.

CONCLUSION

Children with anatomical or neurological feeding dysfunctions have to struggle to maintain their nutritional status from the day they are born. Although modern medicine has devised many methods and formulas to help infants and children survive nutritionally, the most important element in the care of the infant is the ability of the caretaker to consider all the needs of the infant. Professionals who integrate both physiological and emotional needs into therapy seem to have the best results. An evaluation that acknowledges the individual characteristics of the child and makes adjustments for the altered demands of the handicapping condition is essential. The complexities of management require the involvement of an interdisciplinary team working in an atmosphere of mutual respect to formulate a feeding technique and envision a total treatment program.

ACKNOWLEDGMENTS

The author wishes to acknowledge the assistance of the Plastic Surgical Service and Kenneth J. Welch, M.D., General Surgery, of The Children's Hospital, and Frances A. Lytz.

REFERENCES

1. Euler, A. R. Use of Bethanechol for the treatment of gastroesophageal reflux. *J. Pediatr.* 90:321, 1980.
2. Euler, A. R., et al. Recurrent pulmonary disease in children: A complication of gastroesophageal reflux. *Pediatrics* 63:47, 1979.
3. Finnie, N. R. *Handling the Young Cerebral Palsied Child at Home.* New York: Dutton, 1975. Pp. 113–140.
4. Holder, T. M., and Ashcroft, K. W. *Pediatric Surgery.* Philadelphia: Saunders, 1980. Pp. 266–281.
5. Howard, R. B., and Herbold, N. H. (Eds.). *Nutrition in Clinical Care.* McGraw-Hill, 1982. Pp. 227–238, 594–628.
6. Jolley, S. G., et al. Postcibal gastroesophageal reflux in children. *J. Pediatr. Surg.* 16:487, 1981.

7. Pryor, H., and Thelander, H. Growth deviations in handicapped children; an anthropometric study. *Clin. Pediatr. (Phila.)* 6:501, 1967.
8. Ravitch, M. M., et al. *Pediatric Surgery.* Chicago: Year Book, 1979. Pp. 233–248, 262–272, 446–491.
9. Schatzlein, M., et al. Gastroesophageal reflux in infants and children. *Arch. Surg.* 114:505, 1979.
10. Winter, H. S. Delayed acid clearance and esophagitis after repair of esophageal atresia. *Gastroenterology* 80:1317, 1981.
11. Woolley, M. M. Esophageal atresia and tracheoesophageal fistula: 1939–1979. *Am. J. Surg.* 139:771, 1980.

12. Home Total Parenteral Nutrition in Infants and Children

Marvin E. Ament

Total parenteral nutrition (TPN) has to be considered one of the most important advances in medical care of critically ill patients in this century. Although in use for only slightly more than a decade, it has rapidly become accepted worldwide as a major technique for supporting critically ill patients in the hospital who, for a variety of reasons, cannot or should not use their gastrointestinal tracts.

In 1971, 3 years after the development of inpatient parenteral nutrition, Dr. Belding Scribner, the developer of the artificial kidney, devised a technique for providing parenteral nutrition at home for patients whose primary reason for remaining in the hospital was nutritional support. Dr. Scribner's first attempt at long-term parenteral support on an outpatient basis was with the use of arteriovenous shunts. For reasons that are not clear, the shunts frequently clotted, and the technique was not successful.

This problem led to the development of semipermanent catheters made of Silastic, which could be placed in the central venous circulation for prolonged intervals of time. Dr. Scribner, in conjunction with Dr. John Broviac, developed the Broviac Silastic catheter. The advantages of this catheter over others lay in its unique construction. The catheter had a Dacron cuff at its midpoint that, when placed in a subcutaneous tunnel on the chest or abdomen, caused a fibrous reaction to develop around it, resulting in adherence of the catheter to the chest or abdominal wall and prevented the catheter from becoming dislodged. In addition, the catheter had a Luer-Lok connection that allowed a screw cap to be placed over the end when the catheter was not being used.

Dr. Scribner and Dr. Broviac also developed techniques for aseptically cleaning the catheter when starting and discontinuing parenteral nutrition (as a means for utilizing it in cyclical TPN). They recognized that the catheter would have to be heparinized before it could be used for long-term therapy.

Two of the first patients who were sent home in 1972 on parenteral nutrition were children. One was a 10-year-old child who had systemic mast cell disease with involvement of the entire gastrointestinal tract, and the other was a 4-year-old child who had end-stage acrodermatitis enteropathica. In 1975, we instituted home parenteral nutrition for infants for the first time and in 1977, instituted parenteral nutrition for long-term home care in infants less than 3 months of age. The delay in developing such a program for young infants was caused by the lack of a miniature Silastic catheter for long-term support. However, in 1977, a miniature version of the Broviac catheter was developed for infants; it differed only in its length and its internal diameter from the standard catheter. Until that time, we had not gained sufficient experience with our adult patients to be confident of our success in getting infants to gain weight and grow normally while receiving cyclical TPN. This chapter describes for the practitioner the indications and technique of home hyperalimentation [6].

HOME TOTAL PARENTERAL NUTRITION IN INFANTS AND CHILDREN

The indications for home total parenteral nutrition in infants and children are summarized in Table 12-1.

In patients with short bowel syndrome, the physician must discuss with the surgeon the amount of intestine that is capable of absorption and determine if the patient has a good chance of adapting. It is known that infants who have at least 20 cm of small intestine plus an intact ileocecal valve have greater than a 50 percent chance of having intestinal adaptation and being able to discontinue total parenteral nutrition. Infants who have 40 cm of small intestine plus an intact ileocecal valve have greater than a 90 percent chance of adaptation. Infants who lack an ileocecal valve and have less than 20 cm of small intestine almost never adapt their enteral function; they will probably always be on parenteral nutrition. Therefore, the pediatric surgeon

Table 12-1. Indications for Home Parenteral Nutrition in Infants and Children

1. Short bowel syndrome in which the intestine will ultimately adapt and allow complete enteral support
2. Short bowel syndrome in which the intestine may ultimately adapt for complete enteral support
3. Short bowel syndrome in which the intestine is too short to ever support a patient by means of the enteral route
4. Chronic idiopathic intestinal pseudo-obstruction syndrome
5. Secondary pseudo-obstruction syndrome secondary to scleroderma
6. Mucosal injury severe enough to cause malabsorption syndrome
7. Mucosal injury secondary to severe gastrointestinal allergy
8. Severe mucosal injury secondary to viral invasion
9. Mucosal injury from unknown causes
10. Crohn's disease of the small intestine, which results in a short bowel syndrome or in which there is a failure of all medical therapy
11. Cystic fibrosis as a means to provide supplemental nutrition when an insufficient amount may be taken enterally
12. In cases of diffuse radiation injury of the small intestine

and pediatrician must confer on the likelihood that the patient with short bowel syndrome will adapt.

Patients with chronic idiopathic intestinal pseudo-obstruction syndrome may follow one of three patterns: those with the congenital variety of the disease who lack motility at birth may never develop any functional emptying of the stomach, small intestine, and/or colon. Another group who may appear clinically the same as the first group at birth may later develop motility in the digestive tract and be able to tolerate a limited amount of eating and drinking without being symptomatic. The third group includes infants in whom the condition develops suddenly, who have a limited period of bowel dysfunction, but who do have partial recovery of function with the passage of time and the use of parenteral support.

Patients with cystic fibrosis may benefit from the use of parenteral nutrition as a means of supplementing their limited caloric intake. It has been well established that parenteral nutrition in cystic fibrosis patients can have a major impact on their growth, weight gain, and maturation and improve pulmonary function. The use of parenteral nutrition in these patients helps ameliorate morbidity of the disease, which in part is secondary to nutritional deficiencies.

The physician is obligated to discuss with the family the prognosis, the odds of adaptation, the real costs, the potential complications, the potential mortality, and the benefits of long-term parenteral support [11]. Similarly, in patients with mucosal injury from recognized causes, the physician can counsel parents on the likelihood of full mucosal recovery after a period of prolonged bowel rest. A physician cannot be as confident when the source of the mucosal injury or failure of the mucosa to function in a normal fashion is unrecognized. Patients with Crohn's disease who have failed medical treatment and are not candidates for surgery should be told that parenteral support offers them a chance to maintain normal weight and rate of growth and possibly to gain a remission in a substantial number of cases. The family must then decide whether they want their child supported parenterally.

There are no absolute contraindications to the use of a home total parenteral nutrition program. The physician, however, must think carefully before offering it to a family when the child is severely impaired. When there are no family members who wish to care for an infant or child requiring home TPN, the physician must decide whether or not foster homes are available. Local government support also must be assured with the recognition that the child may need lifetime parenteral support. Thus far in our experience, only one set of parents decided against home parenteral nutrition. Their child had a midgut volvulus with a duodenal transverse colonic anastomosis. The parents felt that going through life without eating and drinking plus having the restrictions of a catheter was too much for their child. They chose no support for their infant. This was more than half a decade ago, and it is doubtful whether they would make such a choice today because of the relatively normal growth and weight gain induced by TPN and the limited difficulties in adaptation [4].

TECHNIQUE

The first step in establishing a patient on a home total parenteral nutrition program involves the placement of a central venous catheter into the circulation [5]. Any number of sites may be chosen for placement of the catheter. At our medical center, the external and internal jugular veins are the most commonly used; however, the femoral and

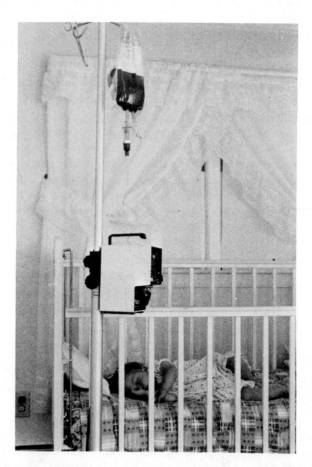

Figure 12-1. With the development of sophisticated infusion devices, the transition to home hyperalimentation is facilitated. (Photo courtesy of Enid Gillman, R.N., New England Critical Care, Inc.)

saphenous veins can also be used and are more easily reached, are less noticeable, and seem to be at no greater risk for clotting or becoming infected than catheters in the veins in the upper half of the torso.

An infant Broviac catheter is placed in all infants under 6 months of age, and a standard Broviac catheter is placed in infants between ages 6 months and 2 years [8]. After infancy, a Hickman catheter, which is a larger version of the Broviac catheter, is more typically used; it may be used for blood withdrawal as well as the administration of TPN and antibiotics. These catheters are typically placed by the surgical staff in the operating room under aseptic conditions. Two incisions are made on the chest and neck (or abdomen and thigh when femoral or saphenous veins are used). One is made to isolate a vein and the other is made in order to establish a subcutaneous tunnel through which the catheter is placed in order to establish it in a central vein. Once the catheter is established, the patient's parenteral nutrition program is started (Fig. 12-1).

NUTRITIONAL NEEDS

The physician must determine the nutritional needs of all patients on parenteral nutrition [1]. The fluid requirements of infants and children are summarized in Table 12-2.

Protein is provided in the form of an amino acid solution. The requirements are summarized in Table 12-3. Typically, amino acid solutions appropriately balanced for infants and children are used. Usu-

Table 12-2. Fluid Requirements for Infants and Children

Weight (kg)	Fluid (ml/kg/day)
0–10	100
11–20	100 (1st 10 kg)
	50 (2nd 10 kg)
21–up	100 (1st 10 kg)
	50 (2nd 10 kg)
	20 (after 20 kg)

Table 12-3. Protein Requirements

Age (yr)	Protein (gm/kg/day)
1 mo to 1 yr	2
1–3	1.5–2.0
4–6	1.5
7–10	1.0–1.5
11–18	1

Table 12-4. Caloric Requirements

Age (yr)	Kcal/kg/day
Term newborn infants	100–120
1–3	70–100
4–10	70–100
11–14	50–100
15–18	50–70

ally a 2% solution is provided. Standard solutions are used when possible to minimize the cost. Presently, no amino acid solution is truly better than any other.

Caloric needs are met by the solution (requirements are summarized in Table 12-4). The carbohydrate source of the solution is dextrose, which supplies 3.4 kcal/gm. TPN is generally started with a 10% dextrose solution and increased in concentration by 5% increments until the appropriate concentration provides the necessary calories. In cases where there is a restriction in the volume of fluid that may be administered safely, it is not uncommon to use a 30% or 35% dextrose solution in cases that require restriction of volume.

Intravenous fat is provided for two purposes: (1) to provide a concentrated energy source, and (2) to provide essential fats for metabolism and prevent essential fatty acid deficiency. Currently, there is a controversy as to whether linoleic acid is the only essential fatty acid; it is believed by some that linolenic acid is also essential. Typically, a minimum of 20 to 30 percent of the calories is preferred as lipid emulsion. Opinions vary concerning the superiority of one lipid preparation to the other. This relates to the relative deficiency of linolenic acid in the safflower oil emulsion. One case of linolenic acid deficiency has been described in a child on a long-term total parenteral nutrition program. Until this suspected deficiency can be clarified, the use of a soy oil emulsion is advised when possible. For those who fail to tolerate this, the use of limited amounts of corn oil given orally is recommended. In patients who tolerate intravenous lipids, 20 to 30 percent of calories are given as lipid in 10% or 20% solution depending on the availability and tolerance for fluid volumes. For patients who have no difficulty in handling fluid volumes, a 10% solution is used because it is less expensive. Electrolytes are provided in the concentrations recommended in Table 12-5. Bicarbonate is not given because it causes generation of CO_2 in the TPN solutions. Trace metals are also provided in the solution in the amounts summarized in Table 12-6.

Vitamin requirements are provided according to the RDA. For neonates, infants, and children, the entire vial typically is diluted in the volume of TPN solution. A pediatric multivitamin infusion is used

Table 12-5. Electrolyte Requirements

Electrolyte	Requirement
Sodium	2.5 mEq/100 kcal (plus replacement of losses from ostomies)
Potassium	1–2 mEq/100 kcal
Magnesium	0.3 mEq/kg
Phosphate	2 mmol/kg
Chloride	as sodium chloride or potassium chloride
Calcium (elemental)	
Infants	400–500 mg/day
Adolescents	600–700 mg/day

Table 12-6. Trace Metals

Trace Metal	Infants and Children (mg/kg/day)	Adolescents
Zinc	150–300	2–3 mg/day
Copper	20–40	0.5–1.5 mg/day
Chromium	0.1–0.4	10–20 mg/kg/day
Manganese	2–10	0.1–0.8 mg/day
Selenium	Not known	200 µg/day

that contains all recognized water- and fat-soluble vitamins including vitamins K, B_{12}, folic acid, and biotin.

HOME TOTAL PARENTERAL NUTRITION ROUTINE

Once a patient has had his or her formula formulated for parenteral nutrition, the infusion is begun over a period of 24 hours. After the maximal concentration of dextrose to be used is reached, the number of hours of infusion is decreased by 1 per day and the rate of infusion is increased proportionally. At the completion of the infusion, the rate of infusion is reduced by 50 percent for 15 minutes and then is reduced 50 percent again for an additional 15 minutes. The catheter is occluded, aseptically scrubbed at the site where the intravenous tubing joins the catheter, and disconnected. A heparin flush is given to ensure that the catheter does not become occluded during the hours when the infusion is not being given. A dose of 50 units of heparin per kilogram diluted to a volume of 3 ml is used to flush the catheter. Once the flushing procedure is completed, the syringe is disconnected and the catheter is capped either with a screw cap or an occlusion plug.

Some individuals prefer to use the injection or occlusion cap on the end of their catheters because this does not require as many steps in cleaning and potentially may lessen the risk of contamination. However, this has not definitely been established. The injection caps that may be used on the Broviac or Hickman catheters are disposable and should be changed at least once per week. Disposable Broviac catheter caps are available and may be discarded on a daily basis; one problem with them is they may leak. The disposable caps allow disposal of the 1½% formalin solution that these caps are usually kept in to prevent them from becoming contaminated.

Most infants and children tolerate a rapid rate of parenteral nutrition and typically receive all their nutritional needs over a period of 10 to 12 hours. Occasional patients are intolerant of the rapid rate of infusion and may require a longer period in which to administer the parenteral nutrition solution. These are typically patients who have either pulmonary and/or cardiac disease.

In patients who develop cardiopulmonary symptoms from the rapid infusion of the parenteral nutrition solutions, the physician may choose to do one of two things: (1) give the infusion over a longer period of time, or (2) decrease the volume of parenteral nutrition solutions given by increasing the concentration of the nutrients in the solution. This may be successful in a patient with cardiac or pulmonary disease who might not have been able to tolerate more dilute solutions in larger volumes. Some physicians believe that a period of 10 to 12 days for adaptation to the rapid infusion of the parenteral nutrition solutions is excessive and that adaptation can be achieved more rapidly. We were able to bring about adaptation in as little as 1 week in a selected group of patients. Unfortunately, these patients were found to be at greater risk for developing hyperglycemia and glycosuria. The 10- to 12-day period of adaptation typically required to reach the maximal rate of infusion actually has an advantage: it is compatible with the amount of time it takes to train parents and/or youngsters to do the home TPN care.

Both parents should learn the routines for home TPN care so that one may assist the other and in case one of the parents becomes ill. It is also advisable to try and teach TPN techniques to other family members such as older siblings, grandparents, aunts, uncles, and cousins who may take an active interest in the patient and want to help provide his or her care. These family members can relieve exhausted parents of some of their responsibility. By having other family members able to do this care, the parents are able to take nights, weekends, and/or vacations away from their child if they so choose. This is important because home parenteral nutrition can be a tiring and time-consuming task that goes on day after day, month after month, and possibly indefinitely. The respite care that can be provided by other family members ensures that the patient will receive more optimal care from his or her parents.

In certain instances when no family members are available to care for the youngsters and/or to provide respite care, home health care agencies may have trained nurses come in and care for the child in order to give parents a rest from the routines. We strongly urge physicians who place patients on home TPN to develop plans for care in case the parents are not always able to care for their youngsters.

HOME TEACHING OF PARENTERAL NUTRITION TECHNIQUES

The training of families for home parenteral nutrition should involve didactic sessions given by a nurse, pharmacist, or physician who is expert in the techniques of home care. Reading pamphlets and/or books developed by the hospital or home health care agencies on these techniques will also be helpful.

The parents of our patients see a TV tape showing each one of the steps required for connecting and disconnecting the patient from parenteral nutrition that demonstrates all techniques. The family has the opportunity to see the nurse perform the techniques on a mannequin and can practice on the mannequin themselves while the nurse offers advice and assistance to perfect the technique.

The practice is done on a daily basis under the supervision of a parenteral nutrition care nurse who must ensure that the patient's central line is not jeopardized by family members as they are being trained. After the training nurse certifies that family members can do the techniques flawlessly in her presence for at least 2 days, we would then encourage the parent or other family members to do the care for at least 5 to 7 days in the hospital unattended by nursing personnel; family members should understand that the nurse will provide assistance if it is needed.

Once the training nurse certifies the competence of family members with home techniques, the patient is ready for discharge. Prior to discharge, the medical social worker must determine the financial eligibility of the family in order to learn who is going to pay for the home health care. Fortunately, in most states, this is paid for by private medical insurance, major medical insurance, Medicaid, and by social security insurance. Few children are financially ineligible for home care. It is important to establish financial responsibility early in order to avoid stress caused by the cost factors in home care.

The social worker must also determine if the family has adequate space for the parenteral support supplies and should visit the home to determine whether or not the household is clean and orderly. Within 24 hours of discharge, a visiting nurse trained in home parenteral nutrition techniques should visit the home in order to detect any problems with the home TPN techniques. It is his or her job to report whether or not things are satisfactory to the physicians who care for these youngsters.

The family must decide whether they wish to have the solutions delivered directly to their homes or come to the hospital as the source. Currently there are three methods for obtaining home parenteral nutrition supplies and equipment. The patient's hospital may directly mix the solutions for the patient and provide them on a weekly or monthly basis. The solutions typically contain all the nutrients except vitamins, which are added just before the solutions are administered. Any patient who may also require insulin or other drugs typically has them added just before they are to be used.

Some patients' families may elect to have all supplies and solutions delivered directly to the home. Reputable home parenteral nutrition companies are currently in business throughout the United States. Some offer a variety of services, including home delivery, nursing care, and counseling; others offer very little except delivery of supplies and solutions.

The third method is to have the patient's family mix their own solutions. This is the cheapest method, but it takes 30 to 60 minutes to mix the solution, thereby reducing the time family members have to work or do other household chores.

Physicians must remember that home health care agencies are not doctors, and it remains the physician's responsibility to care for the patients. All problems of these patients must be directed back to the physician to ultimately resolve or concur with decisions regarding changes in formulation, changes in feeding, and complications.

OUTPATIENT MANAGEMENT

In the case of infants and children, doctors see home parenteral nutrition patients on a weekly basis in the first month after discharge. Throughout the remainder of the first year of life, these youngsters are seen on a monthly basis. Beyond the first year of life, patients are seen on a quarterly basis. Of course, the frequency of visits must be flexible, and some patients may require more frequent visits depending on the problems parents may have in dealing with home parenteral nutrition.

At each visit, weight and height are recorded, the mid-arm muscle circumference and triceps skinfold thickness are measured, and blood chemistries are obtained for electrolytes, calcium, magnesium, total protein, and albumin. Liver function tests are also performed and a complete blood count is taken.

Trace metal determinations need to be done quarterly or semiannually. At each visit, the physician or the TPN team associates must sit down and calculate the number of milliliters of fluid the patient receives per day, the number of calories per kilogram, the number of grams of protein per kilogram, the number of grams of fat, and the concentrations of all the other nutrients. The physician then determines whether the growing child should have an increase in the volume and/or a change in the concentration of the various nutrients. With attention to height, weight, and blood chemistry, the patient can be adequately monitored and normal growth and weight gain can be achieved.

At each clinic visit, the members of the home support team see and talk with the parents and/or examine the patient. The home parenteral nutrition nurse asks if there are any problems with the techniques being used by the patient and the family. The pharmacist discusses with the family any problems concerning solution delivery and/or composition of the solutions [2]. Each patient is given a card that lists the solutions they receive and the nutrient concentrations of the solutions so that this information is readily available at each visit. The social worker also visits with the family and determines whether there are any financial problems and/or social problems caused by the youngster's illness and if parenteral support is needed. The social worker's job is also to determine whether there are any family problems [7].

It is the physician's role to examine the patient, review the laboratory data obtained, and to look at the nutrients provided to determine if and how the formulation should be changed.

CLINICAL EXPERIENCE WITH HOME TPN

The numbers, ages, and major diagnoses of our home TPN population are summarized in Table 12-7. Prior to the start of home parenteral nutrition therapy, 20 patients with Crohn's disease had been treated

Table 12-7. Clinical Profile of Home TPN Patients

Clinical Aspects	Number of Patients
Total	54
Sex distribution	
Males	37
Females	17
Age of placement of central venous catheter	
<6 months	9
1 yr–<10 yr	10
10 yr–<15 yr	18
15 yr–<21 yr	17
Major diagnosis	
Crohn's disease	20
Short bowel syndrome	16
Chronic idiopathic intestinal pseudo-obstruction syndrome	8
Mucosal injury of unknown etiology	4
Congenital failure of villous development	4
Cystic fibrosis	2

with Azulfidine, adrenocorticosteroids, and/or previous surgical resections. Four of the eight patients with chronic idiopathic intestinal
pseudo-obstruction syndrome developed obstructive symptoms and/
or diarrhea in the neonatal period. In two, home parenteral nutrition
was started within the first 3 months of life, while the other patients
were hospitalized intermittently during infancy and/or did not develop
their symptoms until later childhood. The patients with mucosal injury
had chronic diarrhea from virtually the first day of life, and three of
the cases had evidence of hypoplasia of the intestinal mucosa; they
had almost no villous development and virtually no mitotic figures
in the crypt epithelium. The others, including two with combined
immune deficiency disease, developed chronic diarrhea in the last
half of the first year of life and require parenteral nutrition on a daily
basis even now. They are now 3 and 5 years of age.

Two patients had complete healing of their intestinal mucosa but
it took nearly 18 months for this to occur. Of the patients with short
bowel syndrome, the etiology in most was secondary to jejunal-ileal
atresia or necrotizing enterocolitis. Two patients developed midgut
volvulus after age 1 year, one had a traumatic injury to the bowel
secondary to a pool-sweep accident, and the remainder were born
with congenitally short small intestines. Adaptation has occurred in
half of this group. One patient with 14 cm of small intestine plus an
intact ileocecal valve now receives three-quarters of his nutrition enterally; it is very likely he will soon adapt completely.

Two patients with cystic fibrosis have used parenteral support both
for antibiotics and supplemental nutrition. These patients were post-
pubertal and had severe chronic lung disease. The use of the catheter
enabled them to stay home and receive antibiotics rather than being
repeatedly hospitalized.

Of the patients with Crohn's disease, primary complications leading
to initiation of home parenteral nutrition was growth failure in nine,
enterocutaneous fistula in four, steroid unresponsive diffuse disease
in two, obstructive symptoms in two, short bowel syndrome in one,
severe rectal fissure with incontinence in one, and chronic pancreatitis
in one [10].

All those with diffuse small bowel disease unresponsive to medical
therapy went into clinical remission. No patients who had an obstructive lesion had a reversion of the stricture. The parenteral support
did not seem to result in healing of perianal fissures or fistulas, and
these patients required surgery for this problem. Of the patients with
pseudo-obstruction syndrome, some remarkable observations were
made. Patients who at the time of birth had no intestinal motility had
gradual development of motility with the passage of time. They began
to have ostomy output and began to eat and drink. Some of the
youngsters who began home TPN in the neonatal period now take

one-third to one-half of their calories enterally. It is interesting to note that if, for any reason, the parenteral nutrition solutions are withdrawn, their motility gradually fails and they develop obstructive symptoms. It is not known if there is some specific substance or substances in the parenteral support responsible for this phenomenon. Unfortunately, there are some infants with pseudo-obstruction syndrome at birth who do not develop motility.

The average catheter life per patient was in excess of 1,220 days. The average catheter required repair for breakage every 400 to 500 days. The most common complication in patients on home support was the development of chronic liver disease, especially in patients who received 90 percent or more of their nutrition parenterally. In patients with short bowel syndrome where TPN was necessary, all developed some degree of hepatic fibrosis and/or cirrhosis after 1 or more years on parenteral support.

Cholelithiasis developed in more than 40 percent of all patients who received parenteral nutrition for more than 3 months. This is an astounding figure in view of the patients' ages, because the risk of cholelithiasis in this age group is less than 1 in 16,000 at autopsy.

Death has occurred in eight of the 54 patients. Overwhelming sepsis was responsible for six of the deaths, two deaths were caused by end-stage liver disease, and one patient died of an unknown cause. Rare complications have occurred, such as superior vena cava thrombosis in three patients and perforation of the brachial vein in one patient. Perforation of the vena cava occurred in one patient.

The organisms most commonly associated with septic death have been *Staphylococcus aureus* and *Candida*. In instances where few, if any, catheter sites remain available, the physician may choose to treat the catheter with systemic antibiotics. The catheters may be treated for up to 1 month if the organism is susceptible to treatment. At the end of 1 month, the antibiotics are discontinued and cultures are repeated after 48 hours. Treating patients with *Candida* infections of their central line has not been successful; the line is always removed, and the patient is treated with amphotericin.

CONCLUSION

Home parenteral nutrition for children has demonstrated that youngsters can grow and gain weight normally and live a near-normal life. Testing of the youngsters appears to demonstrate that intelligence has been at the appropriate level within each family [9]. Psychosocial problems are apparent in a few of the children, but these have not yet been well defined [3].

All school-age children attend regular schools with regular classes. All preschool-age children attend appropriate nurseries. Only two of all the children are retarded; one of these had multiple congenital facial anomalies, imperforate anus, and absence of a stomach at the time of birth.

Bowel adaptation has occurred in all infants with at least 14 cm of small intestine and an intact ileocecal valve. However, the final outcome for these children is still in question because their survival depends on the continued maintenance of venous access and their avoiding long-term complications of sepsis and progressive liver disease.

REFERENCES

1. Cannon, R. A., Byrne, W. J., Ament, M. E., Gates, B., O'Connor, M., and Fonkalsrud, E. W. Home parenteral nutrition in infants. *J. Pediatr.* 96:1098, 1980.
2. Karnack, C. M., Gallina, J. N., and Jeffrey, I. P. Pharmacist involvement in home parenteral nutrition programs. *Am. J. Hosp. Pharm.* 38(2):215, 1981.
3. Ladefoged, K. Quality of life in patients on permanent home parenteral nutrition. *J.P.E.N.* 5(2):132, 1981.
4. Lees, C. D., Steiger, E., Hooley, R. A., Montague, N., Srp, F., Gulledge, A. D., Wateska, L. P., and Frame, C. Home parenteral nutrition. *Surg. Clin. North Am.* 61(3):621, 1981.
5. Maksimak, M., Ament, M. E., and Fonkalsrud, E. W. Comparison of the pediatric broviac silastic catheter with a standard no. 3 french silastic catheter for central venous alimentation. *J. Pediat. Gastroenterol. Nutr.* 1:227, 1982.
6. Parfitt, D. M., and Thompson, V. D. Pediatric home hyperalimentation: Educating the family. *Matern. Child Nurs. J.* 5(3):196, 1980.
7. Perl, M., Hall, R. C., Dudrick, S. J., Englert, D. M., Stickney, S. K., and Gardner, E. R. Psychological aspects of long-term home hyperalimentation. *J.P.E.N.* 4(6):554, 1980.
8. Pollack, P. F., Kamden, M., Byrne, W. J., Fonkalsrud, E. W., and Ament, M. E. 100 patient years experience with the broviac silastic catheter for central venous nutrition. *J.P.E.N.* 5(1):32, 1981.
9. Roslyn, J. J., Berquist, W. E., Pitt, H. A., Mann, L. L., Kangarloo, H., DenBesten, L., and Ament, M. E. Increased risk of gallstones in children receiving total parenteral nutrition. *Pediatrics* 71:784, 1983.
10. Strobel, C. T., Bryne, W. J., and Ament, M.E. Home parenteral nutrition in children with Crohn's disease: An effective management alternative. *Gastroenterology* 77:272, 1979.
11. Wateska, L. P., Sattler, L., and Steiger, E. Cost of a home parenteral nutrition program. *J.A.M.A.* 244:2303, 1980.

Appendixes

Thalia Metalides

Appendix 1. Recommended Nutrient Intakes

A. Recommended Daily Dietary Allowances
B. Mean Heights and Weights and Recommended Energy Intake
C. Estimated Safe and Adequate Daily Dietary Intakes of Selected Vitamins and Minerals
D. Average Energy Intakes (0–3 years)

A. Recommended Daily Dietary Allowances

	Age (years)	Weight kg	lb	Height cm	in.	Protein gm	Fat-soluble vitamins Vitamin A µg RE[b]	Vitamin D µg[c]	Vitamin E mg α-TE[d]	Vitamin C mg	Thiamine mg
Infants	0.0–0.5	6	13	60	24	kg × 2.2	420	10	3	35	0.3
	0.5–1.0	9	20	71	28	kg × 2.0	400	10	4	35	0.5
Children	1–3	13	29	90	35	23	400	10	5	45	0.7
	4–6	20	44	112	44	30	500	10	6	45	0.9
	7–10	28	62	132	52	34	700	10	7	45	1.2
Males	11–14	45	99	157	62	45	1000	10	8	50	1.4
	15–18	66	145	176	69	56	1000	10	10	60	1.4
	19–22	70	154	177	70	56	1000	7.5	10	60	1.5
	23–50	70	154	178	70	56	1000	5	10	60	1.4
	51 +	70	154	178	70	56	1000	5	10	60	1.2
Females	11–14	46	101	157	62	46	800	10	8	50	1.1
	15–18	55	120	163	64	46	800	10	8	60	1.1
	19–22	55	120	163	64	44	800	7.5	8	60	1.1
	23–50	55	120	163	64	44	800	5	8	60	1.0
	51 +	55	120	163	64	44	800	5	8	60	1.0
Pregnant						+30	+200	+5	+2	+20	+0.4
Lactating						+20	+400	+5	+3	+40	+0.5

[a]Designed for the maintenance of good nutrition of practically all healthy people in the United States. The allowances are intended to provide for individual variations among most normal persons as they live in the United States under usual environmental stresses. Diets should be based on a variety of common foods in order to provide other nutrients for which human requirements have been less well defined. See Appendix 1-B for weights and heights by individual year of age and for suggested average energy intakes.

[b]Retinol equivalents. 1 retinol equivalent = 1 µg retinol or 6 µg β carotene.

[c]As cholecalciferol. 10 µg cholecalciferol = 400 IU of vitamin D.

[d]α-Tocopherol equivalents. 1 mg d-α tocopherol = 1 α-TE.

[e]1 NE (niacin equivalent) is equal to 1 mg of niacin or 60 mg of dietary tryptophan.

[f]The folacin allowances refer to dietary sources as determined by Lactobacillus casei assay after treatment with enzymes (conjugases) to make polyglutamyl forms of the vitamin available to the test organism.

[g]The recommended dietary allowance for vitamin B_{12} in infants is based on average concentration of the vitamin in human milk. The allowances after weaning are based on energy intake (as recommended by the American Academy of Pediatrics) and consideration of other factors, such as intestinal absorption.

[h]The increased requirement during pregnancy cannot be met by the iron content of habitual American diets nor by the existing iron stores of many women; therefore the use of 30–60 mg of supplemental iron is recommended. Iron needs during lactation are not substantially different from those of nonpregnant women, but continued supplementation of the mother for 2–3 months after parturition is advisable in order to replenish stores depleted by pregnancy.

Source: Food and Nutrition Board, *Recommended Daily Dietary Allowances*, Revised 1980, National Academy of Sciences, National Research Council.

Water-soluble vitamins					Minerals					
Ribo-flavin mg	Niacin mg NE[e]	Vitamin B_6 mg	Folacin[f] μg	Vitamin B_12 μg	Calcium mg	Phos-phorus mg	Magne-sium mg	Iron mg	Zinc mg	Iodine μg
0.4	6	0.3	30	0.5[g]	360	240	50	10	3	40
0.6	8	0.6	45	1.5	540	360	70	15	5	50
0.8	9	0.9	100	2.0	800	800	150	15	10	70
1.0	11	1.3	200	2.5	800	800	200	10	10	90
1.4	16	1.6	300	3.0	800	800	250	10	10	120
1.6	18	1.8	400	3.0	1200	1200	350	18	15	150
1.7	18	2.0	400	3.0	1200	1200	400	18	15	150
1.7	19	2.2	400	3.0	800	800	350	10	15	150
1.6	18	2.2	400	3.0	800	800	350	10	15	150
1.4	16	2.2	400	3.0	800	800	350	10	15	150
1.3	15	1.8	400	3.0	1200	1200	300	18	15	150
1.3	14	2.0	400	3.0	1200	1200	300	18	15	150
1.3	14	2.0	400	3.0	800	800	300	18	15	150
1.2	13	2.0	400	3.0	800	800	300	18	15	150
1.2	13	2.0	400	3.0	800	800	300	10	15	150
+0.3	+2	+0.6	+400	+1.0	+400	+400	+150	[h]	+5	+25
+0.5	+5	+0.5	+100	+1.0	+400	+400	+150	[h]	+10	+50

B. Mean Heights and Weights and Recommended Energy Intake*

Category	Age (years)	Weight		Height		Energy needs (with range)		
		kg	lb	cm	in.	kcal		MJ
Infants	0.0–0.5	6	13	60	24	kg × 115	(95–145)	kg × 0.48
	0.5–1.0	9	20	71	28	kg × 105	(80–135)	kg × 0.44
Children	1–3	13	29	90	35	1300	(900–1800)	5.5
	4–6	20	44	112	44	1700	(1300–2300)	7.1
	7–10	28	62	132	52	2400	(1650–3300)	10.1
Males	11–14	45	99	157	62	2700	(2000–3700)	11.3
	15–18	66	145	176	69	2800	(2100–3900)	11.8
	19–22	70	154	177	70	2900	(2500–3300)	12.2
	23–50	70	154	178	70	2700	(2300–3100)	11.3
	51–75	70	154	178	70	2400	(2000–2800)	10.1
	76+	70	154	178	70	2050	(1650–2450)	8.6
Females	11–14	46	101	157	62	2200	(1500–3000)	9.2
	15–18	55	120	163	64	2100	(1200–3000)	8.8
	19–22	55	120	163	64	2100	(1700–2500)	8.8
	23–50	55	120	163	64	2000	(1600–2400)	8.4
	51–75	55	120	163	64	1800	(1400–2200)	7.6
	76+	55	120	163	64	1600	(1200–2000)	6.7
Pregnancy						+300		
Lactation						+500		

*The data in this table have been assembled from the observed median heights and weights of children shown in Appendix 1-A. The mean heights of men (70 in.) and women (64 in.) between the ages of 18 and 34 years as surveyed in the U.S. population (HEW/NCHS data).

The energy allowances for the young adults are for men and women doing light work. The allowances for the two older age groups represent mean energy needs over these age spans, allowing for a 2-percent decrease in basal (resting) metabolic rate per decade and a reduction in activity of 200 kcal/day for men and women between 51 and 75 years, 500 kcal for men over 75 years, and 400 kcal for women over 75 years. The customary range of daily energy output is shown in parentheses for adults and is based on a variation in energy needs of ± 400 kcal at any one age, emphasizing the wide range of energy intakes appropriate for any group of people.

Energy allowances for children through age 18 are based on median energy intakes of children of these ages followed in longitudinal growth studies. The values in parentheses are 10th and 90th percentiles of energy intake, to indicate the range of energy consumption among children of these ages.

Source: Food and Nutrition Board, *Recommended Daily Dietary Allowances*, Revised 1980, National Academy of Sciences, National Research Council.

C. Estimated Safe and Adequate Daily Dietary Intakes of Selected Vitamins and Minerals[a]

Vitamins

Age (years)	Vitamin K (µg)	Biotin (µg)	Pantothenic Acid (mg)
Infants			
0–0.5	12	35	2
0.5–1.0	10–20	50	3
Children and adolescents			
1–3	15–30	65	3
4–6	20–40	85	3–4
7–10	30–60	120	4–5
11+	50–100	100–200	4–7
Adults	70–140	100–200	4–7

Trace Elements[b]

Age (years)	Copper (mg)	Manganese (mg)	Fluoride (mg)	Chromium (mg)	Selenium (mg)	Molybdenum (mg)
Infants						
0–0.5	0.5–0.7	0.5–0.7	0.1–0.5	0.01–0.04	0.01–0.04	0.03–0.06
0.5–1.0	0.7–1.0	0.7–1.0	0.2–1.0	0.02–0.06	0.02–0.06	0.04–0.08
Children and adolescents						
1–3	1.0–1.5	1.0–1.5	0.5–1.5	0.02–0.08	0.02–0.08	0.05–0.1
4–6	1.5–2.0	1.5–2.0	1.0–2.5	0.03–0.12	0.03–0.12	0.06–0.15
7–10	2.0–2.5	2.0–3.0	1.5–2.5	0.05–0.2	0.05–0.2	0.10–0.3
11+	2.0–3.0	2.5–5.0	1.5–2.5	0.05–0.2	0.05–0.2	0.15–0.5
Adults	2.0–3.0	2.5–5.0	1.5–4.0	0.05–0.2	0.05–0.2	0.15–0.5

Electrolytes

Age (years)	Sodium (mg)	Potassium (mg)	Chloride (mg)
Infants			
0–0.5	115–350	350–925	275–700
0.5–1.0	250–750	425–1275	400–1200
Children and adolescents			
1–3	325–975	550–1650	500–1500
4–6	450–1350	775–2325	700–2100
7–10	600–1800	1000–3000	925–2775
11+	900–2700	1525–4575	1400–4200
Adults	1100–3300	1875–5625	1700–5100

[a]Because there is less information on which to base allowances, these figures are not given in the main table of RDA and are provided here in the form of ranges of recommended intakes.

[b]Since the toxic levels for many trace elements may be only several times usual intakes, the upper levels for the trace elements given in this table should not be habitually exceeded.

Source: Food and Nutrition Board, *Recommended Daily Dietary Allowances*, Revised 1980, National Academy of Sciences, National Research Council.

D. Average Energy Intakes (0–3 years)

Age Range (yr/mo)	Number	Mean	SD	Total Calories Percentiles					Calories/kg Body Weight Percentiles			Calories/cm Body Height Percentiles		
				10th	25th	50th	75th	90th	10th	50th	90th	10th	50th	90th
MALES														
0/0–0/1	33	405	110	275	315	400	480	580	88	115	150	5.7	7.7	10.7
0/1–0/2	39	575	86	465	515	565	635	680	108	131	157	8.7	10.3	12.0
0/2–0/3	42	630	107	505	545	625	715	795	93	116	139	8.4	10.8	13.3
0/3–0/4	44	655	97	550	590	640	715	785	90	103	124	9.1	10.4	12.7
0/4–0/5	46	710	124	550	625	675	810	885	88	101	122	8.9	10.5	13.5
0/5–0/6	45	760	138	615	670	740	850	960	81	100	122	9.4	11.0	14.3
0/6–0/9	46	845	135	710	760	820	895	1020	82	100	123	10.1	11.8	14.5
0/9–1/0	49	985	196	795	845	925	1070	1230	81	101	137	10.6	12.5	17.7
1/0–1/3	47	1060	277	745	845	990	1240	1430	71	98	138	9.6	13.0	19.2
1/3–1/6	46	1165	276	850	935	1135	1350	1480	78	103	136	10.6	14.3	18.6
1/6–1/9	45	1215	271	855	1000	1220	1425	1565	75	102	136	10.3	14.3	19.0
1/9–2/0	44	1260	265	895	1050	1255	1415	1560	73	108	127	10.6	14.9	18.2
2/0–2/3	45	1320	298	965	1135	1290	1475	1705	75	103	135	10.8	14.8	19.2
2/3–2/6	44	1385	294	1055	1205	1375	1560	1840	81	104	136	11.6	14.8	20.6
2/6–2/9	45	1420	312	1050	1150	1435	1625	1850	73	102	129	11.4	15.4	20.0
2/9–3/0	43	1480	286	1175	1275	1430	1635	1975	78	103	129	12.1	15.2	20.0

FEMALES

0/0–0/1	23	385	86	290	310	375	440	510	84	115	144	5.8	7.7	9.7
0/1–0/2	30	530	105	415	445	510	580	700	100	131	160	7.6	9.6	13.0
0/2–0/3	32	565	90	455	510	580	645	675	98	115	133	8.0	10.1	11.4
0/3–0/4	34	620	84	515	575	615	665	730	97	111	130	8.8	10.5	12.1
0/4–0/5	37	665	85	540	615	675	725	775	89	104	120	8.8	10.7	12.5
0/5–0/6	38	715	93	610	635	690	770	840	89	104	127	9.6	10.8	12.7
0/6–0/9	41	770	122	620	690	760	825	915	76	97	122	9.2	11.1	14.3
0/9–1/0	44	885	149	705	755	890	950	1125	80	97	129	9.8	12.0	15.8
1/0–1/3	45	985	216	720	820	980	1095	1245	79	98	136	9.9	12.7	17.2
1/3–1/6	45	1080	212	810	880	1075	1250	1355	79	104	139	10.4	14.2	17.7
1/6–1/9	44	1140	214	915	970	1080	1290	1430	79	103	135	11.0	13.4	17.7
1/9–2/0	45	1195	215	945	1015	1165	1330	1485	78	103	134	11.1	14.0	17.7
2/0–2/3	47	1230	248	945	1075	1200	1330	1545	78	99	135	11.0	13.8	17.8
2/3–2/6	48	1235	232	945	1070	1210	1375	1515	75	96	131	10.8	13.8	17.3
2/6–2/9	46	1245	261	970	1095	1210	1345	1585	74	94	124	10.6	13.4	17.5
2/9–3/0	45	1300	296	990	1125	1250	1460	1765	72	93	124	10.6	13.3	19.0

Source: McGammon, R. W. *Human Growth and Development.* Springfield, Illinois: Charles C Thomas, 1970.

Appendix 2. Growth Charts

A. Normal Growth Charts
B. Down Syndrome Growth Charts

A. Normal Growth Charts

These charts to record the growth of the individual child were constructed by the National Center for Health Statistics in collaboration with the Center for Disease Control. The charts are based on data from the Fels Research Institute, Yellow Springs, Ohio. These data are appropriate for young [boys and girls] in the general U.S. population. Their use will direct attention to unusual body size, which may be due to disease or poor nutrition.

MEASURING

Take all measurements with the child nude or with minimal clothing and without shoes. Measure length with the child lying on [his or her] back fully extended. Two people are needed to measure recumbent length properly. Use a beam balance to measure weight.

RECORDING

First take all measurements and record them. Then graph each measurement on the appropriate chart. Find the child's age on the horizontal scale; then follow a vertical line from that point to the horizontal level of the child's measurement (length, weight, or head circumference). Where the two lines intersect, make a cross mark with a pencil. In graphing weight for length, place the cross mark directly above the child's length at the horizontal level of his or her weight. When the child is measured again, join the new set of cross marks to the previous set by straight lines.

INTERPRETING

Many factors influence growth. Therefore, growth data cannot be used alone to diagnose disease, but they do allow you to identify some unusual children.

Each chart contains a series of curved lines numbered to show selected percentiles. These refer to the rank of a measure in a group of 100. Thus, when a cross mark is on the ninety-fifth percentile line of weight for age it means that only five children among 100 of the corresponding age and sex have weights greater than that recorded.

Inspect the set of cross marks you have just made. If any are particularly high or low (for example, above the ninety-fifth percentile or below the fifth percentile), you may want to refer the child to a physician. *Compare* the most recent set of cross marks with earlier sets for the same child. If he or she has changed rapidly in percentile levels, you may want to refer him or her to a physician. Rapid changes are less likely to be significant when they occur within the range from the twenty-fifth to the seventy-fifth percentile.

Department of Health, Education, and Welfare, Public Health Service Health Resources Administration, National Center for Health Statistics, and Center for Disease Control

363

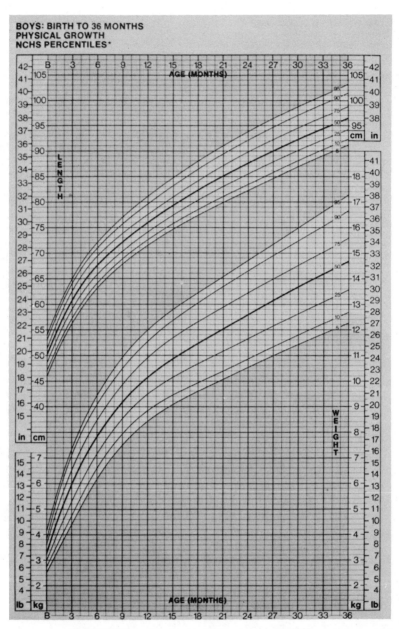

Figure 2A-1. Boys, birth to 36 months: length and weight. (From United States National Center for Health Statistics Monthly Vital Statistics Report 25 No. 3 Supplement NCHS Growth Charts, 1976. Hyattsville, Md.: Public Health Administration, June 1976 [DHEW Publication No. (HRA) 76-1120].)

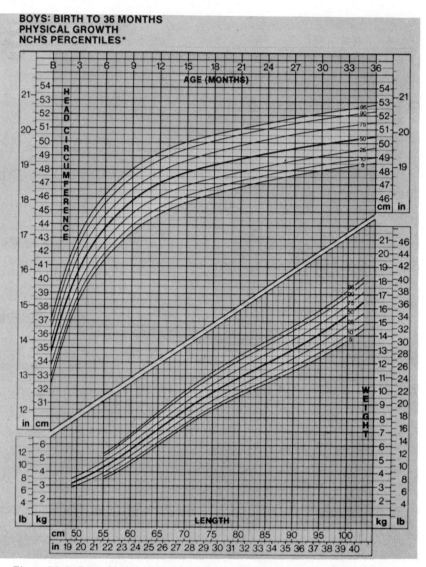

Figure 2A-2. Boys, birth to 36 months: head circumference and weight. (From United States National Center for Health Statistics Monthly Vital Statistics Report 25 No. 3 Supplement NCHS Growth Charts, 1976. Hyattsville, Md.: Public Health Administration, June 1976 [DHEW Publication No. (HRA) 76-1120].)

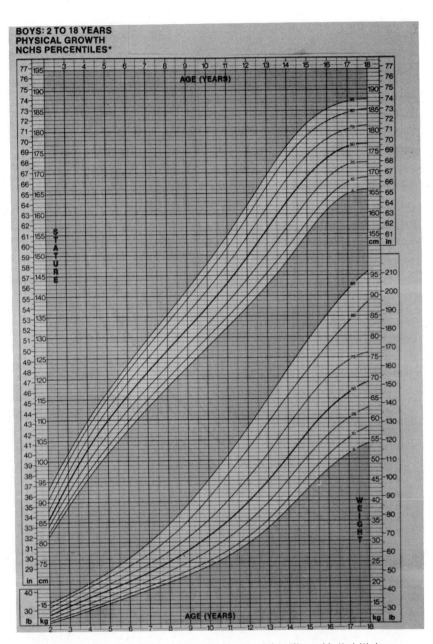

Figure 2A-3. boys, 2 to 18 years: stature and weight. (From United States National Center for Health Statistics Monthly Vital Statistics Report 25 No. 3 Supplement NCHS Growth Charts, 1976. Hyattsville, Md.: Public Health Administration, June 1976 [DHEW Publication No. (HRA) 76-1120].)

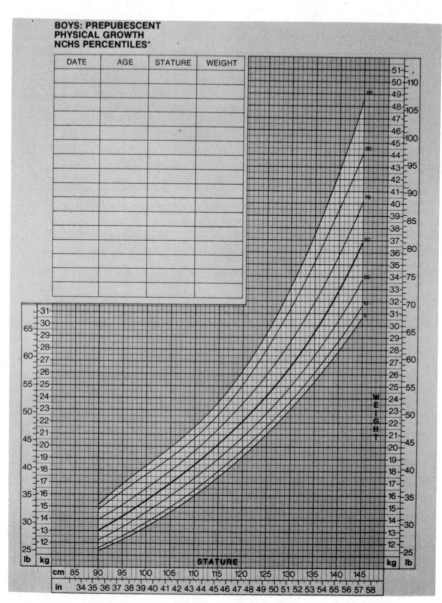

Figure 2A-4. Boys: prepubescent physical growth. (From United States National Center for Health Statistics Monthly Vital Statistics Report No. 3 Supplement NHCS Growth Charts, 1976. Hyattsville, Md.: Public Health Administration, June 1976 [DHEW Publication No. (HRA) 76-1120].)

GIRLS: BIRTH TO 36 MONTHS
PHYSICAL GROWTH
NCHS PERCENTILES*

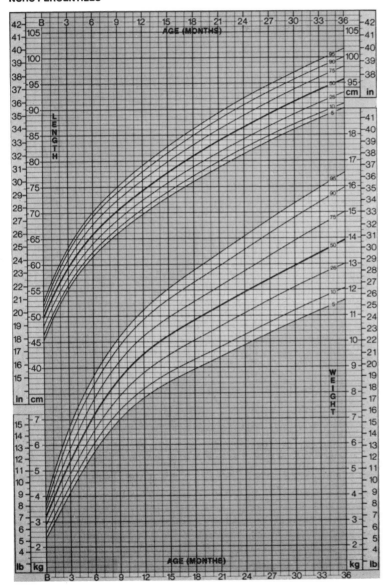

Figure 2A-5. Girls, birth to 36 months: length and weight. (From United States National Center for Health Statistics Monthly Vital Statistics Report No. 3 Supplement NCHS Growth Charts, 1976. Hyattsville, Md.: Public Health Administration, June 1976 [DHEW Publication No. (HRA) 76-1120].)

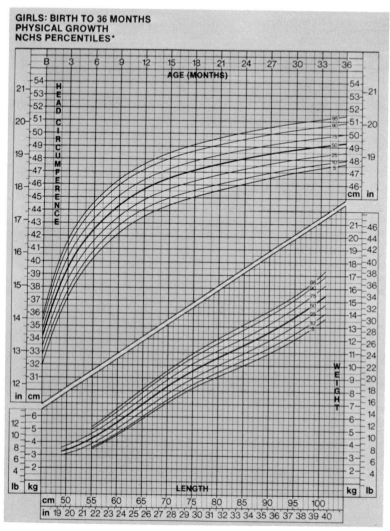

Figure 2A-6. Girls, birth to 36 months: head circumference and weight. (From United States National Center for Health Statistics Monthly Vital Statistics Report No. 3 Supplement NCHS Growth Charts, 1976. Hyattsville, Md.: Public Health Administration, June 1976 [DHEW Publication No. (HRA) 76-1120].)

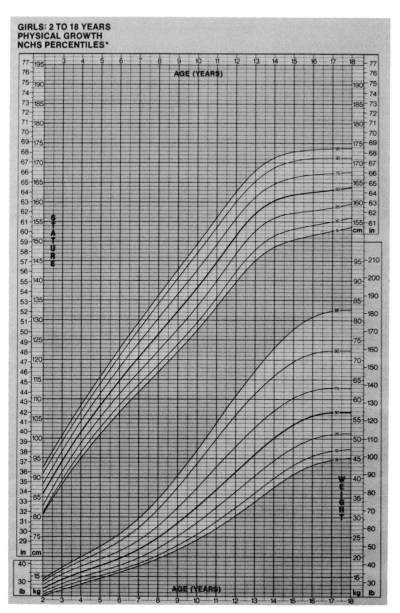

GIRLS: 2 TO 18 YEARS
PHYSICAL GROWTH
NCHS PERCENTILES*

Figure 2A-7. Girls, 2 to 18 years: stature and weight. (From United States National Center for Health Statistics Monthly Vital Statistics Report No. 3 Supplement NCHS Growth Charts, 1976. Hyattsville, Md.: Public Health Administration, June 1976 [DHEW Publication No. (HRA) 76-1120].)

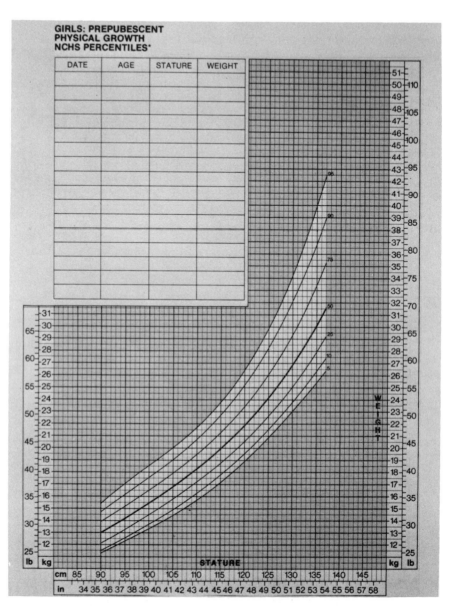

Figure 2A-8. Girls: prepubescent physical growth. (From United States National Center for Health Statistics Monthly Vital Statistics Report No. 3 Supplement NCHS Growth Charts, 1976. Hyattsville, Md.: Public Health Administration, June 1976 [DHEW Publication No. (HRA) 76-1120].)

B. Down Syndrome Growth Charts

Ninety children with Down syndrome were measured for recumbent length and weight from birth to age 36 months at The Children's Hospital, Boston, Ma. At birth, means for both length and weight were reduced by about 0.5 SD from the control group means. By 36 months, mean recumbent length was greater than 2 SD below that for the control group, while the mean for weight was reduced by about 1.5 SD from the control group mean. Growth velocity for both length and weight was most deficient within the first two years of life. About 30 percent of the sample demonstrated excess weight for length relations by 36 months. Children with moderate or severe heart disease were significantly smaller than those without heart disease or those with mild cardiac problems at all times after birth. Measurements of a subsample of children at 4, 5, and 6 years of age suggested that growth velocity after 3 years of age may be within the normal range.

Assessment of growth of the child with Down syndrome may be carried out with reference to charts plotting tenth to ninetieth percentiles based on these data. These charts are helpful to determine how children with Down syndrome are growing in relationship to other children with Down syndrome. They should not be used to determine ideal body weight. (From Down's syndrome, growth, growth standards. *Pediatrics* 61:564, 1978. Based on data from the Developmental Evaluation Clinic, The Children's Hospital, Boston, Ma.)

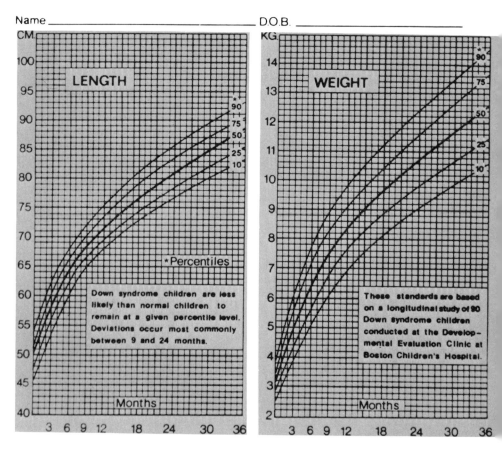

Figure 2B-1. Down syndrome boys. (Courtesy of Christine E. Cronk, Sc.D., Developmental Evaluation Clinic, The Children's Hospital, Boston, Ma.)

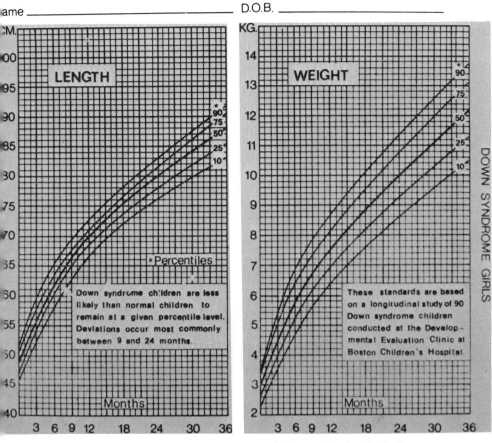

Figure 2B-2. Down syndrome girls. (Courtesy of Christine E. Cronk, Sc.D., Developmental Evaluation Clinic, The Children's Hospital, Boston, Ma.)

Appendix 3. Therapeutic Diets

A. Corn-free Diet
B. Dye-free Salicylate-free Diet
C. Egg-free Diet
D. Gluten-free Diet
E. Wheat-free Diet
F. Milk Protein- and Lactose-free Diet
G. Soy-free Diet
H. Sucrose-free Diet
I. Fructose-free Diet
J. Low-Cholesterol Diet
K. Low-Fat Diet
L. No Added Salt Diet
M. Recipe Information for Therapeutic Diets
N. Infant Formula Concentration
O. Recipes for High-Energy Supplements

Note: All diets should be adapted to the child's individual needs and tolerances with special attention given to possible deficiencies due to dietary restrictions. (See Table 7-18.)

A. Corn-free Diet
Avoid: Corn, cornstarch, corn syrup, corn oil, corn sweeteners

Food	Allowed	Avoid
Beverages	Milk; unsweetened fruit juices, sugar-free soft drinks; Ovaltine; cocoa (made from milk and plain cocoa powder); coffee; tea	Instant Breakfast; carbonated beverages; quick-mix powdered drinks (e.g., Kool-Aid, Tang); prepared chocolate milk; Swiss Miss
Breads	French, Italian, Vienna, and Syrian breads; Norwegian flatbread; plain doughnuts	All other breads; English muffins; corn bread; corn muffins; corn pone; pancake mixes; taco shells; Shake 'n Bake
Cereals	Puffed wheat; puffed rice; granola; Cheerios; Wheaties; Cream of Wheat; Cream of Rice; Familia	Cornflakes; Corn Chex; Rice Krispies; presweetened cereals; cornmeal; hominy grits
Crackers	Saltines; rye krisp; hard tack; Royal Lunch; zwieback	Graham crackers
Cheese	All	Imitation cheese made with corn oil
Eggs	All	Egg substitutes containing corn oil (e.g., Egg Beaters)
Fats	Butter; margarine made without corn oil; lard; cream; corn-free mayonnaise; pure vegetable oils (e.g., coconut, cottonseed, olive, peanut, safflower, soy, sunflower)	Corn oil; corn oil margarine; salad dressings; salad oils; vegetable shortening made with corn oil; gravies thickened with cornstarch
Meat, fish, poultry	All types plain or prepared with allowed ingredients	Processed meats containing corn syrup solids (e.g., luncheon meats)
Meat alternates	Legumes; nuts; seeds; pure peanut butter; homemade baked beans	Peanut butter with corn syrup solids added; canned baked beans
Potato or substitute	Potato; rice; pastas (e.g., spaghetti, macaroni, noodles)	Commercial spaghetti sauces; pastas made from corn
Vegetables	All *except* corn	Corn; corn on cob; cream style corn; corn niblets; any other vegetable with sweetened sauces
Fruits	All types	Any with corn sweeteners added

A. Corn-free Diet (*Continued*)

Food	Allowed	Avoid
Soups	Homemade soups without corn or cornstarch added	All canned, dried, frozen soups and corn chowder
Desserts	Fruit; Jell-O; homemade puddings (e.g., rice, tapioca); homemade ice cream; homemade cakes; cookies, and pies made without corn or cornstarch; plain yogurt; macaroons	Cornstarch puddings; commercial ice cream, sherbert, fruit ices, Popsicles, Fudgicles; commercial frostings; fruit flavored yogurt
Sweets	Sugar (cane); molasses; honey; pure maple syrup; jams, jellies, and syrups made without corn sweeteners; homemade candies; sugarless candy and gum	Corn syrup (e.g., Karo); commercial flavored syrups; all commercial candies and gum; marshmallows; cranberry sauce
Miscellaneous	Salt; pepper; spices; mustard; pickles (dill and sour only); olives; coconut; baking chocolate; dry roasted peanuts; snack foods *if* prepared without corn (e.g., potato chips prepared with cottonseed oil); pizza made without corn oil	Cornstarch; relish; catsup; sweet pickles; Davis baking powder; pretzels; whipped toppings; gum; popcorn; Cracker Jacks; corn chips; Corn Kurls; tacos; tortillas

Developed by Thalia Metalides while at The Children's Hospital, Boston, Ma.

B. Dye-free Salicylate-free Diet
Avoid: Artificial food dyes (red Nos. 2, 3; yellow Nos. 5, 6; blue Nos. 1, 5),
BHT (butylated hydroxytoluene), tartrazine, preservatives, salicylates

Food	Allowed	Avoid
Beverage	Milk; allowed fruit juices (e.g., homemade lemonade); 7-Up; hot chocolate made with homemade chocolate syrup and milk; coffee	Juices from fruits not allowed; carbonated beverages; cider; Instant Breakfast; quick-mix powdered drinks (e.g., Kool-Aid, Tang); prepared chocolate milk; tea; beer; gin; wine
Breads	All breads except those listed to avoid; baked products without artificial color or flavor (most items must be prepared at home); English muffins made without artificial coloring and flavoring; biscuit mixes; homemade French toast, pancakes, and waffles; saltines	Egg bread; whole wheat bread (usually dyed); all commercial cakes, cookies, pastries, sweet rolls, doughnuts, and pie crusts; packaged baking mixes; prepared poultry stuffing; seasoned bread crumbs
Cereals	Any cereal without artificial colors or flavors (e.g., Puffed Rice, Grapenuts, Shredded Wheat, oatmeal)	All cereals with artificial colors and flavors (e.g., presweetened cereals, Cornflakes); all instant breakfast preparations
Cheese	All natural (white) cheeses (e.g., cream cheese, cottage cheese, feta); Parmesan; white cheddar; white Jack	Colored cheeses (processed, yellow, or orange)
Eggs	All	Egg substitutes
Fats	Sweet butter (not colored or flavored); cream; all cooking oils and fats; shortening; homemade mayonnaise	Colored butter; margarine; commercial mayonnaise and salad dressings; all products using BHT as preservative
Meat, fish, poultry	All unprocessed meats, fish, and poultry (without stuffing); tongue; corned beef without flavoring or coloring	Frozen or canned meats; cured or processed meats (e.g., bologna, salami, frankfurters, sausages, meatloaf, ham, corned beef, pastrami, bacon); barbecued poultry; all "self-basting" turkeys; frozen fish filets and fish sticks that are dyed or flavored

B. Dye-free Salicylate-free Diet (*Continued*)

Food	Allowed	Avoid
Meat alternates	Dried peas, beans, lentils, and nuts	Almonds
Potato or substitute	Potato (white, sweet); rice; pasta (spaghetti, macaroni, noodles)	Commercially prepared potato, rice, or noodle mixtures
Vegetables	Only fresh vegetables	Tomatoes* and all tomato products*; cucumbers; all frozen and canned vegetables
Fruits	Avocado; banana; blueberries; cranberries; dates; figs; grapefruit and grapefruit juice; guavas and guava nectar; fresh lemon; limes; mango; melons; papaya and papaya juice; pears and pear nectar; persimmon; pineapple and pineapple juice	Apples*; apricots*; blackberries*; boysenberries*; cherries*; currants*; gooseberries*; grapes*; nectarines*; oranges*; peaches*; plums*; prunes*; raisins*; raspberries*; strawberries*; frozen and dried juice mixes; fruit juice drinks; all frozen and canned fruits; dried fruits
Soups	Bouillon; chicken broth; beef broth; soups made from allowed vegetables	All canned soups, dried soups
Desserts	Allowed fruit; ice cream, sherbet and ices (only if no artificial coloring or flavoring is added); homemade puddings (cornstarch, tapioca, rice, custard); gelatin desserts made from unflavored gelatin; homemade cakes, cookies, and pies with no artificial coloring or flavoring and with allowed ingredients (e.g., angel cake, lemon or pumpkin pie); plain yogurt	All commercial products and all homemade products containing artificial coloring or flavoring; commercial puddings, junket, and Jell-O; flavored yogurt
Sweets	Sugars, jams and jellies (made from allowed fruits without artificial color or flavor); honey; corn syrup; homemade chocolate syrup; Baker's German sweet chocolate; homemade candies without almonds	All commercial types hard or soft candies (e.g., Life Savers, jelly beans); all mint-flavored items; maple syrup unless pure; commercial chocolate syrup; commercial fruit flavored syrup (e.g., Zarex)

B. Dye-free Salicylate-free Diet (*Continued*)

Food	Allowed	Avoid
Miscellaneous	Salt; pepper; baking powder; baking soda; cream of tartar; cinnamon; pure vanilla; olives; oregano; mixed dry Italian spices; bay leaf; peppercorn; distilled white vinegar; homemade mustard (pure powder and distilled white vinegar); unflavored, uncolored soy sauce; Italian pesto sauce; homemade popcorn; pure caramel; potato chips with no added flavoring or coloring	Cider vinegar; wine vinegar; mustard; soy sauce; barbecued-flavored potato chips; cloves; catsup; chili sauce; pickles*; all mint- and wintergreen-flavored items; gum; also vitamins; aspirin; Bufferin; Excedrin; Alka-Seltzer; Empirin Compound; Anacin; all toothpastes and tooth powders; all mouthwashes; cough drops; throat lozenges; antacid tablets; perfumes; deodorants; shampoo; plastic animals

*Foods that can be reintroduced after 4–6 weeks (if child has shown a favorable response to the diet). Add the foods one at a time with about a 3–4 day interval between additions.
Developed by Thalia Metalides while at The Children's Hospital, Boston, Ma.

C. Egg-free Diet
Avoid: Egg, egg powder, dried egg, egg white, (lact)albumin

Food	Allowed	Avoid
Beverages	Milk; fruit juices; carbonated beverages; Kool-Aid; cocoa; hot chocolate; Instant Breakfast; Quik	Eggnog; root beer if egg white is added to create foam
Breads	White, wheat, rye, oatmeal, pumpernickel breads and rolls; English muffins; French, Italian, and Syrian breads; plain bagels; homemade biscuits	Breads with glazed crust; egg bagels; egg rolls; French toast; waffles; doughnuts; pancakes; muffins; prepared mixes for breads and rolls
Cereals	All	None
Crackers	Plain crackers (e.g., saltines, graham, oyster, soda, Triscuits); taco shells	Zwieback; Royal Lunch
Cheese	All	None
Eggs	None	All fresh, frozen, and powdered eggs used in any form and in cooking; souffles; omelets; quiche; egg substitutes
Fats	Butter; margarine; cream; lard; vegetable oils and shortenings; egg-free mayonnaise; whipped toppings	Mayonnaise; salad dressings containing egg; Hollandaise, tartar, and egg sauces
Meat, fish, poultry	All except poultry; luncheon meat; frankfurters	Poultry, especially chicken; fish sticks or any meat or fish with egg coating; croquettes; any meats using egg as binding agent; hash; sausages
Meat alternates	Legumes; nuts; peanut butter; seeds; baked beans	
Potato or substitute	Potato; rice; pastas (spaghetti, macaroni, plain noodles)	Egg noodles
Vegetables	All fresh, frozen, and canned	Those prepared with egg (e.g., Caesar salad)
Fruits	All fresh, frozen, and canned	None

C. Egg-free Diet (*Continued*)

Food	Allowed	Avoid
Soups	All soups prepared without egg	Chicken broth and bouillon; chicken soup; soups containing noodles; mock turtle soup; egg drop soup; egg foo yong
Desserts	Fruit; Jell-O; junket; puddings prepared without egg (cornstarch, rice, tapioca); ice cream without egg; sherbet, fruit ices, Popsicles, Fudgicles; homemade cakes, cookies, and pies made with allowed ingredients; baking chocolate; yogurt	Angel and sponge cakes; all cakes, cookies, and pies made with egg, boiled frostings; whips; custard; meringues; macaroons; Bavarian cream
Sweets	Limit amount for good dental hygiene: sugars, jams, jellies, honey, molasses, syrups, and hard candy	Marshmallow; fondant; nougats; divinity; cream candies; meringues; shiny coated candies
Miscellaneous	Salt; pepper; spices; Davis baking powder; mustard; relish; catsup; steak sauce; pickles; olives; potato chips; corn chips; popcorn; pretzels; pizza	Virus vaccines made in egg

Developed by Thalia Metalides while at The Children's Hospital, Boston, Ma.

D. Gluten-free Diet

Avoid: Cereal fillers, emulsifiers, flavorings, HVP (hydrolyzed vegetable protein), malt and malt flavoring, stabilizers, starch, vegetable gums unless source is specified (e.g., corn or potato starch)

Food	Allowed	Avoid
Beverages	Milk (skim milk may be better tolerated initially); fruit juices; carbonated beverages; cocoa; Kool-Aid; fruit punch; for adults: tea; coffee; wine; distilled alcohol beverages as permitted	Malted milk; some commercial chocolate drinks; Ovaltine; Postum; ale; beer; gin; vodka; other whiskeys; root beer
Breads, Crackers	Only those made from arrowroot, corn, lima bean, potato, rice, and soybean flours; rice wafers	All breads, rolls, and crackers containing wheat, rye, oats, barley, and graham flours; wheat germ; rye krisp; kasha muffins; biscuits, waffles, pancakes, and other prepared mixes; dumplings; rusk; zwieback; breaded foods; breadcrumbs; matzoh; Pop Tarts; Shake 'n Bake
Cereals	Hot cereals (e.g., cornmeal, hominy grits, cream of rice); cold cereals (e.g., Puffed Rice, Post: Cocoa Pebbles and Fruity Pebbles; Kellogg Sugar Pops; Nabisco Rice Honeys)	All wheat, rye, oat, and barley cereals; grapenuts; bran; kasha; bulgur; wheat germ; millet; malt; graham; cereals containing malt flavoring (including those made from rice and corn); semolina
Desserts	Fruits; gelatin (plain or with fruit); ices; homemade ice cream; custard; junket; homemade cornstarch, rice, tapioca puddings; homemade cakes, cookies, quick breads, and pastries prepared from allowed ingredients; gluten-free macaroons; plain yogurt	Commercial cakes, cookies, pies, and puddings; commercial ice cream unless ingredients are known; ice cream cones; prepared mixes; bread pudding
Fats	Butter; margarine; vegetable oil; cream; bacon; lard; vegetable shortening; mayonnaise; sour cream; gravies and sauces thickened with cornstarch	Commercial salad dressings (unless ingredients are known); gravies and sauces thickened with wheat, rye, oat, and barley flours

D. Gluten-free Diet (*Continued*)

Food	Allowed	Avoid
Meat, fish, poultry	All kinds of fresh meats, fish, and poultry; fish canned in oil or brine; meat, fish, and poultry may be combined or breaded with cornmeal or crumbs from crushed ready-to-eat approved corn and rice cereals; stuffings may be made with cornmeal or rice	Breaded, prepared meats, fish, and poultry that contain wheat, rye, oats, or barley (e.g., luncheon meats: bologna, salami, chicken loaf); frankfurters; sausage; chili con carne; Swiss steak; croquettes; meatloaf unless pure meat; stuffings; commercial hamburgers, which may contain cereal fillers
Eggs	As desired, plain or in allowed prepared dishes	Eggs in sauce made from gluten-containing ingredients (e.g., wheat-based white sauce)
Cheese	All types	Any cheese product containing oat gum as an ingredient
Potato or substitute	All potatoes (white, sweet); yams; hominy; rice; wild rice; special gluten-free noodles (e.g., Aproten from Henkel Corporation)	Regular noodles, spaghetti, and macaroni; barley; some packaged rice mixes; low-gluten products containing wheat starch
Soups	Homemade broth and soups made with allowed ingredients; homemade cream soups and chowders thickened with cream, cornstarch, or allowed flour	Commercially prepared soups containing barley, noodles, macaroni or thickened with wheat, rye, oats, and barley flours
Sweets	Limit amount for good dental hygiene: sugar (brown, white); jam; jelly; corn syrup; molasses; honey; maple sugar; marshmallows; pure cocoa; chocolate; coconut	Candy containing cereal products; candies of unknown content; all licorice (black, red)
Vegetables	All plain, fresh, frozen or canned vegetables; dried beans, peas, lentils	Vegetables prepared with wheat, flour (e.g., creamed or scalloped), or with bread crumbs or matzoh meal; some canned baked beans

D. Gluten-free Diet (*Continued*)

Food	Allowed	Avoid
Fruits	All fresh, canned, dried, and frozen fruits; all fruit juices (include citrus fruit at least once each day)	Canned fruit pie fillings unless ingredients are known
Miscellaneous	Salt; pepper; herbs; spices; vinegar; olives; pickles; peanut butter; coconut; potato chips; plain popcorn	Some dry seasoning mixes; cheese flavored popcorn; monosodium glutamate (MSG); soy sauce; pizza; communion wafers; gum

Note: Diet may be low in B vitamins
Developed by Thalia Metalides while at The Children's Hospital, Boston, Ma.

E. Wheat-free Diet
Avoid: Wheat, bran, durum, wheat germ, flour, semolina, hydrolyzed
vegetable protein (HVP), cereal fillers, emulsifiers, stabilizers

Food	Allowed	Avoid
Beverage	Milk; fruit juices; carbonated beverages; Kool-Aid; cocoa; hot chocolate; Ovaltine	Instant Breakfast; Postum
Breads	Only those made with 100% rye, oatmeal, corn, or rice flour with no wheat added; Norwegian flat bread; taco shells; rice stuffing	White, whole wheat, and cracked wheat breads, rolls, or biscuits; English muffins; waffles; pancakes; doughnuts; dumplings; bread stuffing
Cereals	Any corn, oat, rice, rye cereal that has no wheat flour added (e.g., Puffed Rice, Cornflakes, Rice Krispies, Cream of Rice)	Wheat cereals (e.g., farina, Cream of Wheat, Wheatena, bran, Shredded Wheat, Wheaties, Puffed Wheat)
Crackers	Rye krisp; rice crackers	Crackers made from wheat flour (e.g., saltines, graham, Ritz, Triscuits, Wheat Thins)
Cheese	All	None
Eggs	All	Quiche
Fats	Butter; margarine; vegetable oils; lard; bacon; cream; mayonnaise; gravy thickened with cornstarch	Salad dressings; gravy if thickened with flour
Meat, fish, poultry	All types plain or prepared with allowed ingredients	Breaded meat, fish, and poultry (e.g., fish sticks, chicken croquettes); meats to which fillers have been added (e.g., meatloaf, meatballs)
Meat alternates	Legumes; nuts; seeds; peanut butter; baked beans; tofu	
Potato or substitute	Potato; rice; wheat-free pastas (e.g., Aproten, pastas made from corn)	Pastas made from wheat flour (e.g., spaghetti, macaroni, noodles, pastina)
Vegetables	All	Any prepared with wheat-thickened sauces
Fruits	All	None
Soups	Homemade soups with allowed ingredients	Commercially prepared soups thickened with wheat or containing noodles or macaroni

E. Wheat-free Diet (*Continued*)

Food	Allowed	Avoid
Desserts	Fruit; Jell-O; junket; custard; cornstarch, rice, tapioca puddings; homemade ice cream; homemade cakes, cookies, pies, and pastries prepared from allowed ingredients; macaroons; plain yogurt	Commercial cakes, cookies, pies, and puddings; commercial ice cream unless ingredients are known; ice cream cones; prepared baking mixes; bread pudding
Sweets	Limit amount for good dental hygiene: sugar (brown, white); jam, jelly, corn syrup, molasses; honey; maple sugar; marshmallows; pure cocoa, chocolate; coconut	All licorice (black, red); candy containing cereal products; candies of unknown content
Miscellaneous	Salt; pepper; spices; mustard; catsup; pickles; relish; olives; coconut; baking chocolate; potato chips; popcorn	Beer; pretzels; commercial pizza; gum; Cracker Jacks; communion wafers

Developed by Thalia Metalides while at The Children's Hospital, Boston, Ma.

F. Milk Protein– and Lactose-free Diet
Avoid: Milk, milk solids, buttermilk solids, lactose, curds, whey, casein, lactalbumin

Food	Allowed	Avoid
Beverages	Fruit juices; carbonated beverages; Kool-Aid; cocoa without added milk solids; nondairy creamer; milk substitutes (nondairy products may have added milk solids—read labels); for adults: coffee; tea	Fresh, evaporated, condensed, and dried milk; buttermilk; malted; frappes, ice cream, ice cream sodas and, milk shakes; Instant Breakfast; hot chocolate (e.g., Swiss Miss or cocoa prepared with milk)
Bread, crackers	French, Italian or Vienna bread; bagels; Syrian bread; French toast can be made with allowed breads with eggs but without milk; saltines, graham crackers, oyster crackers, Uneeda Biscuits, and Triscuits	Breads, biscuits, muffins, and rolls made with or enriched with milk solids (e.g., hamburger and frankfurter buns); pancake; waffles; doughnuts; Pop Tarts; stuffing mixes
Cereals	All types (served without milk and eaten dry or with fruit juice)	
Cheese	None	All types
Desserts	Fruit; Jell-O; water ice, Popsicles, and Italian ices; fruit pies (pie crust made without butter or regular margarine); tapioca, homemade cornstarch puddings, and junket made with fruit juice or milk substitute; angel cake; milk-free cookies (e.g., fig bars, gingersnaps, lemonsnaps)	Cakes; cream pie; cookies made with milk; ice cream, milk ice, and sherbert; custard; commercial pudding mixes; instant pudding mixes
Eggs	All	None
Fats	Sweet unsalted Mazola stick margarine, Weight Watcher's diet margarine, Diet Fleishman margarine, and kosher margarine; lard; vegetable oil; cream substitutes (e.g., Coffee Rich, Coffee-mate); mayonnaise	Butter; margarine; sour cream; whipped cream; salad dressing made with milk

F. Milk Protein– and Lactose-free Diet (*Continued*)

Food	Allowed	Avoid
Meat, fish, poultry	All types; kosher hot dogs and cold cuts only (e.g., Morrison and Schiff, Hebrew National); kosher products labeled "Parve" or "Pareve"	Creamed meats; gravies; processed or canned meats (e.g., luncheon meat; sausage, frankfurts unless 100% pure meat, commercial hamburgers)
Potato or substitute	All	Potatoes mashed with milk or butter; canned spaghetti; macaroni and cheese
Soups	Clear soups; broth	Cream soups; chowder
Sweets	Limit amount for good dental hygiene: sugar, jams, jellies, syrups, honey, candies such as gum drops, Canada mints, Planters Jumbo Block, Good and Fruity, Dots, Necco Wafers, Mason's Black Crows, Life Savers (except butterscotch flavor)	Candies made with milk, chocolate, butter or cream, butterscotch, caramels; Pop Rocks
Vegetables	All types	Those in butter or cream sauces
Fruits	All types	None
Miscellaneous	Mustard; relish; catsup; salt; pepper; spices; peanut butter; gravy without added milk or cream; potato chips; pretzels; pickles; olives; corn chips; plain popcorn	Yogurt; pizza; some artificial sweeteners (e.g., Sugarlo)

Note: Calcium supplementation is needed if restriction is longer than 4–6 weeks. Non-dairy milk substitute is not a milk substitute. Milk-free diet is not appropriate for patients with galactosemia.
Developed by Thalia Metalides while at The Children's Hospital, Boston, Ma.

G. Soy-free Diet
Avoid: Soy, soybean, soybean oil, vegetable oils, hydrogenated oils,
lecithin, monosodium glutamate (MSG), textured vegetable protein

Food	Allowed	Avoid
Beverages	Milk; fruit juices; carbonated beverages; Kool-Aid; cocoa; hot chocolate; Ovaltine; for infants: soy-free formula (e.g., Pregestimil, Nutramigen)	Soy-based formula or milk; nondairy creamers containing soy; Instant Breakfast; Nestlé's Quik; cocoa powders containing lecithin; Swiss Miss
Breads	Only those prepared without soy (e.g., Syrian bread); French toast prepared from homemade soy-free bread	Breads prepared with soy; English muffins; doughnuts; pancake mixes; stuffing mixes; seasoned bread crumbs; Shake 'n Bake; taco shells
Cereals	All cereals without soy; Cornflakes; Rice Krispies; Cheerios; Puffed Wheat; Puffed Rice; Wheaties; Cream of Rice; Familia	Presweetened cold cereals; soy grits; granola; Cream of Wheat
Crackers	Only those prepared without soy (e.g., hardtack; Norwegian flatbread; rye krisp)	All those prepared with soy (e.g., graham, Ritz, Royal Lunch, saltines, Triscuits, zwieback)
Cheese	All	Imitation cheeses containing soy
Eggs	All	Imitation eggs containing soy
Fats	Butter; cream; bacon; soy-free margarine; soy-free mayonnaise; lard; pure vegetable oil (e.g., coconut, corn, cottonseed, olive, peanut, safflower, sunflower)	Soybean oil; soy-containing margarine and mayonnaise; salad dressings and salad oils; vegetable shortenings that contain soy; vegetable cooking sprays (greaseless frying compounds)
Meat, fish, poultry	All types plain or prepared with allowed ingredients; water-packed tuna; processed meats; and frankfurters with no fillers added	Soy protein isolates; textured vegetable proteins (e.g., imitation meat and bacon bits); ground meat with extenders; canned chili; tuna packed in oil
Meat alternates	Legumes; nuts; seeds; baked beans; pure peanut butter	Soybeans; peanut butter with hydrogenated oils added; tofu; miso; tempeh

G. Soy-free Diet (*Continued*)

Food	Allowed	Avoid
Potato or substitute	Potato; rice; pastas (spaghetti, macaroni, noodles)	Canned spaghetti; packaged macaroni and cheese
Vegetables	All except soybeans	Soybeans
Fruits	All	None
Soups	Homemade soups made with allowed ingredients without soy	All canned, dried, and frozen soups; bouillon
Desserts	Fruit; Jell-O; junket; homemade puddings (cornstarch, tapioca; rice) ice cream; sherbet; fruit ices; Popsicles; and Fudgicles; homemade cakes, cookies, and pies made with allowed ingredients; baking chocolate; yogurt	Canned puddings; commercial cakes, cookies, and pies containing soy; commercial frostings; desserts made with chocolate bits
Sweets	Limit amount for good dental hygiene: sugar, jams, jellies, honey, molasses; syrups	Chocolate bits; milk chocolate
Miscellaneous	Salt; pepper; spices; mustard; relish; catsup; pickles; olives; coconut; snack foods only if prepared without soy (e.g., potato chips, corn chips, popcorn); dry roasted peanuts; homemade pizza made without soy oil	Soy sauce; MSG; commercial pizza; pretzels; Chinese food

Developed by Thalia Metalides while at The Children's Hospital, Boston, Ma.

H. Sucrose-Free Diet
Avoid: Sugar, invert sugar, sucrose, cane sugar, beet sugar, corn syrup, honey, maple sugar, molasses, sorbitol

Food	Allowed	Avoid
Beverages	Milk; unsweetened cocoa; sugar-free carbonated beverages; Kool-Aid sweetened with dextrose or saccharin	Sweetened condensed milk; milk shakes; sugar sweetened beverages (e.g., Kool-Aid and carbonated beverages)
Breads, cereal, crackers	Homemade breads made with dextrose but without sugar; Syrian bread; farina; oatmeal; hominy; Puffed Rice; Shredded Wheat; crackers that do not contain added sugar (e.g., saltines, soda crackers); rye flour	All other breakfast cereals; wheat germ; rice bran

Note: Patients may be gradually advanced to a *sucrose-restricted diet*. The following foods may then be *added* to the sucrose-free diet.

Food	Allowed	Avoid
Fruits	Limit to 1½ cups/day: blackberries, cherries (fresh or dietetic pack), cranberries, currents, figs, gooseberries, grapes, lemons, loganberries, pomegranates, raspberries, strawberries	All others
Vegetables	Limit to 2 cups/day: string beans, cabbage, cauliflower, celery, corn, cucumber, eggplant, lettuce, potato (white), pumpkin, radishes, squash (butternut, Hubbard), tomatoes	All others
Potato or substitute	White potato; macaroni; rice (brown, white); spaghetti	Sweet potato

Note: Both diets should be supplemented with ascorbic acid, folic acid, iron, thiamine, and niacin. Consult physician for supplements that do not contain sugar.
Developed by Thalia Metalides while at The Children's Hospital, Boston, Ma.

I. Fructose-free Diet
Avoid: Fructose, sucrose, sugar, cane sugar, beet sugar, invert sugar, sorghum, levulose, honey, corn syrup, maple syrup, sorbitol, mannitol, fruit, fruit juice

Food	Allowed	Avoid
Beverages	Milk; evaporated milk; Kool-Aid sweetened with dextrose; unsweetened cocoa; sugar-free sorbitol-free carbonated beverages; coffee; tea	Sweetened condensed milk; milk shakes; fruit drinks; sugar sweetened Kool-Aid; carbonated beverages containing sugar or sorbitol; wine, brandy
Breads	Homemade bread and rolls prepared with dextrose and without sugar (some Jewish bakeries bake their bread without sugar); Syrian bread	Sweet breads; commercially prepared breads and rolls containing prohibited ingredients
Cereals	Cooked cereals (from barley, oats, rye, corn)	Prepared cereals; sugar coated cereals; rice bran; wheat germ
Crackers	Saltines; soda crackers	Those with sugar added
Cheese	All	Some processed cheese spreads
Eggs	All	None
Fats	Butter; margarine; oil; homemade mayonnaise or salad dressing made without sugar; lard	Mayonnaise and salad dressings made with sugar
Meat, fish, poultry	Fresh beef, veal, lamb, pork, chicken, turkey, and fish; ham and bacon not sugar-cured	Ham, bacon, luncheon meats, and any other meat or fish processed with sugar or fillers containing sugar; organ meats, including liver
Meat alternates		Dry beans and peas; lentils; nuts; seeds; peanut butter
Potato or substitute	White potato*; macaroni*; noodles*; spaghetti*	Brown rice; sweet potato
Vegetables	Asparagus; cabbage*; cucumber*; cauliflower*; celery*; green beans*; green pepper; lettuce*; mushrooms; radishes*; spinach	All others
Fruit	None	All fruit, fruit juices, and fruit drinks
Soups	Chicken and beef broth; soups made from allowed vegetables	Bouillon; dried soups

394 Appendix 3. Therapeutic Diets

I. Fructose-free Diet (*Continued*)

Food	Allowed	Avoid
Desserts	Dietetic gelatin, ice cream, pudding, cake, cookies, and pies made with allowed ingredients and without sugar, sorbitol, or fructose; plain gelatin prepared with unsweetened Kool-Aid; plain unflavored yogurt	All desserts containing sugar, fruit, fruit juice, fructose, honey, or sorbitol (e.g., cakes, pies, cookies, pudding, Jell-O, ice cream, sherbert)
Sweets	"Sugarless" candy; gum sweetened with saccharin; dextrose	All candy, gum, jams, jellies, syrups, honey, molasses, and chocolate
Miscellaneous	Salt; pepper; spices (except allspice); herbs; vinegar; corn chips; potato chips; popcorn; homemade baby foods	Catsup, chili sauce, and other condiments containing sugar; soy sauce; sweet pickles; allspice; commercial baby foods containing prohibited ingredients

*These foods contian 0.3 gm (or less) sucrose per 100 gm edible portion.
Note: This diet should be supplemented with ascorbic acid, folic acid, iron, thiamine, and niacin. Consult physician for supplements that do not contain sugar.
Developed by Thalia Metalides while at The Children's Hospital, Boston, Ma.

J. Low-Cholesterol Diet
Avoid: Hydrogenated fats, fried foods, shortening, coconut oil, palm oil

Food	Allowed	Avoid
Beverages	Nonfat milk; skim milk; 99% fat-free milk; fruit juices; carbonated beverages; Kool-Aid; cocoa made with allowed milk; coffee; tea	Whole milk; buttermilk (if 2% fat); commercial chocolate milk; milk shakes; frappes
Breads	All plain breads except those to avoid; English muffins; bagels; Syrian bread; *homemade* biscuits, muffins, waffles, and pancakes prepared with allowed ingredients (e.g., margarine or corn oil in place of butter or shortening)	Butter rolls; cheese breads; egg breads; butter top breads; commercial (store-bought) biscuits, muffins, Danish, doughnuts, and sweet rolls waffles; French toast; Pop Tarts; Shake 'n Bake
Cereals	All hot and cold varieties	Those containing coconut (e.g., certain granola-type cereals)
Crackers	Plain crackers (e.g., saltines, grahams, matzoh, oyster, rye krisp, Uneeda biscuits; melba toast	High fat crackers (e.g., Ritz, Triscuits, Triangle Thins)
Cheese	Cheese made from skimmed or partially skimmed milk (e.g., cottage cheese—uncreamed or low fat type); farmer's, baker's, pot, or hoop cheese; skim milk mozzarella and sapsago cheese; grated Parmesan cheese in limited amounts	Natural and processed; made from whole milk or cream; cheese spreads; cream cheese
Eggs	Egg whites; commercial egg substitutes (e.g., Egg Beaters); limit egg yolks to 3 per week	More than 3 egg yolks per week

J. Low-Cholesterol Diet (*Continued*)

Food	Allowed	Avoid
Fats	Include 1–2 tbsp/day: polyunsaturated oils such as corn oil, cottonseed oil, safflower oil, sesame oil, soybean oil, sunflower seed oil; polyunsaturated margarines (preferably soft-tub type); salad dressings and mayonnaise made from allowed oils; olives	Cream, whipped cream, and toppings; sour cream; gravies made from fat drippings; nondairy creamers; solid fats, and shortenings (e.g., butter, lard, Crisco, salt pork, meat fat, chicken fat); hydrogenated margarine; vegetable shortening; coconut oil, palm oil, and products containing coconut or palm oils
Meat, Fish, Poultry	Choose lean cuts (trim all visible fat and remove skin of poultry before cooking): chicken, turkey, veal, beef, lamb, pork, ham; lean ground beef; fish; shellfish may be substituted for meat occasionally; chicken loaf, turkey loaf; chicken frankfurters may be substituted for meat occasionally	Duck; goose; fatty (marbled) meats; shoulder; spare ribs; mutton; canned meats; bacon; sausage; commercial (store-bought) hamburger unless extra lean; luncheon meats (e.g., bologna, salami, liverwurst, frankfurters, pastrami, corned beef, tongue); organ meats (e.g., liver, kidney, brain, heart, sweet breads); fried and frozen fish; canned main meals (e.g., stews, chili, spaghetti)
Meat alternates	Dried beans and peas (e.g., kidney beans, lima beans, navy beans, pinto beans, red beans, lentils, chick peas, split peas, soybeans); seeds (e.g., pumpkin, sunflower, squash); peanut butter; walnuts	Canned baked beans with pork; macadamia nuts; cashew nuts; coconut
Potato or substitute	Potato; macaroni; rice; spaghetti; plain noodles	Egg noodles; chow mein noodles; canned spaghetti and macaroni products
Vegetables	All	Those in cream or butter sauces
Fruits	All except avocado	Avocado
Soups	Broth; bouillon; clear soups; vegetable soup	Cream soups; chowders

J. Low- Cholesterol Diet (*Continued*)

Food	Allowed	Avoid
Desserts	Fruit; gelatin; ice milk and sherbet; Dairy Queen; ice cream cones; water ices, frozen juice bars, Popsicles, and Fudgicles; puddings made with skim or low-fat milk; angel cake; meringues; low-fat yogurt; low-fat cookies (e.g., animal crackers, vanilla wafers, ginger snaps, fig bars); homemade cakes, cookies, and pies made with polyunsaturated fat and low-fat milk in place of solid shortening and whole milk	Commercial (store-bought) cakes, cookies, pies, and pastries; ice cream; whole milk yogurt; desserts made with whole milk and/or shortening
Sweets	Limit amount for good dental hygiene: sugar, jam, jelly, marmalade, honey, syrups (e.g., corn, maple), molasses, marshmallows, gum drops, hard candy, peanut brittle	Caramels; fudge; candies made with chocolate, butter, or cream
Miscellaneous	Salt; pepper; spices; seasonings; soy sauce; Worcestershire sauce; chili sauce; fat-free gravy; pickles; catsup; mustard; relish; popcorn (made with allowed oil or margarine); pretzels; potato chips may be used occasionally	Pizza

Developed by Thalia Metalides while at The Children's Hospital, Boston, Ma.

K. Low-Fat Diet

Food	Allowed	Avoid
Beverages	Nonfat milk; skim milk; 99% fat-free milk; fruit juices; carbonated beverages; Kool-Aid; cocoa made with low-fat milk (also Swiss Miss, Quik, Instant Breakfast); coffee; tea	Whole milk; chocolate milk; butter milk; frappes; milk shakes
Breads	All plain breads except those to avoid; English muffins; bagels; Syrian bread; homemade biscuits, muffins, pancakes, and waffles using allowed ingredients	Butter-top bread; egg rolls; cheese bread; commercial (store-bought) biscuits, muffins, Danish, doughnuts, French toast, sweet rolls, pancakes and waffles; Pop Tarts; Shake 'n Bake; stuffings
Cereals	All types hot and cold	Those containing coconut (e.g., certain granola-type cereals)
Crackers	Plain crackers (e.g. saltines, graham, matzo, oyster, rye krisp, Uneeda biscuits)	High-fat crackers (e.g., Ritz; Triscuits; Triangle Thins)
Cheese	Cheese made from skimmed or partially skimmed milk (e.g., cottage cheese— preferably uncreamed, farmer's, baker's, pot, or hoop cheese); imitation processed cheeses (those containing less than 5% butterfat)	Cheeses made from cream or whole milk
Eggs	3 whole eggs per week (used as such or in cooking); egg whites; low-fat egg substitutes	More than 3 egg yolks per week
Fats	Diet margarine; imitation mayonnaise; low-calorie dressings	Butter; regular margarine; bacon; cream; shortening; lard; meat fat; salt pork; oils; regular salad dressings; mayonnaise; sour cream; whipped cream and toppings; gravies; nondairy creamers

K. Low-Fat Diet (*Continued*)

Food	Allowed	Avoid
Meat, fish, poultry	Trim all visible fat before cooking; choose fish and poultry more often than meat; choose lean cuts: lean groundbeef, fish, poultry; tuna packed in water	Fatty meats; spare ribs; mutton; ham hocks; frankfurters; sausages; commercial hamburgers; luncheon meats (e.g., bologna, salami, liverwurst, pastrami, corned beef); fish canned in oil; (frozen) fried fish; canned main meals (e.g., stews, chili); duck; goose; skin of chicken or turkey
Meat alternates	Kidney beans; lima beans; lentils; chick peas; split peas	Peanut butter; nuts; canned baked beans with pork added
Potato or substitute	Potato; rice; macaroni; spaghetti; noodles	Potato and macaroni salad; macaroni and cheese
Vegetables	All	Those in butter or cream sauces; fried vegetables
Fruits	All except avocado, coconut	Avocado; coconut
Soups	Clear broth; bouillon; fat-free soups (canned or homemade)	Cream soups; chowders
Desserts	Fruit; gelatin; water ices, ice milk, sherbet, frozen juice bars, Fudgicles, Popsicles, Dairy Queen, and ice cream cones; puddings made with skim milk; angel cake; meringues; low-fat yogurt; low-fat cookies (e.g., animal crackers, vanilla wagers, ginger snaps, fig bars)	Ice cream; whole milk yogurt; puddings made with whole milk; commercial cakes, cookies, and pies containing shortening, chocolate, or nuts
Sweets	Limit amount for good dental hygiene: sugar, jam, jelly, marmalade, honey, marshmallows, molasses, syrups (e.g., corn, maple), gum drops, jelly beans, hard candy, fondant	Caramels; fudge; candies made with chocolate, butter, cream, or nuts

K. Low-Fat Diet (*Continued*)

Food	Allowed	Avoid
Miscellaneous	Salt; pepper; seasonings; soy sauce; Worcestershire sauce; chili sauce; catsup; mustard; relish; pretzels; air-popped popcorn; fat-free gravy	Olives; gravies; peanut butter; potato chips; corn chips; buttered popcorn; nuts; cream sauces; frozen packaged dinners; pizza

Note: When low-fat diet is used for patients with cystic fibrosis, diet should be adapted to individual needs (e.g., child may be able to tolerate more fat).
Developed by Thalia Metalides while at The Children's Hospital, Boston, Ma.

L. No Added Salt Diet
Avoid: Sodium, salt, sea salt, brine, MSG

Food	Allowed	Avoid
Beverages	Milk; fruit juices; carbonated beverages; Kool-Aid; cocoa	Buttermilk; instant cocoa mixes
Breads	White, wheat, rye, oatmeal, or pumpernickel breads and rolls; English muffins; French, Italian, and Syrian breads; bagels; French toast	Breading mixes (e.g., Shake 'n Bake); cheese breads; salted-top rolls and bagels
Cereals	All cereals hot or cold prepared without added salt	All with added salt
Crackers	All unsalted-top crackers	Salted-top crackers; cheese crackers
Cheese	Cottage cheese, cream cheese, and ricotta cheese used in moderation; low sodium cheeses	Processed cheeses or cheese spreads (e.g., American, Swiss, cheddar, blue, feta, Parmesan, Roquefort, Cheez Whiz)
Eggs	Limit to 3 per week	Egg substitutes (e.g., Egg Beaters)
Fats	Regular butter and margarine; oil; lard; shortening; cream and sour cream; mayonnaise; commercial salad dressings used in moderation; homemade gravy	Bacon; salt pork; blue cheese and Roquefort dressings; canned or packaged gravies
Meat, fish, poultry	Unsalted fresh or frozen meat, fish, or poultry	Cured and canned meats (e.g., ham, bacon, Canadian bacon, frankfurters, sausage, corned beef, bologna, salami, liverwurst, chicken loaf, turkey loaf, pastrami); kosher meats; salted or smoked fish (e.g., dried cod, lox, finnan haddie); canned fish packaged in brine (e.g., anchovies, sardines, tuna in oil); frozen fish

L. No Added Salt Diet (*Continued*)

Food	Allowed	Avoid
Meat alternate	Dried beans and peas (e.g., kidney, lima, and navy beans; lentils; soybeans; split peas; chick peas); seeds (e.g., unsalted pumpkin, sunflower, squash seeds); peanut butter; unsalted nuts (e.g., unsalted peanuts, almonds, walnuts)	Canned baked beans; salted or smoked nuts and seeds
Potato or substitute	Potato; macaroni; rice; noodles; spaghetti	Commercially prepared potato or rice products; canned or frozen potato, spaghetti, and macaroni products
Vegetables	All fresh, canned, or frozen vegetables without added salt	Vegetables canned with extra salt; sauerkraut; tomato juice; V-8 Juice
Fruit	All fresh, frozen, canned, or dried fruits; fruit juices	None
Soups	Homemade broth and soups using allowed ingredients	Bouillon cubes; canned, dried, and frozen soups; instant soups
Desserts	Fruit; Jell-O; ice cream, ice milk, sherbet, Popsicles, and Fudgicles; puddings; cakes; cookies; homemade pies made without salt; yogurt	Commercial pies; meringue and chiffon pies
Sweets	Limit amount for good dental hygiene; sugar; jam; jelly; honey; molasses; syrup (e.g., corn, maple); marshmallows; all candies	
Miscellaneous	Pepper; herbs; spices; dry mustard; celery powder; garlic powder; onion powder; raw horseradish; unsalted popcorn; unsalted potato chips	Salt; celery salt; garlic salt; onion salt; catsup; prepared mustard; prepared horseradish; monosodium glutamate (MSG) (e.g., Accent); meat tenderizers; barbecue sauce; chili sauce; steak sauce; pickles; pickle relish; olives; soy sauce; Lite Salt; sea salt; salted popcorn and potato chips; corn chips;

L. No Added Salt Diet (*Continued*)

Food	Allowed	Avoid
		pretzels; other salted snack foods (e.g., cheese puffs, cheese twists); TV dinners; pizza; Chinese food; Italian food; baking soda; "alkalizers" for indigestion (e.g., Alka Seltzer; Brioschi; Rolaids)

Note: A small amount of salt may be used in cooking; use no extra salt at the table. Avoid fast food restaurants, as they usually add large amounts of salt in the preparation of foods. Consult physician before using any "salt substitute."
Developed by Thalia Metalides while at The Children's Hospital, Boston, Ma.

M. Recipe Information for Therapeutic Diets

Allergy Recipes (egg-free, milk-free, wheat-free recipes)
The American Dietetic Association
430 North Michigan Avenue
Chicago, Ill. 60611

Baking for People with Food Allergies (egg-free, gluten-free, milk-free, wheat-free recipes)
Superintendent of Documents
U.S. Government Printing Office
Washington, D.C. 20402

Celiac Disease Recipes (some recipes include oatmeal and wheat starch)
The 5 Fifty 5 Shop
c/o The Hospital For Sick Children
555 University Avenue
Toronto, Canada M5G 1X8

Cooking Without, Recipes for the Allergic Child
Margaret Williams
Tricor Inc.
427 Houston Road
Ambler, Pa. 19002

Delicious and Easy Rice Flour Recipes
Marion Wood
Charles C Thomas, Publisher
Springfield, Ill. 62701

Gluten Intolerance Group Cookbook
Elaine I. Hartsook, R.D.
26604 Dover Court
Kent, Wa. 98031

Good Recipes to Brighten Allergy Diets
Best Foods, A Division of CPC
Consumer Service Department
International Plaza
Englewood, N.J. 07632

Gourmet Food on a Wheat-Free Diet
Marion Wood
Charles C Thomas, Publisher
Springfield, Ill. 62701

Low Gluten Diet with Tested Recipes (barley-free, oat-free, rye-free, wheat-free recipes; some recipes include oats, wheat, and starch)
A.B. French, M.D.
Clinical Research Unit
University Hospital
1405 East Ann Street
Ann Arbor, Mich. 48104

Low Protein Cookery for Phenylketonuria
Virginia E. Schuett
The University of Wisconsin Press
Box 1379
Madison, Wis. 53701

Luncheon With Laurie (barley-free, rye-free, wheat-free recipes)
  Mrs. Carolyn Carpenter
  237 Pinewood Lane
  Rock Hill, S.C. 29730

125 Great Recipes for Allergy Diets (egg-free, gluten-free, milk-free, wheat-free recipes)
  Good Housekeeping
  959 Eighth Avenue
  New York, N.Y. 10019

Special Recipes and Allergy Aids (corn-free, egg-free, gluten-free, milk-free recipes)
  General Foods Consumer Center
  White Plains, N.Y. 10625

The PKU Cookbook (Phenylketonuria)
  Elizabeth Read, Elizabeth Wanz, Roslyn Duffy, Nancy Wellman, Aissa Acosta, and Phyllis Acosta
  University of New Mexico Printing Plant
  Albuquerque, N.M. 87101

Wheat, Milk and Egg-Free Recipes
  The Quaker Oats Company
  Merchandise Mart Plaza
  Chicago, Ill. 60654

N. Infant Formula Concentration

Formula Concentration (kcal/oz)	Formula Type	Water (oz)	Corn Syrup[a]		Polycose[a]		Corn Oil[a]		MCT Oil[a]
25	13 oz concentrate	8	—		—		—		—
25	13 oz concentrate	13	3 tbsp	or	6 tbsp	or	1¼ tbsp	or	1⅓ tbsp
30	13 oz concentrate	8	2 tbsp	or	3 tbsp	or	1 tbsp	or	1 tbsp
30	13 oz concentrate	13	—		10 tbsp		—		—
20	1 cup powder[b] (packed level)	29	—		—		—		—
30	1½ cup powder[b] (packed level)	29	—		—		—		—

Note: Concentration of formula must be increased gradually and the infant watched for symptoms of intolerance.
[a] Energy content of caloric supplements:
Corn syrup = 57 kcal/tbsp
Polycose = 30 kcal/tbsp
Corn oil = 126 kcal/tbsp
MCT oil = 116 kcal/tbsp
[b] e.g., Portagen or Pregestimil.

O. Recipes for High-Energy Supplements

HIGH-ENERGY FRUIT WITH CASEC AND LIPOMUL
Ingredients
1 jar strained peaches (4¼ oz)
2 tbsp Casec
1 tbsp Lipomul

Directions
Mix ingredients well. Serve at room temperature for between-meal
feedings or dessert. Give in small amounts (i.e., 1 tbsp per feeding).

Nutritive value
26 gm CHO
 9 gm PRO (1 gm PRO per tbsp)
10 gm FAT
230 kcal (29 kcal/tbsp)

Considerations
This mixture is used for infants and children capable of taking only small
quantities of food or for those needing to gain weight (e.g., infants
neurologically impaired, with congenital heart disease, or with failure to
thrive).

HIGH-ENERGY FRUIT WITH POWDERED MILK AND CORN OIL
Ingredients
1 jar strained peaches or bananas (4½ oz) or ½ cup regular applesauce
2 tbsp nonfat dry milk solids
1 tbsp corn oil

Directions
Mix ingredients well. Serve at room temperature for between-meal
feedings or dessert. Give in small amounts (i.e., 1 tbsp per feeding).

Nutritive value
30 gm CHO
 3 gm PRO (0.4 gm PRO per tbsp)
14 gm FAT
259 kcal (32 kcal/tbsp)

Considerations
Same as listed for High-Energy Fruit with Casec and Lipomul.

HIGH-ENERGY, LOW-FAT DRINK
Ingredients
½ cup liquid skim milk
½ cup orange juice
1 cup orange sherbet
1 tbsp nonfat dry milk solids
1 package vanilla Instant Breakfast

Directions
Mix well in blender.

Nutritive value
78 gm CHO
13 gm PRO
 2 gm FAT
416 kcal

Appendix 4. Food Composition

A. Amino Acid Content of Foods per 100 gm, Edible Portion
B. Nutritive Value of Selected Foods
C. Iron Content of Selected High-Iron Foods
D. Enteral Products

A. Amino Acid Content of Foods per 100 gm, Edible Portion

Food item	Nitrogen conversion factor	Protein content (%)	Phenylalanine (mg)	Isoleucine (mg)	Leucine (mg)	Valine (mg)	Sulfur-containing Methionine (mg)	Cystine (mg)	Total (mg)	Tryptophan (mg)	Threonine (mg)	Lysine (mg)	Tyrosine (mg)	Arginine (mg)	Histidine (mg)
MILK, MILK PRODUCTS															
Fluid, whole	6.38	3.5	170	223	344	240	86	31	117	49	161	272	178	128	92
Human milk	6.38	1.4	48	68	100	70	25	22	47	18	50	73	61	45	22
Isomil	6.38		105	107	153	92	29	—	29	19	69	91	—	—	53
Cheese, cheddar, processed	6.38	23.2	1244	1563	2262	1665	604	131	735	316	862	1702	1109	847	756
EGGS, WHOLE															
fresh or stored	6.25	12.8	739	850	1126	950	401	299	700	211	637	819	551	840	307
MEAT, POULTRY, FISH															
Hamburger, regular	6.25	16.0	658	837	1311	888	397	202	599	187	707	1398	543	1032	556
Rib roast	6.25	17.4	715	910	1425	590	432	220	652	203	768	1520	590	1122	604
Lamb leg	6.25	18.0	732	933	1394	887	432	236	668	233	824	1457	625	1172	501
Pork loin	6.25	16.4	646	842	1207	853	409	192	601	213	761	1346	585	1005	567
Chicken, fryer	6.25	20.6	811	1088	1490	1012	537	277	814	250	877	1810	725	1302	593
Haddock, raw	6.25	18.2	676	923	1374	930	530	245	775	181	789	1596	492	1025	—
LEGUMES, DRY, AND NUTS															
Bean, red kidney, canned	6.25	5.7	315	324	490	346	57	57	114	53	247	423	220	343	162
Peanuts	5.46	26.9	1557	1266	1872	1532	271	463	734	340	828	1099	1104	3296	749
GRAINS AND GRAIN PRODUCTS															
Bread, white, 4% milk solids	5.70	8.5	465	429	668	435	142	200	342	91	282	225	243	340	192
Rice, white or converted	5.95	7.6	382	356	655	531	137	103	240	82	298	300	347	438	128
VEGETABLES															
Beans, lima, canned	6.25	3.8	197	233	306	246	41	42	83	49	171	240	131	230	125

Data from Orr, M. L., and Watt, B. K., *Amino Acid Content of Foods*, Home Economics Research Report No. 4, U.S. Dept. of Agriculture, Washington, D.C., 1957, Forman, S. J., *Infant Nutrition*, (2nd ed.), Philadelphia: Saunders, 1974. p. 362, and *Handbook of Infant Formulas*, (6th ed.), New York: Charles Pfizer & Co. Inc., J.B. Roerig Division, 1969.

B. Nutritive value of Selected Foods

Food and Approximate Measure	Weight (gm)	Food Energy kcal	Food Energy kJ	Protein (gm)	Fat, total lipids (gm)	Fatty Acids Saturated, total (gm)	Fatty Acids Unsaturated Oleic (gm)	Fatty Acids Unsaturated Linoleic (gm)	Carbohydrate (gm)	Calcium (mg)	Iron (mg)	Vitamin A value (IU)	Thiamine (mg)	Riboflavin (mg)	Niacin (mg)	Ascorbic acid (mg)
MILK, CREAM, CHEESE (RELATED PRODUCTS)																
Milk, cow's																
Fluid, whole (3.5% fat) 1 cup	244	160	672	9	9	5	3	trace	12	288	0.1	350	0.08	0.42	0.1	2
Fluid, nonfat (skim) 1 cup	246	90	378	9	trace	—	—	—	13	298	0.1	10	0.10	0.44	0.2	2
Cheddar, process 1 oz	28	105	441	7	9	5	3	trace	1	219	0.3	350	trace	0.12	trace	0
Cottage, creamed 1 cup	225	240	1008	31	9	5	3	trace	7	212	0.7	380	0.07	0.56	0.2	0
Ice cream, plain, factory packed container 8 fl oz	142	295	1239	6	18	10	6	1	29	175	0.1	740	0.06	0.27	0.1	1
Yogurt, from partially skimmed milk 1 cup	246	120	504	8	4	2	1	trace	13	295	0.1	170	0.09	0.43	0.2	2
EGGS																
Whole, without shell 1 egg	50	80	336	6	6	2	3	trace	trace	27	1.1	590	0.05	0.15	trace	0
MEAT, POULTRY, FISH, SHELLFISH (RELATED PRODUCTS)																
Hamburger (ground beef), broiled, regular 3 oz	85	245	1029	21	17	8	8	trace	0	9	2.7	30	0.07	0.18	4.6	—
Steak, broiled, lean and fat 3 oz	85	330	1386	20	27	13	12	1	0	9	2.5	50	0.05	0.16	4.0	—
Chicken, cooked flesh only, broiled 3 oz	85	115	483	20	3	1	1	1	0	8	1.4	80	0.05	0.16	7.4	—
With bone 3.3 oz	94	155	651	25	5	1	2	1	1	9	1.3	70	0.04	0.17	11.2	—
Lamb leg roasted, lean and fat 3 oz	85	235	987	22	16	9	6	trace	0	9	1.4	—	0.13	0.23	4.7	—

B. Nutritive Value of Selected Foods (*Continued*)

Food and Approximate Measure	Weight (gm)	Food Energy kcal	Food Energy kJ	Protein (gm)	Fat, total lipids (gm)	Saturated, total (gm)	Unsaturated Oleic (gm)	Unsaturated Linoleic (gm)	Carbohydrate (gm)	Calcium (mg)	Iron (mg)	Vitamin A value (IU)	Thiamine (mg)	Riboflavin (mg)	Niacin (mg)	Ascorbic acid (mg)
Pork, fresh, trimmed to retail basis, cooked																
Chop, thick, with bone 3.5 oz	98	260	1092	16	21	8	9	2	0	8	2.2	0	0.63	0.18	3.8	—
Bluefish, baked or broiled 3 oz	85	135	567	22	4	—	—	—	0	25	0.6	40	0.09	0.08	1.6	—
Haddock, fried 3 oz	85	140	588	17	5	1	3	trace	5	34	1.0	—	0.03	0.06	2.7	2
Tuna, canned in oil 3 oz	85	170	714	24	7	—	—	—	0	7	1.6	70	0.04	0.10	10.1	—
MATURE DRY BEANS AND PEAS NUTS, PEANUTS (RELATED PRODUCTS)																
Red beans 1 cup	256	230	966	15	1	—	—	—	42	74	4.6	trace	0.13	0.10	1.5	—
Lima beans, cooked 1 cup	192	260	1092	16	1	—	—	—	48	56	5.6	trace	0.26	0.12	1.3	trace
Cashew nuts, roasted 1 cup	135	760	3192	23	62	10	43	4	40	51	5.1	140	0.58	0.33	2.4	—
Peanut butter 1 tbsp	16	95	399	4	8	2	4	2	3	9	0.3	—	0.02	0.02	2.4	0
Peas, split, dry, cooked 1 cup	250	290	1218	20	1	—	—	—	52	28	4.2	100	0.37	0.22	2.2	—
VEGETABLES AND VEGETABLE PRODUCTS																
Asparagus, canned green 6 spears	96	20	84	2	trace	—	—	—	3	18	1.8	770	0.06	0.10	0.8	14
Snap beans, green, cooked short time in small amount of water 1 cup	125	30	126	2	trace	—	—	—	7	62	0.8	680	0.08	0.11	0.6	16
Broccoli spears, cooked 1 cup	150	40	168	5	trace	—	—	—	7	132	1.2	3,750	0.14	0.29	1.2	135
Carrots, cooked, diced 1 cup	145	45	189	1	trace	—	—	—	10	48	0.9	15,220	0.08	0.07	0.7	9
Peas, green, cooked 1 cup	160	115	483	9	1	—	—	—	19	37	2.9	860	0.44	0.17	3.7	33
Potato, baked, peeled after baking 1	99	90	378	3	trace	—	—	—	21	9	0.7	trace	0.10	0.04	1.7	20

Food	Amount																
Spinach, cooked	1 cup	180	40	168	5	1	—	—	—	6	167	4.0	14,580	0.13	0.25	1.0	50
Squash, winter, baked, mashed	1 cup	205	130	546	4	1	—	—	—	32	57	1.6	8,610	0.10	0.27	1.4	27
Sweet potatoes, boiled, peeled after boiling	1	147	170	714	2	1	—	—	—	39	47	1.0	11,610	0.13	0.09	0.9	25
Tomato juice, canned	1 cup	242	45	189	2	trace	—	—	—	10	17	2.2	1,940	0.13	0.07	1.8	39
FRUITS AND FRUIT PRODUCTS																	
Apple, raw, 2½ in. diameter	1	150	70	294	trace	trace	—	—	—	18	8	0.4	50	0.04	0.02	0.1	3
Fruit cocktail, canned in heavy syrup	1 cup	256	195	819	1	1	—	—	—	50	23	1.0	360	0.04	0.03	1.1	5
Grapefruit, white, raw, medium, 4½ in. diameter	½	285	55	231	1	trace	—	—	—	14	22	0.6	10	0.05	0.02	0.2	52
Orange, raw California, naval, 2⅘ in. diameter	1	180	60	252	2	trace	—	—	—	16	49	0.5	240	0.12	0.05	0.5	75
Orange juice, frozen concentrate, diluted with 3 parts water, by volume	1 cup	248	110	462	2	trace	—	—	—	27	22	0.2	500	0.21	0.03	0.8	112
Raisins, dried	1 cup	160	460	1932	4	trace	—	—	—	124	99	5.6	30	0.18	0.13	0.9	2
Strawberries, raw, capped	1 cup	149	55	231	1	1	—	—	—	13	31	1.5	90	0.04	0.10	1.0	88
Tangerine raw, medium	1	114	40	168	1	trace	—	—	—	10	34	0.3	350	0.05	0.02	0.1	26
BREAD (RELATED PRODUCTS)																	
White bread, enriched	1 slice	23	60	252	2	1	trace	trace	trace	12	16	0.6	trace	0.06	0.04	0.5	trace
Whole-wheat bread, made with 2% nonfat dry milk	1 slice	23	55	231	2	1	trace	trace	trace	11	23	0.5	trace	0.06	0.03	0.7	trace

B. Nutritive Value of Selected Foods (Continued)

Food and Approximate Measure	Weight (gm)	Food Energy kcal	Food Energy kJ	Protein (gm)	Fat, total lipids (gm)	Fatty Acids Saturated, total (gm)	Unsaturated Oleic (gm)	Unsaturated Linoleic (gm)	Carbohydrate (gm)	Calcium (mg)	Iron (mg)	Vitamin A value (IU)	Thiamine (mg)	Riboflavin (mg)	Niacin (mg)	Ascorbic acid (mg)
Macaroni, enriched, cooked, firm stage (8–10 minutes, undergoes additional cooking in a food mixture) 1 cup	130	190	798	6	1	—	—	—	39	14	1.4	0	0.23	0.14	1.9	0
Rice, white (fully milled or polished) cooked, common commercial 1 cup	168	185	777	3	trace	—	—	—	41	17	1.5	0	0.19	0.01	1.6	0
Wheat flakes, with added nutrients 1 oz	28	100	420	3	trace	—	—	—	23	12	1.2	0	0.18	0.04	1.4	0
FATS, OILS																
Butter, pat or square (64 per pound) 1 pat	7	50	210	trace	6	3	2	1	trace	1	0	230	—	—	—	0
Margarine, pat or square (64 per pound) 1 pat	7	50	210	trace	6	1	3	1	trace	1	0	230	—	—	—	0
Corn oil 1 tbsp	14	125	525	0	14	1	4	7	0	0	0	—	0	0	0	0
Mayonnaise 1 tbsp	15	110	462	trace	12	2	3	6	trace	3	1	40	trace	0.01	trace	—
SUGARS, SWEETS																
Candy, fudge plain 1 oz	28	115	483	1	3	2	1	trace	21	22	0.3	trace	0.01	0.03	0.1	trace
Jellies 1 tbsp	20	55	231	trace	trace	—	—	—	14	4	0.3	trace	trace	0.01	trace	1
Sugar, cane or beet, granulated 1 tbsp	12	45	189	0	0	—	—	—	12	0	trace	0	0	0	0	0
BEVERAGES Carbonated																
Cola type 1 cup	240	95	399	0	0	—	—	—	24	—	—	0	0	0	0	0
Ginger ale 1 cup	230	70	294	0	0	—	—	—	18	—	—	0	0	0	0	0
Coffee 1 cup	180	2	8	trace	trace	—	—	—	trace	4	0.2	0	0	trace	0.5	0

Source: U.S. Department of Agriculture, Nutritive Values of Food. Home and Garden Bulletin No. 72, 1971.

C. Iron Content of Selected High-Iron Foods

Food	Measure	Iron (mg)
RED MEATS (COOKED)		
Liver		
Pork	2 oz	16.6
Lamb	2 oz	10.2
Beef, calf, chicken	2 oz	8.1
Liverwurst	2 oz	3.2
Beef, pork, veal (most cuts)	2 oz	1.0–2.6
Lamb (most cuts)	2 oz	0.6–1.0
OTHER ANIMAL PRODUCTS (COOKED)		
Clams, oysters, sardines	2 oz	2.4–4.6
Eggs	1	1.1
CEREAL PRODUCTS (COOKED)		
Enriched Malt-o-Meal	½ cup	1.3
Quick or Instant Cream of Wheat	½ cup	7.8
FORTIFIED DRY CEREALS	(1 oz)	
Wheat Chex	⅔ cup	9.0
40% Bran Flakes	¾ cup	4.2
Raisin Bran	½ cup	6.2
Product 19	1 cup	17.8
Fortified Oat Flakes	⅔ cup	4.7
Total	1½ cups	17.8
Buck Wheats	1 cup	8.0
COOKED DRIED BEANS AND PEAS (LEGUMES)		
Beans		
White, kidney, lima, pinto, soybeans, canned pork and beans	½ cup	2.2–2.7
Peas		
Blackeyed, cowpea, split, and lentils	½ cup	1.3–1.7
LEAFY VEGETABLES		
Greens		
Beets, chard, dandelion, mustard, spinach (cooked)	½ cup cooked	1.8–3.3
MISCELLANEOUS		
Pumpkin and squash kernels	¼ cup	3.9
Wheat germ	½ cup	2.7
Sunflower seeds	¼ cup	2.5
Prunes, cooked	4	1.5
Dates, pitted	5	1.2
Raisins	¼ cup (1½ oz)	1.4
Dried apricots	4 halves	1.0
Dried figs	2	1.2
Nuts, most kinds	1 oz	1.0
Molasses		
Light	1 tbsp	0.9
Blackstrap	1 tbsp	2.3
INFANT FOODS		
Strained beef liver	3½ oz (1 jar)	4.3
Baby cereals		
all kinds	2 tbsp dry	4.7
Strained egg yolk	3½ oz	2.9
Strained beef, chicken, lamb and veal	3½ oz (1 jar)	1.0–1.8

D. Enteral Products

Type (Pharmaceutical)	Nutrient Source			Nutrient Composition (gm/100 ml)				
	Protein	Carbohydrate	Fat	PRO	CHO	FAT	Ca	Fe
NUTRITIONALLY COMPLETE FEEDINGS								
Isocal (MJ)	Calcium, caseinate, sodium caseinate, soy protein isolate	Maltodextrin	MCT 20%, soy oil	3.4	13.2	4.4	0.63	0.
Isocal HCN (MJ)	Calcium caseinate, sodium caseinate	Corn syrup	MCT 30%, soy oil	7.5	22.5	9.1	0.67	0.
Osmolite (Ross)	Sodium caseinate, calcium caseinate, soy protein isolate	Hydrolyzed corn syrup	MCT 50%, corn oil, soy oil	3.7	14.3	3.8	0.05	0.
Compleat-B (Doyle)	Beef puree, nonfat dry milk	Maltodextrin, green bean puree, pea puree, sucrose, peach puree, orange juice, lactose	Corn oil, beef fat	4.3	12.8	4.3	0.07	0.
Ensure (Ross)	Sodium caseinate, calcium caseinate, soy protein isolate	Hydrolyzed corn starch, sucrose	Corn oil	3.7	14.3	3.7	0.05	0.0
Ensure Plus (Ross)	Sodium caseinate, calcium caseinate, soy protein isolate	Hydrolyzed corn starch, sucrose	Corn oil	5.4	19.7	5.3	0.06	0.
Meritene Liquid (Doyle)	Skim milk, sodium caseinate	Corn syrup solids, sucrose, lactose	Corn oil, mono- and di-glycerides	6.0	11.5	3.3	0.13	0.0
Sustacal Liquid (Ross)	Calcium caseinate, soy protein isolate, sodium caseinate	Sucrose, corn syrup	Soy oil	6.1	14.0	2.3	1.0	0.
Vital (Ross)	Partially hydrolyzed soy, whey, meat protein L-amino acids	Glucose and polysaccharides, sucrose	Safflower oil, MCT	4.2	18.5	1.1	0.67	0.
DIETARY SUPPLEMENTS								
Carnation Instant Breakfast (powder mixed with whole milk as directed)	Nonfat milk, calcium caseinate, lactalbumin, whey	Sucrose, corn syrup solids, lactose	Butterfat	6.3	14.6	3.3	0.2	0.0
Sustagen (MJ)	Nonfat milk, powdered whole milk, calcium caseinate	Corn syrup solids, dextrose, lactose	Milk fat	9.8	27.7	1.5	2.95	0.0
Citrotein (Doyle)	Egg white solids	Sucrose, maltodextrin	Mono- and diglycerides	4.4	12.95	0.2	0.11	0.0

Note: Additional water may be needed with certain enteral products. Check manufacturer's literature for additional information and contraindications.

Nitrogen (gm/100 kcal)	kcal/ml	Electrolyte Composition (mEq/liter)			Osmolality (mOsm/kg H$_2$O)	Renal Solute Load mOsm/kg/qt	Considerations, Description
		Na$^+$	K$^+$	Cl$^-$			
20.0	1.06	23	34	30	300	211	Used as a tube feeding when normal ingestion is impaired (e.g., TE fistula, omphalocele repair); also can be used as an oral supplement. Note: Additional water should be given.
22.5	2.0	35	36	34	690	383	Meets the high-calorie, high-nitrogen needs of hypermetabolic patients (e.g., burns, major trauma), of fluid restricted patients (e.g., congestive heart failure, neurosurgery), and of volume restricted patients (e.g., cardiac or cancer.) Note: Additional water should be given as needed.
21.8	1.06	24	26	23	300	—	A low-residue product used as an oral or gavage feeding for patients sensitive to hyperosmotic feedings.
25.1	1.07	7	3	2	405	—	Normal proportions of natural foods (meat, vegetables, milk, and fruit) mixed in blender for patients requiring total or supplemental intake by tube when normal ingestion is impaired (e.g., throat or oral cancer, coma or paralysis).
20.0	1.06	36	40	40	450	306/liter	A low-residue, lactose-free product used as a tube feeding, as a liquid supplement, or as a full liquid diet in patients with inadequate normal food intake and/or inadequate nutrition.
22.5	1.5	49	59	55	600	455/liter	A lactose-free, high-calorie, high-protein liquid food in a limited volume. Used in patients with increased nutritional needs but with limited capacity (e.g., major burns/trauma, severe anorexia). Used as a supplement in patients with inadequate nutrition.
37.5	1.0	40	43	47	—	—	Used as a complete meal replacement or as a supplement (tube or oral) when appetite is diminished (e.g., convalescents, chronically ill, underweight). Note: Additional water should be given.
38.1	1.0	39	51	52	625	364	A lactose-free, low-residue nutritionally complete food for patients with inadequate intake and/or inadequate nutrition (e.g., anorexia, dental, hypermetabolism, oral or throat cancer).
21.3	1.0	17	30	19	460	234	A low-fat, minimal lactose product that can be used as an oral or tube feeding. It has low osmolality, low residue, and provides essential fatty acids. It is indicated after long NPO status.
32.8	1.2	44	76	—	723	—	Used orally as a complete meal replacement or as a supplement. Product is readily available in supermarkets and is low in cost.
38.3	1.6	49	83	71	—	—	A high-calorie, high-protein, low-fat oral supplementary food used in patients with poor appetite, inadequate intake, and/or increased nutritional needs. Note: Supplement with essential fatty acids if used for long periods of time.
39.3	0.7	33	19	28	495	—	A lactose-, cholesterol-, and gluten-free, low-residue, fruit flavored supplement used when appetite or food tolerance is diminished (e.g., anorexia, chronic illness, rapid growth periods).

Appendix 5. Food Additives

A. Nutrients
B. Preservatives (Antimicrobials)
C. Preservatives (Antioxidants)
D. Emulsifiers
E. Stabilizers, Thickeners, Texturizers
F. Leavening Agents
G. pH Control Agents
H. Humectants
I. Maturing and Bleaching Agents, Dough Conditioners
J. Anticaking Agents
K. Flavor Enhancers
L. Flavors
M. Natural/Synthetic (N/S) Colors
N. Sweeteners

A. Nutrients

Purpose: To improve or maintain nutritional value
Functions: Enrich by replacing vitamins and minerals lost in processing or fortify by adding nutrients that may be lacking in the diet

Some Additives	Where You Might Find Them
B vitamins: thiamine, thiamine hydrochloride, thiamine moninitrate, riboflavin, niacin, niacinamide	Flour, breads, cereals, rice, macaroni products
Beta carotene (source of vitamin A)	Margarine
Iodine, potassium iodide	Salt
Iron	Grain products
Alpha tocopherols (vitamin E)	Cereals, grain products
Vitamin A	Milk, margarine, cereals
Vitamin D, D_2, D_3	Milk, cereals
Ascorbic acid (vitamin C)	Beverages, beverage mixes, processed fruit

B. Preservatives (Antimicrobials)

Purpose: To maintain product quality
Functions: Prevent food spoilage from bacteria, molds, fungi, and yeast; extend shelf life; protect natural color and flavor

Some Additives	Where You Might Find Them
Ascorbic acid (vitamin C)	Fruit products, acidic foods
Benzoic acid, sodium benzoate	Fruit products, acidic foods, margarine
Citric acid	Acidic foods
Lactic acid, calcium lactate	Olives, cheeses, frozen desserts, some beverages
Parabens: butylparaben, heptylparaben, methylparaben, propylparaben	Beverages, cake-type pastries, salad dressings, relishes
Propionic acid: calcium propionate, potassium propionate, sodium propionate	Breads and other baked goods
Sodium diacetate	Baked goods
Sodium erythorbate	Cured meats
Sodium nitrate, sodium nitrite	Cured meats, fish, poultry
Sorbic acid: calcium sorbate, potassium sorbate, sodium sorbate	Cheeses, syrups, cakes, beverages, mayonnaise, fruit products, margarine, processed meats

C. Preservatives (Antioxidants)

Purpose: To maintain product quality
Functions: Delay or prevent undesirable changes in color, flavor, or texture
(e.g., enzymatic browning or discoloration due to oxidation); delay or
prevent rancidity in foods with unstable oils

Some Additives	Where You Might Find Them
Ascorbic acid (vitamin C)	Processed fruits, baked goods
BHA (butylated hydroxyanisole), BHT (butylated hydroxytoluene)	Bakery products, cereals, snack foods, fats and oils
Citric acid	Fruits, snack foods, cereals, instant potatoes
EDTA (ethylenediaminetetraacetic acid)	Dressings, sauces, margarine
Propyl gallate	Cereals, snack foods, pastries
TBHQ (tertiary butylhydroquinone)	Snack foods, fats, and oils
Tocopherols (including vitamin E)	Oils and shortening

D. Emulsifiers

Purpose: To aid in processing or preparation
Functions: Help to distribute evenly tiny particles of one liquid into
another (e.g., oil and water); modify surface tension or liquid to establish a
uniform dispersion or emulsion; improve homogeneity, consistency,
stability, and texture

Some Additives	Where You Might Find Them
Carrageenan	Chocolate milk, canned milk drinks, whipped toppings
Lecithin	Margarine, dressings, chocolate, frozen desserts, baked goods
Mono/diglycerides	Baked goods, peanut butter, cereals
Polysorbate 60, 65, 80	Gelatin and pudding desserts, dressings, baked goods, nondairy creamers, ice cream
Sorbitan monostearate	Cakes, toppings, chocolate
Dioctyl sodium sulfosuccinate	Cocoa

E. Stabilizers

Purpose: To aid in processing or preparation
Functions: Impart body, improve consistency, texture; stabilize emulsions; affect appearance, mouth feel of food; many are natural carbohydrates that absorb water in food

Some Additives	Where You Might Find Them
Ammonium alginate, calcium alginate, potassium alginate, sodium alginate	Dessert-type dairy products, confections
Carrageenan	Frozen desserts, puddings, syrups, jellies
Cellulose derivatives	Breads, ice cream, confections, diet foods
Flour	Sauces, gravies, canned foods
Furcelleran	Frozen desserts, puddings, syrups
Modified food starch	Sauces, soups, pie fillings, canned meals, snack foods
Pectin	Jams/jellies, fruit products, frozen desserts
Propylene glycol	Baked goods, frozen desserts, dairy spreads
Vegetable gums: guar gum, gum arabic, gum ghatti, karaya gum, locust (carob) bean gum, tragacanth gum, larch gum (arabinogalactan)	Chewing gum, sauces, desserts, dressings, syrups, beverages, fabricated foods, cheeses, baked goods

F. Leavening Agents

Purpose: To aid in processing or preparation
Functions: Affect cooking results and texture; increase volume; also produce some flavor effects

Some Additives	Where You Might Find Them
Yeast	Breads, baked goods
Baking powder, doubleacting (sodium bicarbonate, sodium aluminum sulfate, calcium phosphate)	Quick breads, cake-type baked goods
Baking soda (sodium bicarbonate)	Quick breads, cake-type baked goods

G. pH Control Agents

Purpose: To aid in processing or preparation
Functions: Control (change or maintain) acidity or alkalinity; can affect
texture, taste, and wholesomeness

Some Additives	Where You Might Find Them
Acetic acid, sodium acetate	Candies, sauces, dressings, relishes
Adipic acid	Beverage and gelatin bases, bottled drinks
Citric acid, sodium citrate	Fruit products, candies, beverages, frozen desserts
Fumaric acid	Dry dessert bases, confections, powdered soft drinks
Lactic acid	Cheeses, beverages, frozen desserts
Calcium lactate	Fruits, vegetables, dry and condensed milk
Phosphoric acid, phosphates	Fruit products, beverages, ices, sherbets, soft drinks, oils, baked goods
Tartaric acid, tartrates	Confections, some dairy desserts, baked goods, beverages

H. Humectants

Purpose: To aid in processing or preparation
Function: Retain moisture

Some Additives	Where You Might Find Them
Glycerine	Flaked coconut
Glycerol monostearate	Marshmallow
Propylene glycol	Confections, pet foods
Sorbitol	Soft candies, gum

I. Maturing and Bleaching Agents, Dough Conditioners

Purpose: To aid in processing or preparation
Functions: Accelerate the aging process (oxidation) to develop the gluten characteristics of flour; improve baking qualities

Some Additives	Where You Might Find Them
Azodicarbonamide	Cereal flour, breads
Acetone peroxide, benzoyl peroxide, hydrogen peroxide	Flour, breads and rolls
Calcium/potassium bromate	Breads
Sodium stearyl fumarate	Yeast-leavened breads, instant potatoes, processed cereals

J. Anticaking Agents

Purpose: To aid in processing or preparation
Functions: Help keep salts and powders free-flowing; prevent caking, lumping, or clustering of a finely powdered or crystalline substance

Some Additives	Where You Might Find Them
Calcium silicate	Table salt, baking powder, other powdered foods
Iron ammonium citrate	Salt
Silicon dioxide	Table salt, baking powder, other powdered foods
Yellow prussiate of soda	Salt

K. Flavor Enhancers

Purpose: To affect appeal characteristics
Functions: Supplement, magnify, or modify the original taste and/or aroma of a food without imparting a characteristic taste or aroma of its own

Some Additives	Where You Might Find Them
Disodium guanylate	Canned vegetables
Disodium inosinate	Canned vegetables
Hydrolyzed vegetable protein	Processed meats, gravy/sauce mixes, fabricated foods
MSG (monosodium glutamate)	Oriental foods, soups, foods with animal protein
Yeast-malt sprout extract	Gravies, sauces

L. Flavors

Purpose: To affect appeal characteristics
Functions: Make foods taste better; improve natural flavor; restore flavors lost in processing

Some Additives	Where You Might Find Them
Vanilla (natural)	Baked goods
Vanillin (synthetic)	Baked goods
Spices and other natural seasonings and flavorings (e.g., clove, cinnamon, ginger, paprika, turmeric, anise, sage, thyme, basil)	No restrictions on usage in foods; found in many products

M. Natural/Synthetic (N/S) Colors

Purpose: To affect appeal characteristics
Functions: Increase consumer appeal and product acceptance by giving a
desired, appetizing, or characteristic color; any material that imparts color
when added to a food; generally not restricted to certain foods or food
classes; may not be used to cover up an unwholesome food or used in
excessive amounts; must be used in accordance with FDA Good
Manufacturing Practice Regulations

Some Additives	Where You Might Find Them
N Annatto extract (yellow-red)	No restrictions
N Dehydrated beets/beet powder	No restrictions
S Ultramarine blue	Animal feed only 0.5% by weight
N/S Canthaxanthin (orange-red)	Limit = 30 mg/lb of food
N Caramel (brown)	No restrictions
N/S Beta-apo-8' carotenal (yellow-red)	Limit = 15 mg/lb of food
N/S Beta carotene (yellow)	No restrictions
N Cochineal extract/carmine (red)	No restrictions
N Toasted partially defatted cooked cottonseed flour (brown shades)	No restrictions
S Ferrous gluconate (turns black)	Ripe olives
N Grape skin extract (purple-red)	Beverages only
S Iron oxide (red-brown)	Pet foods only; 0.25% or less by wt
N Fruit juice/vegetable juice	No restrictions
N Dried algae meal (yellow)	Chicken feed only
N Tagetes (Aztec Marigold)	Chicken feed only
N Carrot oil (orange)	No restrictions
N Corn endosperm (red-brown)	Chicken feed only
N Paprika/paprika oleoresin (red-orange)	No restrictions
N/S Riboflavin (yellow)	No restrictions
N Saffron (orange)	No restrictions
S Titanium dioxide (white)	Limit = 1% by wt
N Turmeric/Turmeric oleoresins (yellow)	No restrictions
*S FD & C Blue No. 1	No restrictions
*S Citrus Red No. 2	Orange skins of mature, green, eating oranges; limit = 2 ppm
*S FD & C Red No. 3	No restrictions
*S FD & C Red No. 40	No restrictions
S FD & C Yellow No. 5	No restrictions

*Synthetic color additives are subject to certification and are inspected and tested for
impurities.

N. Sweeteners

Purpose: To affect appeal characteristics
Function: Make the aroma or taste more agreeable or pleasurable

Some Additives	Where You Might Find Them
Nutritive sweeteners: mannitol (sugar alcohol), sorbitol (sugar alcohol)	Candies, gum, confections, baked goods
Dextrose, fructose, glucose, sucrose (table sugar)	Cereals, baked goods, candies, processed foods, processed meats
Corn syrup, corn syrup solids, invert sugar	Cereals, baked goods, candies, processed foods, processed meats
Nonnutritive sweeteners: saccharin	Special dietary foods, beverages

A–N: Adapted from *FDA Consumer*, HEW Publication No. (FDA) 79–2118, 79–2119, reprinted May–June 1978.

Appendix 6. Drug and Nutrient Interactions

Drug	Chief Ingredient(s)	Trade Name(s)	Possible Nutrient Interactions
Analgesics/antipyretics	Acetylsalicylic acid	Aspirin	Increases urinary loss of ascorbic acid; reduces serum folate levels, especially in patients being treated for rheumatoid arthritis; causes GI bleeding with subsequent iron deficiency anemia
Antacids	Aluminum hydroxide	Amphogel	Can result in phosphate depletion and decreased absorption of vitamin D
	Calcium carbonate	Tums	Decreases absorption of iron and thiamine
	Cimetidine	Tagamet	
Antibacterials (broad-spectrum)	Tetracylines	Sumycin Achromycin	Large doses inhibit bone growth in infants and young children; also decreases endogenous vitamin K production
	Chloramphenicol	Chloromycetin	May increase requirement for folate, B_6, B_{12}, iron, and riboflavin
	Clindamycin	Cleocin	Frequently causes colitis
	Aminoglycosides		Reduce lactose levels; causes malabsorption syndrome
	Amikacin	Amikin	
	Gentamicin	Garamycin	
	Tobramycin	Nebcin	
	Kanamycin	Kantrex	
	Sulfa drugs		
	Sulfamethoxazole	Bactrim Suspension	As above; also causes phenylalanine accumulation and antagonizes folic acid
	Trimethoprim	Septra Suspension	
Anticonvulsants	Phenytoin (diphenylhydantoin)	Dilantin	Causes inactivation of vitamin D; possible antagonist of folic acid
	Phenobarbital	Phenobarbital elixir	Decrease levels of folic acid, vitamins B_{12}, D, K, B_6, calcium, and magnesium; may increase blood glucose levels; may reduce ascorbic acid levels

Category	Drug	Brand name	Effect
Antidiarrheals/ antispasmodics	Phenobarbital (see above)	Donnatal	
	Bismuth subcarbonate	Peptobismol Kaopectate Parepectolin	Reduces absorption of nutrients
Antienuretics	Imipramine	Tofranil	Decreased absorption of nutrients caused by mild gastrointestinal disturbances (e.g., possible anorexia, vomiting)
Antiinflammatory agents	Sulfasalazine	Azulfidine	Reduces serum levels of folic acid
	Steroids	Hydrocortisone	Alters metabolism of carbohydrate, protein, and fat (increases blood glucose and fat deposition and decreases muscle protein; causes retention of sodium chloride and water); growth retardation; decreases levels of ascorbic acid, folic acid, B_6, vitamins A, D, K, and zinc
Bronchodilators	Theophylline	Aminophylline Slo-phyllin	Nausea, vomiting, taste alteration
	Metaproterenol sulfate	Alupent Metaprel	
Chelating agents	Penicillamine	Curamine	Increases zinc excretion; results in vitamin B_6 deficiency
Diuretics	Thiazides	Hydrochlorothiazide	Increases excretion of magnesium and zinc
	Triamterene	Dyrenium	Results in folate deficiency

Drug	Chief Ingredient(s)	Trade Name(s)	Possible Nutrient Interactions
Laxatives			This class of drugs decreases absorption by decreasing transit time; chronic abuse can result in hypocalcemia, hypokalemia, and general malnutrition
	Diocytl sodium sulfosuccinate	Colace	
	Malt soup extract	Maltsupex	Contains barley malt-d (possible allergen)
	Mineral oil	Mineral oil	Reduces absorption of fat soluble vitamins A, D, E, K, and carotene, calcium, and phosphates
	Phenolphthalein	Ex-Lax Feen-A-Mint	Decreases absorption of vitamin D and calcium
	Mineral oil	Agoral	See mineral oil and phenolphthalein above (contains egg albumin, a possible allergen)
	Senna	Senokot	
Psychostimulants	Methylphenidate hydrochloride	Ritalin	Causes anorexia and weight loss (especially in children) that affects growth
Miscellaneous Drugs that reduce taste acuity	Carbamazepine D-penicillamine Sulfasalazine	Digoxin Tegretol Cuprimine Azulfidine	Increases loss of calcium and magnesium
Drugs that leave a bad taste	Chloral hydrate Briscofulvin griseofulvin Ethambutol Metronidazole Penicillin	Chloral Hydrate Fulvicin Grifulvin Myambutol Flagyl Penicilllin VK	Drug-induced taste disorders may cause decreased appetite and nutrient intake
KCL	Slow-release potassium chloride	Slow-K	Reduces vitamin B_{12} absorption

Note: Generally, drugs in liquid form contain sucrose; drugs in table form contain lactose. Children on medications for extended periods should be on vitamin supplements.
Data from Roe, B. A. *Drug-induced Nutritional Deficiencies.* Westport, Conn.: Avi Publishing Co., 1976; March, D. C. *Handbook: Interactions of Selected Drugs with Nutritional Status in Man* (2nd ed.). Chicago: American Dietetic Association, 1978; and Eichelberger, W., personal communication, The Children's Hospital, Boston, Ma., 1982.

Appendix 7. Drugs Excreted in Breast Milk

Celeste Martin Marx, Pharm.D.

GUIDELINES FOR USE OF DATA ON DRUGS IN MOTHERS' MILK

The following summary is intended to guide the practitioner in choice of equally effective therapies for women who require medication while nursing. Specific patient characteristics, particularly extreme prematurity or history of feeding intolerance in the infant, may affect the decision to give milk to the infant, even when the general guideline indicates safety. When milk should be withheld from the baby, one should encourage the mother to continue to express milk to maintain supply, unless chronic infection is anticipated.

The charts in this section contain very rough estimates of the quantity of drug that a baby may ingest when the nursing mother takes a given agent. The data on milk concentrations from which the tables are drawn are frequently lacking in sophistication regarding when the sample was taken with regard to dosing. However, all concentrations are similar to those that would be predicted from knowledge of the drug's chemical characteristics (molecular weight, lipid solubility, pKa, distribution). In estimating the infant dose, an attempt to err on the side of overestimation has been made by: (1) assuming a generous newborn intake of 200 ml/kg/day of milk and (2) calculating as if reported levels were continuously maintained throughout the dosing interval. These data must not be taken as an absolute dose and relied upon for treatment.

Because of the rapid growth in scientific information in this area, when a particular agent is not listed, information may be sought from local hospital drug information centers or the manufacturer of the drug.

Drugs Excreted in Breast Milk

Drug [Reference]	Reported Milk Levels	Estimated Newborn Intake	Newborn dose (%)	Reported Adverse Effects, Cautions, Monitoring
ANTIBIOTICS				
Ampicillin [48] Amoxicillin [38]	0.014–1 µg/ml up to 0.81 µg/ml	2.8–200 µg/kg/day up to 162 µg/kg/day	0.14–0.4 (0.18% of infant dose)	Minimal exposure; may "flavor" milk; monitor for diarrhea, rash, spitting up (very uncommon)
Carbenicillin [56]	0.265 µg/ml	53 µg/kg/day	0.03	Miniscule amount; not well absorbed from GI tract; nurse as planned
Cefadroxil [38]	0.1–1.64 µg/ml	20–324 µg/kg/day	Not used in newborn	Should be subtherapeutic amount; some change in GI flora could possibly occur; monitor for diarrhea, rash
Cephalexin (Keflex) [38, 56]	0.2–0.5 µg/ml	40–100 µg/kg/day	0.04–0.1	Exposure to these drugs is very small, compared to therapeutic doses; this may sensitize the infant, so that allergic reactions may occur with "first prescription"; monitor for rash, spitting up, diarrhea
Cephalothin (Keflin) [38]	0.27–0.47 µg/ml	54–94 µg/kg/day	0.05–0.09	
Cefazolin [81] (Kefzol, Ancef)	1.5 µg/ml	300 µg/kg/day	0.9	
Cefotaxime [37] (Claforan)	0.25–0.52 µg/ml	50–104 µg/kg/day	0.1–0.2	
Cefoxitin [84]	0.5–1.0 µg/ml	100–200 µg/kg/day	Dose not defined	Exposure is small; extensive clinical experience in nursing mothers without reported adverse effect; with long-term high dose therapy, monitor for SGOT, eosinophils, rash
Chloramphenicol [26, 27]	0.26–25 µg/ml	52–5000 µg/kg/day	0.2–25	Because of significant potential dose and risk of bone marrow toxicity, do not nurse until 12 hours after stopping drug; "gray baby syndrome" of toxicity is also possible

Drug				
Clindamycin [73, 51]	0.74–3.8 µg/ml	148–760 µg/kg/day	(1.4–7.6% of child's dose)	Pharmacology in newborns not studied; potentially significant dose and report of GI bleeding in nursed infant; do not nurse for 24 hours after discontinuation
Dicloxacillin	Not studied	Unknown	Unknown	No reported adverse effects; direct administration to newborns appears safe; monitor for spitting up, abdominal distention
Erythromycin [43]	0.4–6.2 µg/ml (animal work)	50–124 µg/kg/day	0.1–0.25	No adverse effects reported in infants who have nursed; monitor for diarrhea, spitting up, abdominal distention
Ethambutol [18]	1.4–4.6 µg/ml	280–920 µg/kg/day	1–3.6	Exposure is small; potential ophthalmic toxicity (macular degeneration); consider whether risk is new or continued from pregnancy
Gentamicin [34]	0.157 µg/ml	47.1 µg/kg/day	0.9	No need to restrict nursing; extremely small dose, not absorbed except from damaged GI tract; monitor for diarrhea
Isoniazid (INH) [67, 80]	6–12 µg/ml	1.2–2.4 mg/kg/day	6.3–25	Significant passage; will not provide reliable dose to infant of mother with active or inactive TB; some consider contraindicated due to anti-DNA effect; avoid nursing or supplement with PVS for vitamin B_6; monitor for anemia, rash, hepatitis

Drugs Excreted in Breast Milk (*Continued*)

Drug [Reference]	Reported Milk Levels	Estimated Newborn Intake	Newborn dose (%)	Reported Adverse Effects, Cautions, Monitoring
Metronidazole [19] (Flagyl)	1–46 µg/ml	0.2–9.2 mg/kg/day	(Adult dose: 30 mg/kg/day)	Potential carcinogen; nursing considered contraindicated
Methenamine [9]	0.22–1.1 µg/ml	44–280 µg/kg/day	Unknown (50–60 mg/kg/day in children)	No reported adverse effects; monitor for albuminuria and hematuria with prolonged exposure
Minocycline [13] (Minocin)	0.8 µg/ml	36–160 µg/kg/day	Not used in newborn	Tetracyclines are considered contraindicated because of potential for tooth staining and inhibition of bone formation
Nitrofurantoin [31, 79]	0.3–0.5 µg/ml	60–100 µg/kg/day	Not used in newborn	No reported adverse effects; should be avoided if baby may be G6PD deficient because hemolysis could occur
Oxacillin, nafcillin	Not studied	Unknown	Unknown	Anecdotal experience without reported adverse effect; drug frequently used in newborns with only rare hepatitis or leukopenia
Penicillin [25, 68]	60–960 U/liter	12–192 U/kg/day	0.4–0.005	Minuscule dose; provides initial exposure for development of allergy (sensitization); monitor for rash
Sulfamethoxazole (Gantanol), Sulfisoxazole [42] (Gantrisin), Bactrim, Septra	Present	18 mg/day reported	Approximately 1.2	Do not nurse newborn; highly bound sulfa drugs can displace bilirubin from protein, increasing risk of kernicterus without changing serum bilirubin

Tetracycline [63]	0.43–8 µg/ml	86–1600 µg/kg/day	Not used in newborn	Generally considered contraindicated due to potential tooth staining and altered bone growth
Trimethoprim [5] (Proloprim, Trimpex), Bactrim, Septra	1.2–5.5 µg/ml	240–1100 µg/kg/day	Not used in newborn	No reports of adverse effects; preferred to sulfa-containing combination; monitor for rash, anemia, spitting up
Vancomycin	Not studied	Unknown	Unknown	Do not restrict nursing; not abosrbed from intact GI tract
ANALGESICS				
Acetaminophen [10, 22] (Tylenol)	1–15 µg/ml	0.2–3 mg/kg/day	0.05–0.7	No need to withhold nursing; exposure is virtually avoided if dosed after feedings
Aspirin [22, 65]	1.12–42.6 µg/ml	<0.224–9.7 mg/kg/day	0.06–2.5	Substantial exposure is possible with mothers taking rheumatoid doses (3–5g/day); exposure is minimized by dosing after feeds; monitor for spitting up, bleeding
Codeine [30]	Traces	<91 µg/kg/day	1.5	Poor data on narcotics; exposure is likely small; if mother is narcotized, let-down may be inhibited; at high dosage, monitor for sedation (too sleepy to eat); reversible with Narcan
Demerol [56]	<1 µg/ml	<200 µg/kg/day	0.3	
Dilaudid	Not studied	Unknown	Unknown	
Morphine [45]	<6 µg/ml	<1.2 mg/kg/day	50	
Motrin (Ibuprofen) [76]	Not found in milk	<0.2 mg/kg/day	Unknown (very small)	Without experience in the neonate; no reports of adverse effects; chronic administration should probably be avoided; short-term use appears as safe as aspirin
Naprosyn (Naproxen, [35] Anaprox)	0.55 µg/ml	110 µg/kg/day	Approximately 1–2	

Drugs Excreted in Breast Milk (*Continued*)

Drug [Reference]	Reported Milk Levels	Estimated Newborn Intake	Newborn dose (%)	Reported Adverse Effects, Cautions, Monitoring
Percodan (oxycodone + ASA)	Not studied	Unknown	Unknown	Exposure to narcotic agent not quantified but with extensive clinical experience appears small; monitor for sedation; reversible with Narcan.
Percocet, Tylox (oxycodone + Tylenol)	Not studied	Unknown	Unknown	
Stadol [62] (Butorphanol)	4 ng/ml	0.8 µg/kg/day	Approximately 1	No adverse effects noted; rapidly eliminated, dose after feeds to minimize exposure
Zomepirac (Zomax)	Not studied	Unknown	Unknown	Potential carcinogen; use alternative analgesic
SEDATIVE/HYPNOTICS				
Benadryl (Diphenhydramine)	Not studied	Unknown	Unknown	Probably present in small amounts; no adverse effects reported with considerable experience; monitor for sedation, agitation
Chloral hydrate [18, 66]	0–15 µg/ml	0–3 mg/kg/day	0–15	Long history of use in children; no reported adverse effects in nurslings; the mother should avoid alcohol when taking chloral hydrate; monitor for sedation, rash

Drug	Milk concentration	Dose	Ratio	Comments
Dalmane (Flurazepam) [80]	Not found	Unknown	Unknown	Although very early study did not find Dalmane in milk, it is very likely present in small concentration; chronic administration is best avoided (accumulation may occur); monitor for sedation
Seconal [56]	Present; not quantified	Unknown	Unknown	With extensive short-term clinical experience, appears not to produce excessive sedation; avoid chronic administration (accumulation may occur); monitor for sedation
Valium (diazepam) [18]	17–100 ng/ml or more (+ 19–85 ng/ml desmethyl-diazepam active metabolite)	3.4–20 µg/kg/day	1–6 or more (+ active metabolite)	Avoid nursing during chronic administration; higher milk levels may accumulate because diazepam is a basic drug with a very long persistence in the body; single doses probably acceptable with monitoring for sedation
Vistaril (Hydroxyzine), Atarax	Not studied	Unknown	Unknown	No reported adverse effects; monitor for sedation
CARDIOVASCULAR DRUGS				
Antiarrhythmics Digoxin [23, 50]	0.2–0.9 ng/ml (equal to serum)	40–180 ng/kg/day	0.06–0.3	Minuscule dose; only most conservative would check digoxin level at two weeks of age; monitor for spitting up, diarrhea, heart rate
Quinidine [29]	6.4–8.2 µg/ml	1.3–1.6 mg/kg/day	3.5–10.0	Significant exposure; monitor for rash, anemias, widening of QRS, arrhythmias; may be best to avoid with chronic dosing due to optic neuritis risk

Drugs Excreted in Breast Milk (*Continued*)

Drug [Reference]	Reported Milk Levels	Estimated Newborn Intake	Newborn dose (%)	Reported Adverse Effects, Cautions, Monitoring
Diuretics				
Hydrochlorothiazide [54] (or chlorothiazide) [83]	<20–430 ng/ml	<4–86 µg/kg/day	<0.2–4.0	No reported adverse effect; potential to increase bilirubin toxicity would occur only at high dose
Lasix (Furosemide)	Unknown	0.2 mg/kg/day Unknown	0.4–1.0 Unknown	Exposure likely to be very small and poorly absorbed; do not restrict nursing except with chronic use; may decrease milk flow sharply at first or with excessive dose
Spironolactone [59] (Aldactone)	47–104 ng/ml	0.4–20.8 µg/kg/day	0.3–6.0	No reported adverse effect; because of endocrinic side effects and question of carcinogenicity, other agents preferred
Anticoagulants				
Heparin [56]	Not passed	None	None	Very large molecule not passed or orally absorbed; nurse as planned
Warfarin (Coumadin) [57]	Not detectable (<25 ng/ml)	Not significant	Not significant	Do not restrict nursing; only most conservative check protime at two weeks
ANTIHYPERTENSIVE MEDICATIONS				
Aldomet (Methyldopa) [17]	0.07–1.36 µg/ml	14–272 µg/kg/day	0.04–2.7	Extensive anecdotal experience without adverse effects; potential for hemolysis and increased liver enzymes

Captopril [15]	4.7 ± 0.7 ng/ml	0.8–1.1 µg/kg/day	0.1	Exposure is minimal, but long-term safety in newborns unknown
Clonidine (Catapres) [52]	0.05–1.24 ng/ml	10–248 ng/kg/day	up to 10	Information from a single patient; potentially toxic to retina; do not nurse
Guanethidine [56] (Ismelin)	Negligible	Unknown, likely microgram quantity	Unknown	No reported adverse effects in nurslings; because this agent is used chronically and rarely alone, may be best avoided
Hydralazine [47] (Apresoline)	762–1263 nmol/liter	0.034 mg/kg/day	0.3–3.0	No reports of adverse effects in many nursed infants; generally allow nursing if intermittent (IM) therapy is being given short term; long-term exposure by chronically treated mother is best avoided
Propranolol (Inderal) [8, 41]	10–150 ng/ml	2–30 µg/kg/day	0.4–6.0	Dose is small, but due to potential adverse effect on growth hormone, best to avoid nursing
Prazosin (Minipress) [52]	5–18 ng/ml	1.0–3.6 µg/kg/day	No experience in newborns	Minimal passage but long-term safety unknown; no untoward effects with short-term use
ANTICONVULSANTS Carbamazepine [40, 55, 66]	0.3–3.5 µg/ml	60–700 µg/kg/day	Not used in newborns (0.6–7% of child's dose for weight)	Best to avoid; risk of bone marrow suppression exists when drug is taken chronically

Drugs Excreted in Breast Milk (*Continued*)

Drug [Reference]	Reported Milk Levels	Estimated Newborn Intake	Newborn dose (%)	Reported Adverse Effects, Cautions, Monitoring
Dilantin (phenytoin) [40, 86]	0.5–6 µg/ml	100–1200 µg/kg/day	2–40	Avoid if possible; fairly large dose present in milk; few adverse effects reported (methemoglobinemia with cyanosis in one baby, GI distress in another); unknown effect of long-term use on infant's cognition must be considered
Ethosuximide [40, 44] (Zarontin)	18.5–24.1 µg/ml	3680–4800 µg/kg/day	Not used in newborn (10–20% of child's dose for weight)	Because of rare occurrence of bone marrow depression (reversible) and GI upset, must weigh benefit of nursing vs. risk; consider whether exposure is new or continued from pregnancy and unknown long-term safety; mother's neurologist may wish to consider whether drug is still needed
Phenobarbital [40, 86]	1–20 µg/ml	0.2–4 mg/kg/day	4–100	May be best to avoid if mother is receiving anticonvulsant dosage; women receiving short-term dosing for preeclampsia very likely have much lower levels and nursing may be safe; monitor for sucking problems, sedation, rashes

Drug				
Primidone [40, 86]	0.1–4.5 µg/ml	20–900 µg/kg/day (+ phenobarbital metabolite)	Unknown	May cause irritability; avoid or monitor for alertness
Valproic acid [16] (Depakene)	0.45–0.47 µg/ml	90–94 µg/kg/day	Not used in newborn	Recommend withholding nursing due to lack of experience in newborn and risk of hepatitis and hemorrhagic pancreatitis

RESPIRATORY MEDICATIONS

Drug				
Antihistamines Brompheniramine (Dimetane) Chlorpheniramine (Chlor-Trimeton) Cyproheptadine (Periactin) Diphenhydramine (Benadryl)	No quantitative data	Unknown	Unknown	Reports of agitation when taken in combination with decongestant; no other adverse effects on infant or milk supply; use short-acting agent if possible (chlorpheniramine or diphenhydramine); monitor for sedation, feeding problems
Bronchodilators Albuterol (Proventil, Ventolin Inhaler) Isoproterenol (Iso-Medihaler, Isuprel) Metaproterenol (Alupent) Terbutaline (Brethine, Bricanyl) [12, 49]	Not studied 2.5–4.6 ng/ml	Unknown 0.50–0.92 µg/kg/day	Unknown Very small	Reports of agitation and spitting up; use of inhaled form, rather than oral, may decrease systemic absorption and minimize infant dose

Drugs Excreted in Breast Milk (*Continued*)

Drug [Reference]	Reported Milk Levels	Estimated Newborn Intake	Newborn dose (%)	Reported Adverse Effects, Cautions, Monitoring
Decongestants Ephedrine Phenylpropanolamine (diet pills) Pseudoephedrine (Sudafed) many others	No quantitative data	Unknown	Unknown	Reports of agitated infants with oral therapy; using topical (nasal) therapy should decrease systemic absorption and amount passed; pseudoephedrine would be least exciting of oral forms
Prednisone [69]	41.5 ng/ml mean, 14.5 ng/ml prednisolone (20 mg daily dose)	7 µg/kg/day	0.25	Extremely small dose; nursing need not be interrupted for short-term therapy; safety of long-term therapy not established
Theophylline [87] (or aminophylline)	2–4 µg/ml	400–800 µg/kg/day	6.7–20.0	Generally no problems seen; monitor GI upset, agitation, heart rate; check infant blood level after one week of nursing when mother takes theophylline chronically; probably unnecessary with short-term treatment of occasional exacerbations
GASTROINTESTINAL MEDICATIONS				
Cimetidine (Tagamet) [72]	4.88–6.00 µg/ml	0.96–1.20 mg/kg/day	Approximately 2.0–2.5	Relatively concentrated in mother's milk; no studies of long-term safety to endocrine systems so best to avoid exposure

Sucralfate	Not studied; likely to be nil because drug is not systemically absorbed	Unknown (likely none)	Likely none	Because drug is not absorbed into mother's blood, none should appear in milk; however, not conclusively proven
PSYCHOTHERAPEUTIC AGENTS				
Antianxiety agents				
Chlorazepate [1]	Unknown	Unknown	Not used	Use studied alternative
Chlordiazepoxide [6] (Librium)	Reportedly present	Unknown	Not used	In general, an occasional dose does not contraindicate nursing; avoid nursing if use is chronic; monitor for sedation, weight gain
Diazepam (Valium) [18]	17–100 ng/ml or more (+19–85 ng/ml desmethydiazepam active metabolite)	3.4–20 µg/kg/day +	1–6 or more + active metabolite	
Hydroxyzine (Vistaril)	Not studied	Unknown	Unknown	
Meprobamate (Miltown) [28]	Predicted to be 2–4 times concurrent plasma concentration	10–120 mg/kg/day	96	Because of potential for pharmacological sedation, may be best to use studied alternative (i.e., Diazepam)
Oxazepam (Serax)	Not studied	Unknown	Unknown	In general, an occasional dose does not contraindicate nursing; avoid nursing if use is chronic; monitor for sedation, weight gain; may be safest to use alternative
Phenobarbital (See anticonvulsants)				
See also Sedative/Hypnotics				
Antipsychotic drugs				

Drugs Excreted in Breast Milk (*Continued*)

Drug [Reference]	Reported Milk Levels	Estimated Newborn Intake	Newborn dose (%)	Reported Adverse Effects, Cautions, Monitoring
Chlorpromazine (CPZ) (Thorazine) [11, 85]	7–290 ng/ml	1.4–58 µg/kg/day	0.0005–0.03	Several babies who nursed on CPZ were developmentally normal at age 5; for other agents, long-term safety is unknown; the probably small amount of drug received is not a new risk for those who received the drug antenatally, but is a continued and avoidable one; must monitor for growth disorders, sedation, liver function tests, dystonia
Mesoridazine (Serentil) [56]	All reportedly present	Unknown	Unknown	
Piperacetazine (Quide) [56]				
Prochlorperazine (Compazine) [56]				
Thioridazine (Mellaril) [4]				
Trifluoperazine (Stelazine) [43]				
Haloperidol (Haldol) [74, 82]	2–23 ng/ml	0.4–4.6 µg/kg/day	1.3–46.0 of child's dose per kg	No reported adverse effect; because of large potential dose and chronic therapy, other agents preferred
Lithium [71, 77]	0.12–0.6 mEq/liter	24–120 µEq/kg/day	Unknown	Produces serum level in baby as high as 30% of mother's level; although not absolutely contraindicated, safest to avoid; if nursing is allowed, monitor serum Li^+ and Na^+, growth and development

Stimulants				
Amphetamine [6]	Not measured	Unknown	Unknown	No stimulation or insomnia observed in 103 infants whose mothers received amphetamine for depression
Caffeine [70]	8.2 µg/ml 4 hr after 1 cup of coffee (100 mg)	1.6 mg/kg/day per cup or more	8–30 per cup or more	Potential for therapeutic caffeine dose; monitor for agitation; consider caffeine levels in theophylline-treated premature infants
Antidepressants, Tricyclic				
Amitriptyline (Elavil, others) [7]	135–151 ng/ml + 52–59 ng/ml nortriptyline	27–30 µg/kg/day		There is no information about usual dose or safety in the newborn population. However, because early studies were unable to detect the antidepressants in milk, babies have been nursed without reported adverse effect. However, because psychotherapeutic agents are taken chronically, the uncertainty of long-term safety must be considered when a woman wishes to nurse her baby while requiring medication. It should be remembered that, while the small amount of drug ingested during lactation is not a new risk for the child exposed antenatally, it is a continued and avoidable one. If nursing is decided upon, scrupulous follow-up on infant growth and development is necessary
Amoxapine [24]	<20 ng/ml, 115–168 ng/ml active metabolite	23–34 µg/kg/day metabolite		
Desipramine	Unknown	Unknown		
Imipramine [20]	Reportedly present, not quantified	Predicted to be 0.04 mg/kg/day of milk-plasma levels		
Nortriptyline [3]	Although reportedly not detected after a small dose, excretion seen after amitriptyline	Unknown		

Drugs Excreted in Breast Milk (*Continued*)

Drug [Reference]	Reported Milk Levels	Estimated Newborn Intake	Newborn dose (%)	Reported Adverse Effects, Cautions, Monitoring
MAO Inhibitors				
Phenelzine (Nardil) [58]	Unknown	Unknown	}	Avoid because of lack of adequate study and potential for hypertensive crisis
Tranylcypromine (Parnate) [56]	Too low to affect child	Unknown		
OTHER MEDICATIONS WITH OBSTETRIC USAGE				
Magnesium sulfate [14, 53]	60% of concurrent serum level; normal by 12–24 hours after end of infusion	If true milk produced during infusion, approximately 16 mg/kg/day	300% normal or less during infusion	Unless mother produces true milk volumes during infusion, exposure is likely to be insignificant; for woman still on infusion, document presence of bowel sounds in infant if baby was exposed to $MgSO_4$ antenatally. Monitor for sedation, reflexes, tone, bowel movements until 24 hours after end of infusion
Methylergonovine [21] (Methergine)	Unknown	Unknown	Unknown	Does not suppress lactation; although earlier crude ergot preparations were commonly associated with infant vomiting, diarrhea, weak pulse, and unstable blood pressure, no similar problems reported with use of the synthetic; monitor baby for above effects during short-term (<7 days) use

449

Drug				Comments
Oral contraceptives [2]	Estrogen content not significantly different from that of untreated women; progestogen present but does not appear to accumulate		Unknown	No change in quantity of milk if started after the immediate postpartum period; quality of milk not clearly demonstrated to be altered; long-term safety unknown; does not contraindicate nursing if only reliable contraceptive option; avoid if infant has high bilirubin levels
Oxytocin (Syntocinon)	Presumably too large to be excreted	None	None	Enhances let-down reflex
DIAGNOSTIC AGENTS				
Metrizamide [32, 33]	1.7–21.4 µg/ml	1 mg over 48 hours after single intrathecal dose	0.02 of total adult dose	
Diatrizoate (Hypaque, Reno-M-60)	Not studied	Unknown	Unknown	
Technetium [60, 61]	Radioactivity present	Unknown	Unknown	Two studies indicate that infant would be exposed to no excessive radiation if nursing began 48 hours after a 20-mCi dose to the mother or 24 hours after a 4-mCi dose
Gallium 67 [46]	Radioactivity present	Unknown	Unknown	Radioactivity persists for more than 5 days after maternal dose

450

Drugs Excreted in Breast Milk (*Continued*)

Drug [Reference]	Reported Milk Levels	Estimated Newborn Intake	Newborn dose (%)	Reported Adverse Effects, Cautions, Monitoring
LAXATIVE AGENTS: SUMMARY [18]				
The following agents are reported to be present in milk and associated with increased infant bowel motility:				
Aloe				
Cascara				
Danthron				
Pehnolphthalein				
The following agents were either not detected in milk or reported to have no effect on infant bowel function:				
Milk of magnesia				
Mineral oil				
Rhubarb				
Senna (Senokot)				
There is no information regarding adverse effects on the infant from nursing after maternal use of the following:				
Dulcolax (bisacodyl)				
ENDOCRINE MEDICATIONS				
Thyroid hormones [78]	Normal milk content: T_3: <0.5–0.8 µg/dl T_4: <0.5–1.3 µg/dl	<4.5–9.6 µg/day <4.5–15.6 µg/day	Therapeutic dose is 19–25 µg/day for thyroid replacement	Because thyroid hormone is naturally found in mother's serum and milk, use does not contraindicate nursing; it would be expected that women treated to euthyroid state would have only normal milk levels; however, should not be relied upon to treat hypothyroid infant; monitor growth and development, thyroid function as necessary

Antithyroid drugs			
Propylthiouracil [39] 200–600 mg/day	0.5–0.7 µg/ml	1.2–5 of adult weight corrected dose	Although exposure to these drugs in milk is probably too low to affect thyroid function, serious side effects (bone marrow suppression, rash) may occur; if pediatric follow-up is scrupulous, use may not contraindicate nursing; monitor growth and development, thyroid function tests, blood counts; PTU is probably preferred drug
Methimazole [36, 75]	22–70 ng/ml	1.5–5 of adult weight corrected dose studied on low maternal dose (2.5 mg q 12 hr)	
Carbimazole [36]	100–200 µg/ml of methimazole	7–14 of adult weight corrected dose	
Iodides [64] (SSKI, topical povidone-iodine solutions or vaginal gels)	Passes freely due to small molecular size; dose highly variable		Goiter due to thyroid suppression may be seen; use as expectorant or antithyroid agent should be avoided while nursing
I^{131} [18]	Passes freely; dose highly variable		Nursing may be reinstated two weeks after a dose of radioactive iodine

REFERENCES

1. Abbott Laboratories. *Physician's Desk Reference, 1982.* Oradell, N.J.: Medical Economics Company, 1982. Pp. 565–566.
2. American Academy of Pediatrics Committee on Drugs. Breast-feeding and contraception. *Pediatrics* 68(1):138, 1981.
3. Anderson, P. O. Drugs and breast-feeding. *Drug Intell. Clin. Pharm.* 11:208, 1977.
4. Arias, I., and Guptner, L. Jaundice in breast-fed neonates. *J.A.M.A.* 218:746, 1971.
5. Arnauld, R., et al. Etude de passage de la trimethoprime dans le lait maternel. *Ouest Med.* 25:959, 1972.
6. Ayd, F. E. (Ed.). Excretion of psychotropic drugs in human breast milk. *International Drug Therapy Newsletter.* 8:33, 1973.
7. Bader, T. F., and Newman, K. Amitriptyline in human breast milk and the nursing infant's serum. *Am. J. Psychiatry* 137(7):855, 1980.
8. Bauer, J. H., Pape, B., Zajicek, J., and Groshong, T. Propranolol in human breast milk. *Am. J. Cardiol.* 43:860, 1979.
9. Berger, H. Excretion of mandelic acid in breast milk. *Am. J. Dis. Child.* 61:256, 1941.
10. Berlin, C. M., Yaffe, S. J., and Ragni, M. Disposition of acetaminophen in milk, saliva and plasma of lactating women. *Pediatr. Pharmacol.* (New York) 1:135, 1980.
11. Blacker, K. H., Weinstein, B. J., and Ellman, G. L. Mother's milk and chlorpromazine. *Am. J. Psychiatry* 119:178, 1962.
12. Boreus, L. O., et al. Terbutaline in breast milk. *Br. J. Clin. Pharmacol.* 13:731, 1982.
13. Brogden, R. N., et al. Minocycline—A review. *Drugs* 9:251, 1975.
14. Cruikshank, D. P., Varner, M. W., and Pitkin, R. M. Breast milk magnesium and calcium concentrations following magnesium sulfate treatment. *Am. J. Obstet. Gynecol.* 143(6):685, 1982.
15. Devlin, R. G., and Fleiss, P. M. Captopril in human blood and breast milk. *J. Clin. Pharmacol.* 21:110, 1981.
16. Dickenson, R. G., et al. Transmission of valproic acid across the placenta: Half-life of the drug in mother and baby. *J. Pediatr.* 94(5):832, 1979.
17. Ericson, A. J., Unpublished observation, 1977.
18. Ericson, A. J. Drug Use During Lactation. In J. P. Cloherty, and A. R. Stark, (Eds.). *Manual of Neonatal Care.* Boston: Little, Brown, 1980.
19. Erickson, H. S., Oppenheim, G. L., and Smith, G. Metronidazole in breast milk. *Obstet. Gynecol.* 57:49, 1981.
20. Erickson, S. H., Smith, G. H., and Heidrich, F. Tricyclics and breast feeding (letter). *Am. J. Psychiatry* 135(11):1483, 1979.
21. Ferris, A. J., Sandoz Pharmaceuticals, Personal communication, July, 1981.
22. Findlay, J. W. A., et al. Analgesic drugs in breast milk and plasma. *Clin. Pharmacol. Ther.* 29(5):625, 1981.
23. Finley, J. P., Waxman, M. B., Wong, P. Y., and Likrish, G. M. Digoxin excretion in human milk. *J. Pediatr.* 93(3):339, 1979.
24. Gelenberg, A. J. Amoxapine, a new antidepressant, appears in human milk. *J. Nerv. Ment. Dis.* 167(10):635, 1979.
25. Greene, H. J., Burkhart, B., and Hobby, G. L. Excretion of penicillin in human milk following parturition. *Am. J. Obstet. Gynecol.* 51:732, 1946.
26. Havelka, J., and Frankova, A. Study of side effects of maternal chloramphenicol in newborns. *Excerpta Medica* 27:258, 1972.
27. Havelka, J., Hejzlar, M., Popov, V., et al. Excretion of chloramphenicol in human milk. *Chemotherapy* 13:204, 1968.

28. Hervada, A. R., Feit, E., and Sagraves, R. Drugs in breast milk. *Perinatal Care* 2:19, 1978.
29. Hill, L. M., et al. The use of quinidine sulfate throughout pregnancy. *Obstet. Gynecol.* 54:366, 1979.
30. Horning, M. G., et al. Identification and quantification of drugs and drug metabolites in human breast milk using GC-MS-COM methods. *Mod. Probl. Paediatr.* 15:73, 1975.
31. Hosbach, R. E., and Foster, R. B. Absence of nitrofurantoin from human milk. *J.A.M.A.* 202:1057, 1967.
32. Ilett, K. F., Hackett, L. P., and Paterson, J. W. Excretion of metrizamide in milk. *Br. J. Radiol.* 54:537, 1981.
33. Ilett, K. F., et al. Excretion of metrizamide in milk. *Clin. Exp. Pharmacol. Physiol.* 8:672, 1981.
34. Ito, T. Studies on the absorption and excretion of gentamicin in newborn infants. *J. Antibiot.* (Tokyo) 23(3):298, 1970.
35. Jamali, F., Tam, Y. K., and Stevens, R. D. Naproxen excretion in breast milk and its uptake by suckling infant. Abstracts of the Third Annual Meeting of the American College of Clinical Pharmacy, June 24–26, 1982, Kansas City, MO. *Drug Intell. Clin. Pharm.* 16:475, 1982.
36. Johansen, K., Andersen, A. N., Kampmann, J. P., Hansen, J. M., and Mortensen, H. G. Excretion of methimaxole in human milk. *Eur. J. Clin. Pharmacol.* 23:339, 1982.
37. Kafetzis, D. A., Lazarides, C. V., Stafas, C. A., et al. Transfer of cefotaxime in human milk, and from mother to fetus. *J. Antimicrob. Chemother.* 6(S):135, 1980.
38. Kafetzis, D. A., Stafas, C. A., Georgakopoulos, P. A., and Papadatos, C. J. Passage of cephalosporins and amoxicillin into the breast milk. *Acta Paediatr. Scand.* 70:285, 1981.
39. Kampmann, J. P., Hansen, J. M., Johansen, K., and Helweg, J. Propyl-thiouracil in human milk: Revision of a dogma. *Lancet* 1:736, 1980.
40. Kaneko, S., Sata, T., and Suzuki, K. The levels of anticonvulsants in breast milk. *Br. J. Clin. Pharmacol.* 7:624, 1979.
41. Karlberg, B., Lundberg, D., and Aberg, H. Excretion of propranolol in human breast milk (letter). *Acta Pharmacol. Toxicol.* (Copenh) 34:222, 1974.
42. Kauffman, R. E., O'Brian, C., and Gilford, P. Sulfisoxazole secretion into human milk. *J. Pediatr.* 97(5):639, 1980.
43. Knowles, J. A. Excretion of drugs in milk: A review. *J. Pediatr.* 66:1068, 1965.
44. Koup, J. R., Rose, J. Q., and Cohen, M. E. Ethosuximide pharmacokinetics in a pregnant patient and her newborn. *Epilepsia* 19:535, 1978.
45. Kwit, N. T., and Hatcher, R. A. Excretion of drugs in milk. *Am. J. Dis. Child.* 49:900, 1935.
46. Larson, S. M., and Schall, G. L. Gallium 67 concentration in human breast milk. *J.A.M.A.* 218:257, 1971.
47. Liedholm, H., Wahlin-Boll, E., Hanson, A., et al. Transplacental passage and breast milk concentrations of hydralazine. *Eur. J. Clin. Pharmacol.* 21:417, 1982.
48. Lohmeyer, L., and Halfpap, E. Pharmacokinetic studies and clinical experiences with ampicillin. *Z. Geburtshife Gynakol.* 164:184, 1965.
49. Lonnerholm, G., and Lindstrom, B. Terbutaline excretion into breast milk. *Br. J. Clin. Pharmacol.* 13:729, 1982.
50. Loughnan, P. M. Digoxin excretion in human breast milk. *J. Pediatr.* 92(6):1019, 1978.
51. Mann, C. F. Clindamycin and breast-feeding. *Pediatrics* 66(6):1930, 1980.

52. Marx, C. M., Unpublished observation, 1981.
53. Marx, C. M., Scavone, J. S., and Epstein, M. E. Colostrum magnesium content during magnesium sulfate therapy (submitted for publication).
54. Miller, R. E., Cohn, R. D., and Burghart, P. H. Hydrochlorothiazide disposition in a mother and her breast-fed infant. *J. Pediatr.* 101(5):789, 1982.
55. Niebyl, J., Blake, D. A., Freeman, J. M., and Luff, R. D. Carbamazepine levels in pregnancy and lactation. *Obstet. Gynecol.* 53(1):139, 1979.
56. O'Brian, T. E. Excretion of drugs in human milk. *Am. J. Hosp. Pharm.* 31:844, 1974.
57. Orme, M. L., Lewes, R. J., DeSwiet, M, et al. May mothers given warfarin breastfeed their infants? *Br. Med. J.* [Clin. Res.] 1:1564, 1977.
58. Parke-Davis, Division of Warner-Lambert, Inc., Personal communication, Nov., 1980.
59. Phelps, D. L., and Karem, A. Spironolactone: Relationships between concentrations of dethioacetylated metabolite in human serm and milk. *J. Pharm. Sci.* 66:1203, 1977.
60. Pittard, W. B., Bill, K., and Fletcher, B. D. Excretion of technetium in human milk. *J. Pediatr.* 94(4):605, 1979.
61. Pittard, W. B., Merkatz, R., and Fletcher, B. D. Radioactive excretion in human milk following administration of technetium Tc 99m macroaggregated albumin. *Pediatrics* 70(2):321, 1982.
62. Pittman, K. A., Smyth, R. D., Losada, M., et al. Human perinatal distribution of butorphanol. *Am. J. Obstet. Gynecol.* 138:797, 1980.
63. Posner, A. C., Prigot, A., and Konkcoff, N. G. Further observations on the use of tetracycline hydrochloride in prophylaxis and treatment of obstetric infection. *Antibiotic Annual*, p. 594, 1954–5.
64. Postellon, D. C., and Aronow, R. Iodine in mother's milk (letter). *J.A.M.A.* 247:463, 1982.
65. Puller, J., Salrahaya, P., and Stockhausen, H. Quantitative bestemung der hauptmetaboliten der acetylsalizylsaure. *Z. Geburtshife Perinatol.* 178:135, 1974.
66. Pynnonen, S., and Sillanpaa, M. Carbamazepine and mother's milk. *Lancet* 1:563, 1975.
67. Ricci, G., and Copaitich, T. Modalita di eliminazione dell'isoniazide somminstrata per via oral attraverso il latte di donna. *Rasse Int. Clin. Ter.* 209:53, 1954–5.
68. Rozansky, R., and Brezezinsky, A. The excretion of penicillin in human milk. *J. Lab. Clin. Med.* 34:497, 1949.
69. Sagraves, R., Kaiser, D., and Sharpe, G. L. Prednisone and prednisolone concentrations in the milk of a lactating mother. Abstracts of the Second Annual Meeting of the American College of Clinical Pharmacy, June 24–26, 1981, Scottsdale, Ariz. *Drug Intell. Clin. Pharm.* 14:484, 1981.
70. Schiff, E., and Wohinz, R. Uber das vorkommen von coffein in der frauenmilch nach genuss von kaffee. *Arch. Gynecol.* 134:201, 1928.
71. Schou, M., and Amdisen, A. Lithium and pregnancy. III. Lithium ingestion by children breast-fed by women on lithium treatment. *Br. Med. J.* [Clin. Res.] 2:138, 1973.
72. Somogyi, A., and Gugler, R. Cimetidine excretion into breast milk. *Br. J. Clin. Pharmacol.* 7:627, 1979.
73. Steen, B., and Rane, A. Clindamycin passage into human milk. *Br. J. Clin. Pharmacol.* 13:661, 1982.
74. Stewart, R. B., Karas, B., and Springer, P. K. Haloperidol excretion in human milk. *Am. J. Psychiatry* 137(7):849, 1980.

75. Tegler, L., and Lindstrom, B. Antithyroid drugs in milk. *Lancet* 2:591, 1980.
76. Townsend, R. J., et al. A study to evaluate the passage of Ibuprofen into breast milk. Abstracts of the Third Annual Meeting of the American College of Clinical Pharmacy, June 24–26, 1982, Kansas City, MO. *Drug Intell. Clin. Pharm.* 16:483, 1982.
77. Tunnesen, W. W., and Hertz, C. G. Toxic effects of lithium in newborn infants: A commentary. *J. Pediatr.* 81(4):804, 1972.
78. Varma, S. K., Collins, M., Row, A., Haller, W. S., and Varma, K. Thyroxine, tri-iodothyronine, and reverse tri-iodothyronine concentrations in human milk. *J. Pediatr.* 93(5):803, 1978.
79. Varsano, I., Fischl, J., and Shochet, S. B. Excretion of orally ingested nitrofurantoin in human milk. *J. Pediatr.* 82:886, 1973.
80. Vorherr, H. Drug excretion in human milk. *Postgrad. Med.* 56(4):97, 1974.
81. Voshioka, H., Cho, K., Takinoto, M., Naruyana, S., and Shimizu, T. Transfer of cefazolin into human milk. *J. Pediatr.* 94:151, 1979.
82. Walley, L. J., Blain, P. G., and Prime, J. K. Haloperidol secreted in breast milk. *Br. Med. J.* [Clin. Res.] 282:1746, 1981.
83. Werthmann, M. W., and Krees, S. V. Excretion of chlorothiazide in human breast milk. *J. Pediatr.* 81:781, 1972.
84. Whalen, J. J. Personal communication, Merck Sharp & Dohme, Inc., March 1981.
85. Wiles, D. H., Orr, M. W., and Kolakowska, T. Chlorpromazine levels in plasma and milk of nursing mothers. *Br. J. Clin. Pharmacol.* 5(3):272, 1978.
86. Wilson, J. T., et al. Drug excretion in human breast milk. *Clin. Pharmacokinet.* 5:1, 1979.
87. Yurchak, A. M., and Jusko, W. J. Theophylline secretion into breast milk. *Pediatrics* 57:518, 1976.

Appendix 8. Alcohol-Free Over the Counter (OTC) Cough Preparations

Atussin DM Expectorant
Baby Cough Syrup
Codimal Expectorant
Conar A Syrup
Conex Liquid
Congespirin Syrup for Children
Destro-Tussin Syrup
Diabetuss in Liquid
Dr. Drahes Cough Syrup
Efo-Tussin Jr. Cough Syrup
Efricon Syrup
Endotussin-DM Syrup
Expectrosed Syrup
Fedahist-C Expectorant
Four Green Syrup
Four Red Syrup
Glycotuss Syrup
Glycotuss DM Syrup
Histalet DM Syrup
Hydriotic Acid Syrup

Ipsatol Syrup
Ipsatol DM Cough Syrup
Mamatuss Syrup
Malotuss Syrup
Maldetuss Syrup
Noratuss Syrup
Orthoxicol Cough Syrup
Pediaquill Syrup
Pinex Concenrate
Pinex Regular Syrup
Romex Syrup
Romilar Children's Syrup
Sedatuss in Liquid
Silence is Golden Syrup
Silexin Cough Syrup
Sorbutuss Syrup
Superatin Syrup
Tolu-Sed DM
Triaminicol Cough Syrup
Tusscapine Syrup
Tussciden Expectorant

Adapted from Petroni, N. C., and Cardoni, A. A. Alcohol content of liquid medicinals. *Drug Ther.* 8:72, 1978.

Appendix 9. Community Nutrition Resources

THE SPECIAL SUPPLEMENTAL FOOD PROGRAM FOR WOMEN, INFANTS, AND CHILDREN (WIC)

SERVICES PROVIDED

USDA provides funds to state and local agencies as an adjunct to health care delivery systems. Through this program supplemental foods (iron-fortified cereal, juices, eggs, milk, and infant formula) are provided to pregnant women, women up to 6 months post partum, nursing mothers up to 1 year, and children up to 5 years who qualify for financial criteria and are at nutritional risk.

These clients must live in a geographically determined low-income area and be eligible for reduced price or free medical care. They must be certified by a WIC staff member who periodically assesses risk status.

WIC has six food package categories:

1. Infants 0 through 3 months
2. Infants 4 through 12 months
3. Children and women with special dietary needs
4. Children 1 to 5 years
5. Pregnant and breast-feeding women
6. Non-breast-feeding postpartum women

The amount and type of food varies with each package. Foods included are: iron-fortified formula; milk (whole, skim, buttermilk, evaporated whole or skim, dry whole, or nonfat/low-fat); cheese (American, Monteray Jack, Colby, Natural Cheddar, Swiss, Brick, Muenster, Provolone, or Mozzarella); cereal (iron-enriched, no more than 21.2 gm of sugar per 100 gm of dry cereal); eggs (fresh or dried egg mix); legumes (peanut butter, mature dry beans, or peas); juice (at least 30 mg vitamin C per 100 ml of juice).

COMMENTS

Local agencies operating WIC programs are required to see that health services are available to WIC participants. Evaluations suggest that the WIC program has had a positive impact on the health status of its participants, including improvements in birth weights, infant and preschool child growth, and iron status.

CHILD CARE FOOD PROGRAM

SERVICES PROVIDED

USDA reimburses participating agencies (public or private nonprofit institutions providing day care services) up to a prescribed amount for the cost of serving breakfast, lunch, and/or supper to children. Provides meals that meet national requirements established by USDA; provides free or reduced-price meals. Agencies can receive donated food or a cash reimbursement for each lunch or supper served to eligible children.

COMMENTS

Contact state Department of Education.

MATERNITY AND INFANT CARE PROGRAMS (MIC); CHILDREN AND YOUTH (C&Y)

SERVICES PROVIDED

The program is federally funded through state and local health agencies. Free health care services (including nutrition services) are provided for pregnant women and children at a clinic affiliated with a specific hospital. Services include screening and assessment of nutritional status, nutrition counseling, education referral to available food programs, other types of assistance programs in the community, and follow-up.

COMMENTS

Contact local or state Department of Health.

EARLY PERIODIC SCREENING, DIAGNOSIS, TREATMENT (EPSDT)

SERVICES PROVIDED

The program provides preventive health care to Medicaid-eligible children under age 21. It includes follow-up services for any problems with diagnosis and treatment if needed. Nutritional assessment must be a routine part of the overall assessment of a child's health.

Also included are a complete physical examination by primary care providers. This includes dental examination, accurate measurement of height and weight, and various laboratory tests to screen for iron deficiency, lead toxicity, and the like.

If there is suggestive evidence of nutritional inadequacy, EPSDT arranges for preventive treatment and follow-up services including nutrition counseling.

COMMENTS

Part of Medicaid program, which is financed by state and federal funds. Medicaid programs (e.g., EPSDT) are usually administered by the state Department of Public Welfare.

HEAD START

SERVICES PROVIDED

Comprehensive education, social, health, and nutrition services are provided to 3- to 5-year-old children from low-income families. Parental involvement is an integral part of the program. Children in part-day programs receive a quantity of food in meals and snacks that provide one-third of daily nutritional needs; children in a full-day program receive one-half to two-thirds of daily nutritional needs. Nutrition assessment and nutrition education for parents and children are required program components.

FOOD STAMP PROGRAM

SERVICES PROVIDED

The USDA reimbursement program, at the state level, is usually run by the Department of Public Welfare. All individuals who meet the financial criteria can purchase food stamps or coupons that are used like money to buy food; this increases the family's food purchasing power.

Each applicant is considered on an individual basis based on the total income, expenses, and number of people being fed in the household. The cost of the stamps will vary according to financial criteria. The individual can select any type of food; food stamps cannot be used to purchase cleaning items, soap, detergent, paper goods, alcohol, tobacco, or pet food.

COMMENTS

Contact local Social Services or Welfare Department.

EXPANDED FOOD AND NUTRITION EDUCATION PROGRAM (EFNEP)

SERVICES PROVIDED

A major outreach program by Cooperative Extension Service of each state for low-income families and children in cities and rural areas.

The program is designed to provide nutrition education to families with the assistance of nutrition aides. The aides teach homemakers in their homes to plan, select, and prepare nutritious, low-cost meals. Normal and preventive nutrition is emphasized.

COMMENTS

USDA provides funds to the Cooperative Extension Service through the land grant university in each of the fifty states.

Note: Programs and/or services provided may change over time. Check with local sponsoring agencies.

Appendix 10. Sources of Additional Nutrition Information

American Dental Association
Bureau of Dental Health Education
211 East Chicago Avenue
Chicago, Ill. 60611

American Dietetic Association
430 No. Michigan Avenue
Chicago, Ill. 60611

American Heart Association
1329 Greenville Avenue
Dallas, Tex. 75231

American Home Economics
Association
2010 Massachusetts Avenue, N.W.
Washington, D.C. 20036

American Public Health Association
1015 Eighteenth Street, N.W.
Washington, D.C. 20036

Center for Science in the Public
Interest
1755 S Street, N.W.
Washington, D.C. 20009

Consumer Information
Pueblo, Colo. 81009

Cooperative Extension Service
Federal Extension Service
Department of Agriculture
Washington, D.C. 20250

National Dairy Council
620 North River Road
Rosemont, Ill. 60018

National Health Systems
P.O. Box 1501
Ann Arbor, Mich. 48106

National Institute of Child Health
and Human Development
U.S. Department of Health and
Human Services
Bethesda, Md. 20014

Society for Nutrition Education
2140 Shattuck Avenue
Suite 110
Berkeley, Calif. 94704

The Nutrition Foundation, Inc.
Office of Education and Public
Affairs
888 Seventeenth St., N.W.
Washington, D.C. 20006

Superintendent of Documents
U.S. Government Printing Office
Washington, D.C. 20402

United States Department of
Agriculture
Food and Nutrition Office
Nutrition and Technical Assistance
Division
500 12th Street, S.W.
G.H.I. Building
Washington, D.C. 20250

Appendix 11. Common Metric Equivalents

1 U.S. fluid ounce	= 29.573 milliliter
1 U.S. liquid pint	= 0.47317 liter
1 U.S. liquid quart	= 0.94633 liter
1 U.S. gallon	= 3.78533 liter
1 U.S. dry quart	= 1.1012 liter
1 avoirdupois ounce	= 28.350 grams
1 avoirdupois pound	= 0.45359 kilogram
1 pound	= 2.2 kilograms
1 inch	= 2.54 centimeter

COMMON CONVERSION

Milligrams to milliequivalents	$\dfrac{mg}{\text{atomic wt}}$	$\times$ valence	= mEq
Milliequivalents to milligrams	$\dfrac{\text{atomic wt} \times mEq}{\text{valence}}$		= mg
Kilocalories to kilojoules	kcal $\times$ 4.184		= kj
Nitrogen to protein	gm nitrogen	$\times$ 6.25	= gm protein
Protein to nitrogen	$\dfrac{\text{gm protein}}{6.25}$		= gm nitrogen
Sodium chloride to sodium	gm NaCl $\times$ 0.4	$\times$ 1000	= mg Na
Sodium to sodium chloride	mg Na $\times$ 2.5		= mg NaCl

Index

Caloric requirements. *See also* Energy
intake
in congenital heart disease, 211
in infants, 72, 78–79, 302–303
in premature babies, 266–267
in renal disease, 213
in toddlers, 144–145
Calorimetric method of infant feeding,
11, 12
Cal-Power, 216
Campylobacter, causing diarrhea, 234,
237
Candy, and toddler preferences, 133
Canned foods, for infants, 120
Carbohydrate
abnormalities in metabolism of, in
renal disease, 216
content in certain foods, 411–414
digestion of in infants, 85–87
in fast foods, 132
infant formulas free of, 78–79
metabolism of, 87
needs
in infants, 67
in premature infants, 268–269
Cardiac failure, 209
Cardiopulmonary symptoms, and
parenteral nutrition, 344
Cardiovascular drugs, excreted in breast
milk, 439–440
Casec, 73
Casein
in cow's milk vs. human milk, 10
in diet free of milk protein, 388–389
in evaporated milk, 16
in human milk, 268
as standard of protein, 80
Casein hydrolysates, 81
Catch-up growth
and congenital heart disease, 210
and diarrhea due to giardiasis, 236
in infectious diarrhea, 238
in premature babies, 267
in renal disease, 213
Celiac disease. *See* Gluten-sensitive
enteropathy
Cereal
for infants, 114
iron-fortified, 265
presweetened, 151
sugar content, 133, 134
Cerebral palsy, 333–334
Cesarean section, and breast-feeding,
109
Chelating agents, interactions with
nutrients, 431
Chemical residues, 137–138
Chewing
and bite reflex, 311
in infants, 34–37

Child abuse, and failure to thrive, 292,
293–294
Child care food program, 457
Children and Youth (C & Y) program,
458
Choanal atresia, 324
Cholelithiasis, and parenteral nutrition,
349
Cholestasis, 225–227
Cholesterol
content of selected foods, 147
diet low in, 395–397
levels of
in nephrotic syndrome, 217
in serum, and fatty acid intake,
85
in vegetarian toddlers, 161
Cholestyramine, 227
Chromosomal abnormalities, and
abnormal growth, 196
Citrotein, 416–417
Cleft lip and cleft palate, 318–321
Clinitest, in infectious diarrhea, 239
Clostridium difficile, causing diarrhea,
234, 237
Cognitive development, 23
Colic
and infant feeding behavior, 44
infantile, 109, 250–252
and maternal diet, 98–99
Colon, in fetus, 60
Colonic function, in infants, 63
Colors, food, 426–427
Colostrum, 106
immunological factors, 96, 97
Compleat-B, 416–417
Congenital anomalies
alimentary canal malformations
esophageal atresia or
tracheoesophageal fistula, 325–329
evaluation, 310–314
gastroesophageal reflux, 329–332
and breast-feeding, 100
and failure to thrive, 286
neuromuscular disorders
cerebral palsy, 333–334
myelodysplasia, 334–335
oral-facial
cleft lip and cleft palate, 318–319
evaluation, 304–314
hemifacial microsomia, 322–323
partial airway obstruction, 324–325
Pierre Robin syndrome, 321–322
Congenital heart disease, 209–212
nutritional management, 211–212
Constipation, 252–255
causes, 254
dietary management, 255
Contraceptives, oral, excreted in breast
milk, 449